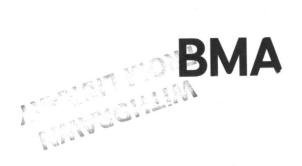

**Textbook of Female Sexual Function and Dysfunction**
*Diagnosis and Treatment*

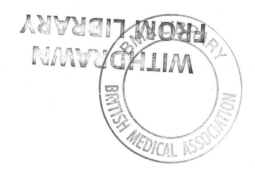

# Textbook of Female Sexual Function and Dysfunction

*Diagnosis and Treatment*

*Edited by*

**Irwin Goldstein, MD, IF**
*Sexual Medicine*
*Alvarado Hospital*
*Department of Surgery*
*University of California, San Diego*
*San Diego Sexual Medicine*
*San Diego, CA, USA*

**Anita H. Clayton, MD, IF, FAPA, FASCP**
*Department of Psychiatry and Neurobehavioral Sciences*
*University of Virginia School of Medicine*
*Charlottesville, VA, USA*

**Andrew T. Goldstein, MD, FACOG, IF**
*Department of Obstetrics and Gynaecology*
*The George Washington University School of Medicine and Health Sciences*
*Centers for Vulvovaginal Disorders*
*Washington, DC, USA*

**Noel N. Kim, PhD, IF**
*Institute for Sexual Medicine*
*San Diego, CA, USA*

**Sheryl A. Kingsberg, PhD, IF**
*Division of Behavioral Medicine*
*Department of OB/GYN*
*University Hospitals Cleveland Medical Center*
*Departments of Reproductive Biology and Psychiatry*
*Case Western Reserve University School of Medicine*
*Cleveland, OH, USA*

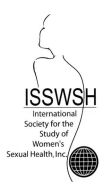

ISSWSH
International
Society for the
Study of
Women's
Sexual Health, Inc.

**WILEY** Blackwell

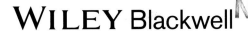

*Registered Office(s)*
John Wiley & Sons, Inc., 111 River Street, Hoboken, NJ 07030, USA
John Wiley & Sons Ltd, The Atrium, Southern Gate, Chichester, West Sussex, PO19 8SQ, UK

*Editorial Office*
9600 Garsington Road, Oxford, OX4 2DQ, UK

For details of our global editorial offices, customer services, and more information about Wiley products visit us at www.wiley.com.

Wiley also publishes its books in a variety of electronic formats and by print-on-demand. Some content that appears in standard print versions of this book may not be available in other formats.

*Library of Congress Cataloging-in-Publication Data*

Names: Goldstein, Irwin, editor. | Clayton, Anita H., editor. |
    Goldstein, Andrew, M.D., editor. | Kim, Noel N., editor. | Kingsberg, Sheryl A., editor.
Title: Textbook of female sexual function and dysfunction : diagnosis and treatment/edited by
    Irwin Goldstein, Anita H. Clayton, Andrew T. Goldstein, Noel N. Kim, Sheryl A. Kingsberg.
Description: Hoboken, NJ : Wiley, 2018. | Includes bibliographical references and index. |
Identifiers: LCCN 2017055314 (print) | LCCN 2017056729 (ebook) | ISBN 9781119266112 (pdf) |
    ISBN 9781119266150 (epub) | ISBN 9781119266136 (oBook) | ISBN 9781119266099 (cloth)
Subjects: | MESH: Sexual Dysfunction, Physiological–diagnosis | Sexual Dysfunction, Physiological–therapy |
    Women | Sexuality–physiology
Classification: LCC RC556 (ebook) | LCC RC556 (print) | NLM WP 610 | DDC 616.85/83–dc23
LC record available at https://lccn.loc.gov/2017055314

Cover Design: Wiley
Cover Image: © Vectorig/Getty Images

Set in 10/12pt Warnock by SPi Global, Pondicherry, India
Printed in Singapore by C.O.S. Printers Pte Ltd

10  9  8  7  6  5  4  3  2  1

# Contents

# List of Contributors

*Stanley E. Althof, PhD, IF*
Center for Marital and Sexual Health of
South Florida
West Palm Beach, FL, USA

*Sophie Bergeron, PhD*
Département de Psychologie
Université de Montréal
Montréal, QC, Canada

*Johannes Bitzer, MD, IF*
University Hospital Basel
Multidisciplinary Center for Sexual
Medicine
Basel, Switzerland

*Karen Brandon, DSc PT WCS, BCB-PMD*
Kaiser Permanente
Fontana, CA, USA

*Anita H. Clayton, MD, IF, FAPA, FASCP*
Department of Psychiatry and
Neurobehavioral Sciences
University of Virginia School of Medicine
Charlottesville, VA, USA

*Leonard R. Derogatis, PhD*
Maryland Center for Sexual Health
Towson, MD, USA

*Melissa A. Farmer, PhD*
Department of Physiology
Feinberg School of Medicine
Northwestern University
Chicago, IL, USA

*Eleni Frangos, PhD*
Pain and Integrative Neuroscience Branch
NCCIH–NIH
Bethesda, MD, USA

*Andrew T. Goldstein, MD, FACOG, IF*
Department of Obstetrics and Gynecology
The George Washington University School
of Medicine and Health Sciences
Centers for Vulvovaginal Disorders
Washington, DC, USA

*Irwin Goldstein, MD, IF*
Sexual Medicine
Alvarado Hospital
Department of Surgery
University of California, San Diego
San Diego Sexual Medicine
San Diego, CA, USA

*Sue W. Goldstein, CSE, CCRC, IF*
San Diego Sexual Medicine
San Diego, CA, USA

*Emmanuele A. Jannini, MD*
Department of Systems Medicine
University of Rome Tor Vergata
Rome, Italy

*Sherri L. Jones, PhD*
Douglas Mental Health University Institute
Department of Psychiatry, McGill University
Montreal, QC, Canada

**Susan Kellogg Spadt, PhD, CRNP, IF, FCST, CSC**
Center for Pelvic Medicine
Bryn Mawr, PA, USA

**Noel N. Kim, PhD, IF**
Institute for Sexual Medicine
San Diego, CA, USA

**Sheryl A. Kingsberg, PhD, IF**
Division of Behavioral Medicine
Department of OB/GYN
University Hospitals Cleveland Medical
Center
Departments of Reproductive Biology and
Psychiatry
Case Western Reserve University School of
Medicine
Cleveland, OH, USA

**Barry R. Komisaruk, PhD**
Department of Psychology
Rutgers University
Newark, NJ, USA

**Tuuli M. Kukkonen, PhD, CPsych**
Department of Family Relations and Applied
Nutrition
University of Guelph
Guelph, ON, Canada

**Fiona McMahon, PT, DPT**
Beyond Basics Physical Therapy, LLC
New York, NY, USA

**Sara Nasserzadeh, PhD, DipPST**
Relationship & Sexual Health Consultants
Palo Alto, CA, USA

**Sharon J. Parish, MD, IF**
Department of Medicine in
Clinical Psychiatry
Department of Clinical Medicine
Weill Cornell Medical College
New York, NY, USA

**Kwangsung Park, MD, PhD, IF**
Department of Urology
Chonnam National University Medical
School
Gwangju, Republic of Korea

**James G. Pfaus, PhD, IF**
Center for Studies in Behavioral
Neurobiology
Department of Psychology, Concordia
University
Montréal, QC, Canada

**Caroline F. Pukall, PhD, CPsych**
Department of Psychology
Queen's University
Kingston, ON, Canada

**Tami Serene Rowen, MD, MS, IF**
Department of Obstetrics, Gynecology and
Reproductive Sciences
University of California, San Francisco
San Francisco, CA, USA

**Sara K. Sauder, PT, DPT**
Austin, TX, USA

**Isbelia Segnini, MSc, CCRC, C-AASECT**
Clinical El Cedral
Caracas, Venezuela

**James A. Simon, MD, CCD, NCMP, IF, FACOG**
IntimMedicine Specialists™
George Washington University School of
Medicine
Washington, DC, USA

**Amy Stein, DPT, BCB-PMD, IF**
Beyond Basics Physical Therapy, LLC
New York, NY, USA

**Linda Vignozzi, MD**
Sexual Medicine and Andrology Unit
Department of Experimental and Clinical
Biomedical Sciences
University of Florence
Florence, Italy

**Nan Wise, PhD**
Department of Psychology
Rutgers University
Newark, NJ, USA

# Foreword

It is a unique honor and privilege for me to introduce readers to this outstanding new volume on female sexual function and dysfunction from the International Society for the Study of Women's Sexual Health (ISSWSH). The depth and breadth of coverage of this complex and rapidly evolving area of women's health is impressive, to say the least, and the inclusion of much new research and clinical data attests to the enormous energy and dedication of growing numbers of researchers and clinicians dedicated to studies in female sexual health. This latest textbook is truly comprehensive in its coverage of both physical and psychological sexual disorders, in addition to providing up-to-date, basic science formulations of underlying mechanisms and processes; all from a consistent and coherent biopsychosocial perspective. As a psychologist and former sex therapist, it is especially gratifying to see this biopsychosocial model applied increasingly across female sexual disorders and problems, regardless of etiology or treatment approaches. The editors have done the field a great service in balancing these perspectives both within and across chapters. The textbook is unique also in the depth of scholarship and extensive reference lists provided with each of the chapters – what a resource for graduate students, residents and fellows!

This new textbook is also a testament to the success of ISSWSH, which, in the 18 years since it was founded, has become the major professional society with a unique focus on female sexual health. Many of us recall the first meeting of the society in Boston in 2000, at which the initial mission statement was drafted and officers elected. The organization has grown in leaps and bounds since then, and this textbook provides impressive testimony to the expanding knowledge base and clinical interests of the society. Since its inception, ISSWSH has benefited greatly from the devotion and energy of its founding members and officers; with special credit due to Sue and Irwin Goldstein, Sharon Parish, Sheryl Kingsberg, Anita Clayton, Stan Althof, Len Derogatis, Jim Simon, Noel Kim, Annamaria Giraldi, and others. I would like to acknowledge also a special debt to my late friend and colleague, Sandra Leiblum, who served as the first president of ISSWSH. Her contributions are cited throughout this volume, and her spirit and energy did much to inspire her colleagues, students and others to pursue clinical or research interests in women's sexuality. Sandy was also a dedicated educator who taught human sexuality and women's sexual health to literally thousands of students and residents during her 40 year career at Rutgers. Her spirit lives on in these pages!

Finally, a special word of appreciation is due to Sue Goldstein – associate editor of this volume and much loved "mother hen" of the society. No one has taken on more roles for the society, or worked as tirelessly as Sue in achieving the goals of ISSWSH. This volume is finally a testament to Sue's enduring and much appreciated contributions to the field. Thank you Sue on behalf of all!

*Raymond C. Rosen, PhD*
*Chief Scientist, New England Research Institutes*
*Former Professor of Psychiatry, Rutgers Medical School*
*Co-Director, Human Sexuality Program*

# Preface

The International Society for the Study of Women's Sexual Health (ISSWSH) is an international, multidisciplinary, academic, clinical and scientific organization dedicated to providing opportunities for communication among scholars, researchers and practitioners about women's sexual health; to support the highest standards of ethics and professionalism in research, education and clinical practice of women's sexual health; and to provide the public with accurate information about women's sexual health.

ISSWSH strongly emphasizes and fervently supports the biopsychosocial management of women with sexual dysfunction. With that encompassing mission and scientific focus in mind, the ISSWSH *Textbook of Female Sexual Function and Dysfunction: Diagnosis and Treatment* has been written by ISSWSH members primarily to help healthcare providers in the various disciplines involved in women's sexual health, including sex therapy, pelvic floor physical therapy and medical therapy, better manage women with distressing sexual health issues. Since ISSWSH is the largest society comprised of specialists in women's sexual health, the idea for an ISSWSH textbook to provide the optimal scientific, multidisciplinary clinical practice guidelines for use by providers was natural. With millions of women needing help, ISSWSH members can provide accurate data for the providers in the various disciplines caring for women with sexual health concerns. By writing a textbook on female sexual dysfunction based on published laboratory and clinical research and

expert clinical experience, ISSWSH is able to further its mission of communication, professionalism and disseminating information.

The multidisciplinary field of women's sexual health has come a long way since the inaugural meeting of ISSWSH in 2000. For almost two decades, ISSWSH has fostered research in the study, nosology, diagnosis and treatment of women with sexual health disorders. ISSWSH funds research projects in women's sexual health, especially important in an era where government funds are lacking. ISSWSH supports numerous educational opportunities including annual meetings, educational courses, and publications from consensus-based panels resulting in nomenclature, white paper and process of care documents. ISSWSH, an affiliate member society of the International Society for Sexual Medicine (ISSM), has three official journals: *The Journal of Sexual Medicine*, *Sexual Medicine*, and *Sexual Medicine Reviews*. Using these and other journals that publish in women's sexual health, ISSWSH has helped grow scientific peer-reviewed publications in women's sexual health, expanding from 273 scientific peer-reviewed publications found in PubMed in 2000 (by using the key phrase "female sexual dysfunction") to 772 in 2016 – almost tripling available literature, much of which has been authored by ISSWSH members.

This ISSWSH textbook is intended to provide clinical practice guidelines for both novice and expert practitioners treating women with sexual health concerns. In the ten years since the publication of the first multidisciplinary textbook in the field, *Women's Sexual Function and Dsyfunction*, our knowledge has expanded and medications for treating various sexual dysfunctions have been added in some countries to the nonpharmacologic treatment strategies already available. As an official publication of the society, this material has been vetted by the editors on behalf of ISSWSH. Four of the editors (Clayton, I. Goldstein, A. Goldstein, Kingsberg) have been presidents of the society while the fifth (Kim) is president-elect. We have all given of our time freely because of our passion for the field and our passion for ISSWSH, as has the associate editor, Sue W. Goldstein. In particular, Sue spent countless hours as the central communicator, tracker of progress, and editorial associate, guiding this book from initial development to final publication. We would also like to thank Gail Goldstein for her time and efforts in helping to edit the pain section.

It is imperative that clinicians understand the various conditions impacting sexual desire, arousal, orgasm, and pain, how to make a correct diagnosis, the therapeutic options available, and the science behind the various treatments, in order to provide optimal patient management and improve patient quality of life. All women have the right to health, including sexual health. The *Textbook of Female Sexual Function and Dysfunction: Diagnosis and Treatment* will serve as a valuable tool to all those involved in helping women maintain or restore their sexual health.

For ease of use, the text is divided into four basic sections: Hypoactive Sexual Desire Disorder, Arousal Disorders, Orgasm Disorders, and Sexual Pain Disorders. Within each section there is content on the nosology and epidemiology, anatomy and physiology, and diagnosis and treatment from both psychologic and biologic points of view, including musculoskeletal management where appropriate.

It is anticipated that ISSWSH will update this textbook as needed. The field of women's sexual medicine is rapidly evolving and ISSWSH members have been influential in paving the way for expansion of knowledge in the field of female sexual dysfunction – this textbook reflects current understanding. We hope that you agree and find the *Textbook of Female Sexual Function and Dysfunction* to be an essential resource in caring for women and their sexual health.

*Irwin Goldstein, MD, IF*
*Anita H. Clayton, MD, IF*
*Andrew T. Goldstein, MD, IF*
*Noel N. Kim, PhD, IF*
*Sheryl A. Kingsberg, PhD, IF*

# 1

# History of the International Society for the Study of Women's Sexual Health (ISSWSH)

*Sue W. Goldstein*

## Abstract

The International Society for the Study of Women's Sexual Health (ISSWSH) emanated from a course assembling experts in different disciplines, becoming the model for the society. Seventeen years later the society remains multidisciplinary, with annual meetings featuring state of the art lectures, symposia on controversial topics, and abstracts judged on scientific merit. Educational efforts expanded from a half day precourse to a fall course and another in conjunction with the National Association of Nurse Practitioners in Women's Health annually. Evidence-based conferences have included consensus panels for nomenclature for desire, arousal, and orgasm; pain; genitourinary syndrome of menopause (GSM); clinical guidelines for identification of sexual health problems; and a process of care for the management of hypoactive sexual desire disorder. ISSWSH is now established as the leading organization for disseminating valuable information to providers, researchers and educators regarding management of distressing sexual dysfunction in women.

**Keywords:**  *ISSWSH; women's sexual health; female sexual dysfunction; multidisciplinary; desire; arousal; orgasm; pain; GSM; nomenclature*

The International Society for the Study of Women's Sexual Health (ISSWSH) is the only professional organization dedicated to women's sexual function and dysfunction. The society was founded less than two decades ago. Therefore, the history of the society is directly linked to the history of the field.

The approval of sildenafil in 1998 by regulatory agencies and a publication in the *New England Journal of Medicine* [1] led women to call urologist Irwin Goldstein to demand a medication for their sexual health problems. There was a paucity of information about the physiology of sexual function and the pathophysiology of sexual dysfunction in women, but Goldstein wanted to change that. Under the auspices of Boston University School of Medicine, he developed a course entitled New Perspectives in Female Sexual Dysfunction, assembling experts in different disciplines to share their information in an effort to piece together available knowledge. This became the model on which the society was developed three years later.

The course was held in the Boston area in 1998, 1999 and 2000. The first year there were over 200 registrants from around the world. Associated with the 1998 course, the American Foundation for Urologic Diseases sponsored a consensus conference with 19

*Textbook of Female Sexual Function and Dysfunction: Diagnosis and Treatment*, First Edition. Edited by
Irwin Goldstein, Anita H. Clayton, Andrew T. Goldstein, Noel N. Kim, and Sheryl A. Kingsberg.
© 2018 John Wiley & Sons Ltd. Published 2018 by John Wiley & Sons Ltd.

international experts, resulting in the development of nomenclature for use in women's sexual dysfunction [2]. Prior to this time all nomenclature was based on the Diagnostic and Statistical Manual of Mental Disorders (DSM) of the American Psychiatric Association [3]. With the recognition of biologic components to sexual function, and the need to understand sexual dysfunction in women, the course was lengthened and podium and poster sessions added. Attendance doubled in 1999 with many returning registrants. When queried about interest in initiating a society, the response was negative. The following year, however, the group had an overwhelmingly positive response and the Female Sexual Function Forum was born.

The society was developed in a multidisciplinary manner with by-laws designating that each committee and the board of directors be balanced in terms of gender, geography, and discipline. All disciplines with an interest in women's sexual health would be welcome in the society, with all active members having equal import, regardless of profession, specialty or degree. Many members of the inaugural board continue to be active members, a testament to both the strength of and need for the organization. One of the first society benefits was the start of a moderated on-line forum (ISSWSHNET) for difficult cases that facilitated communication among people from various locations, disciplines, and perspectives. Having gone through multiple iterations, ISSWSHNET remains a benefit for society members.

The format of the first meeting set the tone for future meetings, with state of the art lectures, symposia on controversial topics, and abstracts judged on scientific merit for podium or poster presentation. The hot topic through the first several annual meetings was the use of androgens in women, transitioning later to oral contraceptives and sexual dysfunction. The first business meeting and election were held on 28 October 2000, with Sandra Leiblum voted in as the first president (Figure 1.1).

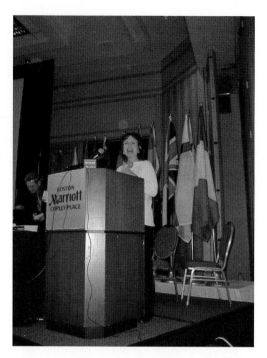

**Figure 1.1** Sandra Leiblum, PhD, first president of the International Society for the Study of Women's Sexual Health, presiding over the business meeting. (*See plate section for color representation of the figure*)

After a year as the Female Sexual Function Forum it was noted that the word "female" could refer to animals, so, in 2001, the organization was renamed the International Society for the Study of Women's Sexual Health. Alessandra Graziottin from Italy ascended to the presidency but the board remained stable to help the fledging society. Only active or honorary members could serve on the board or as committee chairs, as affiliate members were associated with industry. The society struggled financially but survived through the fierce passion of the board and the support of its management company.

Nearly 400 people attended the 2002 meeting in Vancouver – the first time this group met away from Boston. Held shortly after the publication of the widely publicized Women's Health Initiative [4], the leadership responded by adding a lunch seminar to disseminate accurate information and help dispel myths propagated by the press. Symposia were designed to span both the biological and psychological realms in the basic science and clinical arenas. While moving the 2003 meeting to Amsterdam was exciting, it put the society at risk, with a decrease in attendance and increase in meeting costs. Under Cindy Meston's leadership, a development committee was established to seek industry support to help underwrite the conference, as is common among many other societies, with the long term goal of financial stability.

Lorraine Dennerstein put her presidential stamp on the society by recruiting young researchers in an attempt to grow both the society and the field. With the return to the United States in 2004 the society collaborated with the National Institutes of Health, cosponsoring the meeting "Vulvodynia and Sexual Pain Disorders in Women" held the day before the Atlanta ISSWSH meeting [5]. For the first time, several pharmaceutical companies arranged their advisory board meetings around the annual meeting, thus supporting ISSWSH financially and giving increased visibility to the young society. A half-day precourse on the "Practical Management of Women's Sexual Dysfunction" preceded the annual meeting, a response to the increasing demand for instruction for both the novice and advanced health-care provider. The precourse enrollment that first year exceeded expectations with 160 attendees. The board responded by naming an education committee to develop a program of educational courses during the annual meeting, as well as a free-standing three-day course to be held at another time of year.

With these changes ISSWSH was beginning to make its true mark on the field of medicine. In 2005, ISSWSH was under the leadership of its first male president, Stan Althof, and in 2006 the annual meeting moved from October to February, in an attempt to find a dedicated time slot not conflicting with other societies, leaving the October time available for the three-day educational "Fall Course". The rotation of east coast, west coast, Europe for annual meetings would continue for a few years (Table 1.1), until it made more financial sense

to stay in the United States, as attendees and drug development programs were based in the United States, allowing for growth of sponsorship opportunities.

In 2011, the term of president (and consequently both president elect and past president) was changed from one to two years, allowing leadership to develop projects and see them through fruition. With the approval by the Food and Drug Administration of medications for women with various sexual dysfunctions, industry support grew and the society became fiscally sound. The ability to obtain unrestricted educational grants meant the society could fund educational projects outside of the annual meeting. Under the leadership of Andrew Goldstein a new nomenclature for pain was developed in conjunction with International Society for the Study of Vulvovaginal Disease and International Pelvic Pain Society [6], and at a consensus meeting with the North American Menopause Society vulvovaginal atrophy was renamed as genitourinary syndrome of menopause or GSM [7], which is now the accepted term. President Sharon Parish assembled a nomenclature consensus conference to define disorders of desire, arousal, and orgasm [8, 9], and coordinated a meeting sponsored by ISSWSH to ensure these definitions would be considered as part of the new ICD-11 coding [10]. Irwin Goldstein supported the global development committee, securing grants for projects, including a white paper on hypoactive sexual desire disorder [11], and a process of care for the management of women with generalized, acquired hypoactive sexual desire disorder [12]. For the first time, the society was finally able to set aside money in an investment account in 2015 and to use its funds to offer grants to trainees and researchers early in their careers, resulting in future presentations at ISSWSH annual meetings.

With ISSWSH dedicated solely to women's sexual health, other organizations have turned to the society for education. ISSWSH has co-sponsored a course with the National

**Table 1.1** Dates and locations of ISSWSH annual meetings and the presidents at that time.

| Term | President | Meeting location |
| --- | --- | --- |
| 2000–2001 | Sandra R. Leiblum, PhD | Boston, MA (10/01) |
| 2001–2002 | Alessandra Graziottin, MD | Vancouver, Canada (10/02) |
| 2002–2003 | Cindy M. Meston, PhD, IF | Amsterdam, The Netherlands (10/03) |
| 2003–2004 | Lorraine Dennerstein, MBBS, PhD, DPM, IF | Atlanta, GA (10/04) |
| 2004–2005 | Stanley E. Althof, PhD, IF | Las Vegas, NV (10/05) |
| 2005–2006 | Anita H. Clayton, MD, IF, FAPA | Lisbon, Portugal (03/06) |
| 2006–2007 | Anita H. Clayton, MD, IF, FAPA | Lake Buena Vista, FL (02/07) |
| 2007–2008 | Annamaria Giraldi, MD, PhD, IF | San Diego, CA (02/08) |
| 2008–2009 | Rosella E. Nappi, MD, PhD | Florence, Italy (02/09) |
| 2009–2010 | Sheryl A. Kingsberg, PhD, IF | St. Petersberg, FL (02/10) |
| 2010–2011 | Alan Altman, MD, IF | Scottsdale, AZ (02/11) |
| 2011–2012 | Alan Altman, MD, IF | Jerusalem, Israel (02/12) |
| 2012–2013 | Andrew T. Goldstein, MD, IF, FACOG | New Orleans, LA (02/13) |
| 2013–2014 | Andrew T. Goldstein, MD, IF, FACOG | San Diego, CA (02/14) |
| 2014–2015 | Sharon J. Parish, MD, IF, NCMP | Austin, TX (02/15) |
| 2015–2016 | Sharon J. Parish, MD, IF, NCMP | Charleston, SC (02/16) |
| 2016–2017 | Irwin Goldstein, MD, IF | Atlanta, GA (02/17) |
| 2017–2018 | Irwin Goldstein, MD, IF | San Diego, CA (02/18) |

Association of Nurse Practitioners in Women's Health since 2014, providing educational content. The society has taught CME courses at the International Society for Sexual Medicine, American College of Obstetrics and Gynecology, and the International UroGynecology Association, providing evidence-based content to non-ISSWSH members and spreading awareness of women's sexual function and dysfunction.

In recent years, the society has moved into advocacy and has developed useful tools, including publication of clinical pearls and assembling an official educational slide-set, both benefits for members. Online content for both providers and patients has been and will continue to be developed. Consensus panels have convened to establish clinical guidelines in different aspects of sexual dysfunction in women. ISSWSH is now established as a leading organization in disseminating valuable information to providers, researchers, and educators in order to improve management of distressing sexual dysfunction in women.

## References

1 Goldstein I, Lue T, Padma-Nathan H, *et al.* Oral sildenafil in the treatment of erectile dysfunction. *New Engl J Med.* 1998;338:1396–1404.

2 Basson R, Berman J, Burnett A, *et al.* Report of the international consensus development conference on female sexual dysfunction: definitions and classifications. *J Urol.* 2000;163(3):888–893.

3 American Psychiatric Association. Diagnostic and Statistical Manual of Mental Disorders IV, Text Revision (DSM-IV-TR).

American Psychiatric Association, Washington, DC. 2003.

4 Rossouw J, Anderson GL, Prentice RL, *et al.* Risks and benefits of estrogen plus progestin in healthy postmenopausal women: principal results from the Women's Health Initiative randomized controlled trial. *JAMA.* 2002;288(3):321–333.

5 Bachmann G, Rosen R, Pinn VW, *et al.* Vulvodynia: a state-of-the-art consensus on definitions, diagnosis and management. *J Reprod Med.* 2006;51(6):447–456.

6 Bornstein J, Goldstein AT, Stockdale CK, *et al.* 2015 ISSVD, ISSWSH, and IPPS Consensus Terminology and Classification of Persistent Vulvar Pain and Vulvodynia. *J Sex Med.* 2016;13(4):607–612.

7 Portman D, Gass M, Kingsberg S, *et al.* Genitourinary syndrome of menopause: new terminology for vulvovaginal atrophy from the International Society for the Study of Women's Sexual Health and the North American Menopause Society. *Menopause.* 2014;21:1063–1068.

8 Derogatis L, Sand M, Balon R, *et al.* Toward a more evidence-based nosology and nomenclature for female sexual dysfunctions – Part I. *J Sex Med.* 2016;13(12):1881–1887.

9 Parish SJ, Goldstein, AT, Goldstein, SW, *et al.* Toward a More Evidence-Based Nosology and Nomenclature for Female Sexual Dysfunctions – Part II. *J Sex Med.* 2016;13(12):1888–1906.

10 Reed GM, Drescher J, Krueger, RB, *et al.* Disorders related to sexuality and gender identity in the ICD-11: Revising the ICD-10 classification based on current scientific evidence, best clinical practices, and human rights considerations. *World Psychiatry.* 2016;15(3):295–321.

11 Goldstein I, Kim NN, Clayton AH, *et al.* Hypoactive sexual desire disorder: International Society for the Study of Women's Sexual Health (ISSWSH) Expert Consensus Panel Review. *Mayo Clin Proc.* 2017;92(1):114–128.

12 Clayton A, Goldstein I, Kim NN, *et al.* The International Society for the Study of Women's Sexual Health Process of Care for Management of Hypoactive Sexual Desire Disorder in Women. *Mayo Clin Proc.* 2018;93.

# 2

# Sexual Medicine Education and Training

*Sharon J. Parish and Johannes Bitzer*

### Abstract

Sexual health care is part of general medical care and is needed throughout the life cycle of women. Education and training for clinicians is based on a biopsychosocial model of sexual health and should progress from undergraduate level through postgraduate and specialist training programs. The curriculum for each level must be competency based and include learning objectives; describe the knowledge, skills and attitudes; and include methods of monitoring the acquisition of new skills and knowledge. Undergraduate training must include general knowledge about the human sexual response, diagnostic categories and classifications, and skills to communicate about sexuality. Postgraduate and specialized training should provide a broader understanding of the biological, psychological, and social factors contributing to sexual dysfunction; the basis for comprehensive diagnosis; the ability to establish a therapeutic plan in collaboration with the patient; and the capacity to perform interventions or refer.

**Keywords:** *sexual health education; female sexual dysfunction; sexuality communication skills; sexual medicine competencies*

---

Sexual health care is part of general health care and is needed throughout the life span of women and men.

Education and training for health-care professionals are based on a biopsychosocial model of sexual health and should start at undergraduate level and be included in postgraduate and specialist training programs.

The program of each level must include learning objectives; describe the knowledge, skills and attitudes from a competency perspective; and include methods of monitoring the learning process.

---

## Introduction

Sexual problems and sexual dysfunctions have a high prevalence worldwide. As sexual health is part of general health, women consider health-care professionals as the "right persons" to help. The high prevalence and high complexity of sexual health problems create the need for services from both primary care clinicians and sexual medicine specialists. This array of needs implies that all physicians should receive basic education and training in sexual medicine and that a subgroup with interest and commitment in the field should receive specialized postgraduate training [1].

Many institutions in different countries have tried to develop concepts about the learning objectives and competencies in sexual medicine for undergraduate, graduate

*Textbook of Female Sexual Function and Dysfunction: Diagnosis and Treatment*, First Edition. Edited by Irwin Goldstein, Anita H. Clayton, Andrew T. Goldstein, Noel N. Kim, and Sheryl A. Kingsberg.
© 2018 John Wiley & Sons Ltd. Published 2018 by John Wiley & Sons Ltd.

and postgraduate levels [2]. Based on the analyses of these programs and the literature about patients' needs, we propose a model of three levels of competence in female sexual dysfunction (FSD) that should be achieved through education and training programs (Table 2.1) [3].

## Undergraduate (level 1)

Education and training for medical students is based on the transference of knowledge about human sexuality, prevalence of sexual problems, and principles and skills related to communication about sexuality, including strategies and techniques to help patients to disclose problems and difficulties in this intimate and vulnerable domain of life [4]. The core framework for sexuality education focuses on knowledge, skills, and attitudes [5, 6]. Attitudinal training primarily focuses on the development of self-awareness and the cultivation of nonjudgmental behavior and professionalism when interacting with patients with sexuality concerns [6].

Knowledge includes:

- anatomy of sexual organs;
- basics of endocrine, central nervous system, neurological, and neuromuscular processes involved in central and peripheral sexual response;
- models of human sexual response;
- contraception, sexually transmitted diseases, safer sex practices.

Skills incorporate:

- how to encourage patients to ask questions about sexuality and talk about (disclose) difficulties;
- attitude toward discussing and managing sexual problems;
- openness towards the wide spectrum of sexual expression and sexual life styles;
- how to discuss and explain treatment plans, discuss benefits and risks.

Expert recommendations for enhancement of sexual health education in medical schools call for a multidimensional approach that

**Table 2.1** Competencies for undergraduate, graduate and generalist physicians, and postgraduate specialists.

| | Competence level 1: undergraduate | Competence level 2: graduate and generalist physicians | Competence level 3: postgraduate specialists |
|---|---|---|---|
| Female sexual dysfunctions (low desire, arousal dysfunction, orgasmic disorders, sexual pain disorders) | Know definition Screen, diagnose Know about contributing factors and therapeutic options | Diagnose based on standards Assess contributing factors Establish descriptive and comprehensive diagnosis (biopsychosocial model) Elaborate treatment options | Hormonal & drug treatment Sensate focus Couples therapy Physiotherapy |
| Oncologic diseases | Know impact and prevalence Ask and screen | Establish a comprehensive diagnosis including pre-existing factors, disease related factors, and emotional, cognitive and behavioral responses Develop treatment plan Conservative treatment | Specialized surgical interventions Mechanical intervention Hormonal intervention Physiotherapy |
| Metabolic and neurologic diseases | Know impact and prevalence Ask and screen | Establish a comprehensive diagnosis including pre-existing factors disease related factors, and emotional, cognitive and behavioral response Develop treatment plan Conservative treatment | Modified sensate focus Mechanical intervention Drug therapy Physiotherapy |

incorporates curricular reform and innovation aimed at educational infrastructure [7]. Elements include developing a skills-based curriculum, establishing multidisciplinary teams, integrating sexual health content across core curriculum courses and longitudinally throughout medical school, creating mandatory blocks and electives, and including assessment of sexual health knowledge in licensing examinations [7]. Ideally, at least one "champion" should be involved at each institution to ensure that sexuality education is included and effectively integrated into the entire curriculum [6].

Sexuality education should be multidisciplinary and include psychiatry, gynecology, urology, and primary care, and also may incorporate sex therapists, psychologists, epidemiologists, and sexologists. Sexual medicine content is optimally delivered through an array of interactive modalities that enable skills training and assessment. These include didactics, panel discussions, small group case-based seminars, role play, standardized patients, observed structured clinical examinations with direct and immediate feedback, community/peer education, and immersion/desensitization activities [5, 6].

A recent survey regarding lesbian, gay, bisexual, and transgender-related content in United States and Canadian allopathic and osteopathic medical schools reported that dedicated content hours to these topics was small and that the perceived quality was variable. Suggested improvements included increased curricular time dedicated to lesbian, gay, bisexual, and transgender-related health and disparities, instruction about the difference between behavior and identity, and faculty engagement to teach these topics [8].

### Graduate and Postgraduate (Level 2 and 3)

Graduate and generalist physicians, as well as medical specialists, should be able to understand the sexual suffering of their patients and translate it into a descriptive and a comprehensive diagnosis as the basis for a preliminary or more elaborate treatment plan.

The treatment plan may include education and behavioral advice or more specialized interventions, such as hormonal and other pharmacological treatment, surgery, physiotherapy, and specialized psychotherapeutic interventions. The latter competencies need special training (level 3) [9, 10].

The International Consultation in Sexual Medicine published a review of the current state and future educational needs in graduate and postgraduate sexual health education. The key points summarized that: (i) sexual medicine has grown as a specialty in the recent decades; but regulatory aspects of training, assessment, and certification are lagging behind scientific developments and clinical knowledge; (ii) examples of curricula and associated assessments may be related to high quality sexual medicine care; (iii) competency assessment has been applied to surgical training (primarily male), reflecting increased interest in simulation for skills training; (iv) although curriculum development has been primarily executed in medical training, interest is emerging in similar standards for training allied health professionals [2].

Despite the emergence of some training opportunities employing varied methodologies, objective measures of the impact of graduate and postgraduate physician training in sexual health on patient satisfaction and objective health outcomes are lacking [11].

## Education and Training in Female Sexual Health Care for Practicing Clinicians

To provide patients with competent sexual health care, professionals need to train and develop knowledge, skills and attitudes related to the following key principles [12]:

- Sexuality is an intimate part of the patient's identity, self-esteem, shame, and vulnerabilities. Therefore, talking about sexuality requires openness, empathy, a nonjudgmental approach, and a respectful attitude focusing on resources and not on deficits.

- Sexual problems and dysfunctions are usually the result of an interaction of factors that are best identified using the biopsychosocial model. This means that physicians have to be open to, and interested in, different perspectives, ranging from physiology/pathophysiology to psychology/psychopathology to social psychology and sociology [13].
- Solutions to sexual problems and treatment of dysfunctions may be a long-term process and, invariably, require the active collaboration of the patient or couple. This implies that clinicians frequently need to include partners in the process, involve patients in decision making, and adapt strategies that match the resources and capacities of the patient [14].

Incorporating these premises, we have developed a semi-structured approach to patients with sexual problems and dysfunctions that includes the elements that form the core education and training for generalist physicians [4].

## Elements of a Structured Approach to a Patient with Sexual Problems and Dysfunctions

The consultation in sexual medicine is characterized by the following elements:

- Patient-centered: the patient with her needs, subjective suffering, questions, and priorities is at the center of the consultation; she is empowered by knowledge and insight. To achieve this, communication should include active listening, mirroring, summarizing, responding to emotions, and providing information in a language the patient can understand. The doctor–patient relationship should be nonjudgmental and based on respect, aimed at establishing a relationship of mutual trust and confidence.
- Diagnosis and treatment are based on the biopsychosocial understanding of human sexuality. The diagnostic workup integrates biological and psychosocial factors contributing to the sexual problem, understanding these factors as interactive. Based on a shared understanding between the clinician and patient, therapeutic options should be reviewed together, individualizing treatment according to the individual needs of the patient.

## Basic Structured Approach to a Patient Presenting with a Sexual Problem [14]

- Listen to the patient's story (narrative) and practice patient-centered communication.
  - Utilize communications skills: active listening, reflection, mirroring, summarizing, responding to emotions, reframing.
- Ask differentiating questions.
  - Enable differentiation of a sexual problem into primary versus secondary, situational versus global, abrupt beginning versus slow process.
- Explore a typical sexual encounter or experience (behavioral interactive sequence).
  - "What happened last time when you were sexually active?"
- Elaborate a descriptive diagnosis (using classification systems).
  - Disorder/dysfunction according to DSM-5 [15], International Consultation on Sexual Medicine classification [16, International Society for the Study of Women's Sexual Health (ISSWSH) nomenclature [17], ICD-10.
  - Use of questionnaires for screening and diagnosis.
- Explore conditioning and risk factors contributing to the clinical problem.
  - Medical (history, examination).
  - Individual psychological (sexual biography, major life events, lifecycle), sexual learning.
  - Interactional: partner communication and dynamics.
  - Sociocultural: sexual norms and concepts.

- Elaborate a comprehensive explanatory diagnosis as a working model to be shared with the patient.
  - Construct individualized nine-field table of conditioning factors (Table 2.2).
- Develop a treatment plan.
  - Use nine-field table (Table 2.2) [18] results to address possible therapeutic interventions.
  - Practice shared decision making:
    o discuss benefit/risk or advantages/disadvantages of different options in relation to patient's values and needs;
    o make treatment decision transparent and shared.

A useful instrument for training this approach is the use of the graphic summary of the comprehensive explanatory diagnosis in the form of a modified nine-field diagram (Table 2.2) [18]. The horizontal axis includes biomedical, psychological, and sociocultural factors; the vertical axis incorporates predisposing (distant, indirect), precipitating (triggering), and maintaining (proximate factors).

In addition, sexual health care for patients with various medical conditions has to take into account disease and treatment specific factors that have an impact on the sexual function. For the most common conditions, the algorithm shown in Figure 2.1 incorporates the specific medical condition (oncologic, metabolic and neurological disorders, etc.) [3].

Algorithms and structured approaches form the basis for education and training in female sexual disorders in general and in the context of disease and treatment of disease.

Regarding the disease and therapy specific factors, eight different levels through which a disease or a therapy can have an impact on sexual function can be outlined (Table 2.3) [3].

## Education and Training in Female Sexual Health Care for Sexual Medicine Specialists

Based on these schemas, sexual medicine societies and institutions have developed educational and training programs defining knowledge, skills, attitudes, and evaluation methods for defined sexual dysfunctions. These training programs are designed for specialists in sexual medicine. The European Society for Sexual Medicine (ESSM) and the International Society for the Study of Women's Sexual Health have intensive courses that provide didactic, experiential, and hands-on training in an interactive format.

The European Society for Sexual Medicine designed such a curriculum that

**Table 2.2** Modified nine-field diagram [10] for the comprehensive explanatory diagnosis.

| | Biomedical | | Psychological | | Sociocultural |
|---|---|---|---|---|---|
| | *Chronic diseases and drugs* | *Hormonal factors* | *Intraindividual* | *Interpersonal* | |
| Predisposing Distant Indirect | | | | | |
| Precipitating Factors Trigger | | | | | |
| Maintaining Proximate Direct | | | | | |

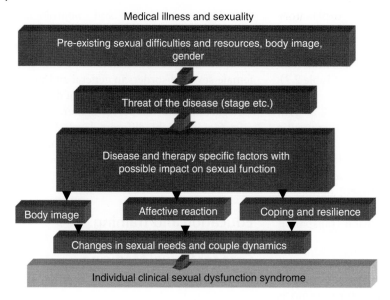

**Figure 2.1** Algorithm incorporating the specific medical condition. (*See plate section for color representation of the figure*)

**Table 2.3** Disease and therapy specific factors having an impact on female sexual function [3].

| | |
|---|---|
| Danger | The subjectively experienced threat |
| Destruction | Destruction of sexual organs |
| Disfigurement | Visible changes of the body |
| Disability: handicap and pain | Loss of mobility, chronic pain |
| Dysfunction | Loss of neurovegetative and neuromuscular function |
| Dysregulation | Hormonal and central nervous disruptions |
| Disease load | Accompanying symptoms (incontinence etc.) |
| Drugs | Many secondary effects of drugs on sexual function |

includes detailed and proscriptive approaches to the spectrum of sexual problems and includes an array of educational and assessment methods. Core components of the ESSM curriculum are the assessment and management of desire, arousal, and orgasm disorders; assessment methods are summarized in Tables 2.4, 2.5, and 2.6.

Objectives for management of each disorder include required knowledge, skills and attitudes.

## Conclusion

Generalist physicians should be able to address sexuality in the context of a medical consultation, assess sexual health problems, offer help or refer women to specialized colleagues. Undergraduate training must include general knowledge about the human sexual response as well as the diagnostic categories and classifications, and skills to communicate about sexuality. Postgraduate and specialized training should be competency based and provide:

- a broader understanding of the biological, psychological and social factors contributing to sexual health and sexual dysfunction in general and in clinical conditions;
- the basis for comprehensive diagnosis;
- the capacity to establish a therapeutic plan shared with the patient;
- the guidance to perform interventions according to individual competence or refer to specialists.

**Table 2.4** Management of the patient with desire disorder [9, 19, 20].

| Objective | | Assessment |
|---|---|---|
| Knowledge | *Anatomy*<br>Anatomy of the brain, enhancing and inhibiting pathways and networks | Multiple choice questions (MCQ) |
| | *Physiology of sexual desire*<br>Endocrine and neurotransmitter pathways and actions involved in the experience of desire | |
| | *Pathology*<br>Definitions in ISSWSH nomenclature and ICD-10<br>Pathophysiological mechanisms of dysfunction (stimulating and inhibiting pathways) | |
| | *Risk and contributing factors*<br>Biological, medical<br>● Diseases and drugs<br>● Hormonal changes<br>Psychological<br>● Understanding the sexual biography (negative sexual learning, traumatic life events, vulnerability, sexual temperament)<br>Relational<br>● Partner conflicts about different needs, communication difficulties<br>Sociocultural<br>● Lack of sex education<br>● Rigid sexual norms, role definitions | Single best answer (SBA) |
| | *Therapeutic options*<br>Sexual counseling<br>Hormonal treatment<br>Drug treatment (centrally acting)<br>Body centered sex therapy<br>Modified sensate focus | |
| Clinical skills | Be able to:<br>● Perform a structured diagnostic interview including listening to the woman's story, (narrative), summarizing, and establishing a comprehensive diagnosis with contributing elements and risk factors (nine-field diagram)<br>● Differentiate between primary and secondary dysfunction | Extended matching questions (EMQ) Objective structured clinical examination (OSCE) |
| | Perform a gynecologic examination with special focus on colposcopy of the vulva, examination of the vagina | |
| | Develop a treatment plan together with the patient based on shared decision making<br>Assess indication for medication treatment taking into account contraindications etc.<br>Psychotherapy – cognitive behavioral therapy and mindfulness-based therapy<br>Systemic couple therapy | |
| Attitudes | Empathic listening, encouraging to talk<br>Offer feedback opportunities, encourage questions<br>Schedule follow up<br>Be patient regarding change | Role play |

**Table 2.5** Management of the patient with arousal disorder [9, 21].

| Objective | | Assessment |
|---|---|---|
| Knowledge | *Anatomy*<br>Anatomy of the vulva, vagina and clitoris<br>Differentiated knowledge about tissues, vascularization, hormonal receptors | MCQ |
| | *Physiology of sexual arousal*<br>Central and peripheral mechanisms of arousal including lubrication | |
| | *Pathology of arousal dysfunction*<br>Definitions of ISSWSH nomenclature and ICD 10<br>Pathophysiological mechanisms | |
| | *Risk and contributing factors*<br>Biological, medical<br>• Sex hormone deficiency<br>• Diabetes/vascular factors<br>• Smoking<br>• Pelvic floor disorders<br>• Lower urinary tract symptoms (LUTS)<br>• Pelvic surgery<br>• Neurological diseases<br>• Drugs: antihormones, hormonal contraceptives, chemotherapy, antidepressants<br>Psychological<br>• Anxiety, depression<br>• Lack of knowledge and experience (masturbation etc.)<br>• Traumatic sexual biography (separation, violence, abuse)<br>Relational<br>• Conflict about needs and expectations<br>• Lack of communication skills to negotiate about differences<br>Sociocultural<br>• Poverty/low income<br>• Working conditions<br>• Sexual norms | SBA |
| | *Therapeutic options*<br>Sexual counseling<br>Local and/or hormonal treatment<br>Drug treatment (PDE-5-inhibitors)<br>Body-centered sex therapy<br>Modified sensate focus | |
| Clinical skills | Be able to perform a structured diagnostic interview including listening to the woman's story, (narrative), summarizing, establishing a comprehensive diagnosis with contributing and risk factors<br>(nine-field diagram) | EMQ, OSCE |
| | Perform a gynecologic examination with special focus on colposcopy of the vulva, examination of the vagina<br>Detect (exclude) vulvovaginal disease | |
| | Develop a treatment plan together with the patient based on shared decision making<br>Assess indication for medication taking into account contraindications<br>Sensate focus, body centered psychotherapy, physiotherapy, masturbation exercises, systemic couple therapy | |
| Attitudes | Empathic listening, encouraging to talk<br>Offer feedback opportunities, encourage questions<br>Schedule follow-up<br>Be patient regarding change | Role play |

**Table 2.6** Management of the patient with orgasmic disorder.

| Objective | | Assessment |
|---|---|---|
| Knowledge | *Anatomy*<br>Anatomy of the brain, enhancing and inhibiting pathways and networks; anatomy and physiology of the vagina and the pelvic floor | MCQ |
| | *Physiology of orgasm*<br>Vascular and muscular response, woman's experience | |
| | *Pathology*<br>Definitions of ISSWSH nomenclature and ICD 10<br>Pathophysiological mechanisms (excitatory and inhibitory pathways) | |
| | *Risk and contributing factors*<br>Biological, Medical<br>● Factors contributing to orgasm disorder<br>● Antidepressant medication<br>Psychological<br>● Lack of education, experience<br>● Partner conflict<br>● Performance anxiety<br>Relational<br>● Inadequate stimulation<br>Sociocultural<br>● Lack of sex education<br>● Rigid sexual norms | SBA |
| | *Therapeutic options*<br>Sexual counseling<br>Masturbation exercises<br>Working with fantasies, sex toys<br>Body centered psychotherapy<br>Physiotherapy pelvic floor | |
| Clinical skills | Be able to:<br>Perform a structured diagnostic interview including listening to the woman's story, (narrative), summarizing, establishing a comprehensive diagnosis with contributing and risk factors (nine-field diagram)<br>Differentiate between primary and secondary | EMQ, OSCE |
| | Consider a gynecologic examination of the vulva, vagina if inadequate arousal is contributing or orgasmic dysfunction | |
| | Develop a treatment plan together with the patient based on shared decision making<br>Assess indication for medication treatment taking into account contraindications etc.<br>Sensate focus, body-centered psychotherapy, sex toys, physiotherapy masturbation exercises<br>Systemic couple therapy | |
| Attitude | Empathic listening, encouraging to talk<br>Offer feedback opportunities, encourage questions<br>Schedule follow up<br>Be patient regarding change | Role play |

## References

1 Reisman Y, Eardley I, Porst H, the Multidisciplinary Joint Committee on Sexual Medicine (MJCSM). New developments in education and training in sexual medicine. *J Sex Med.* 2013;10:918–923.

2 Eardley I, Reisman Y, Goldstein S, *et al.* Existing and future educational needs in graduate and postgraduate education. *J Sex Med.* 2017;14:475–485.

3 Bitzer J, Platano G, Tschudin S, Alder J. Sexual counseling for women in the context of physical diseases: a teaching model for physicians. *J Sex Med.* 2007;4:29–37.

4 Brandenburg U, Bitzer J. The challenge of talking about sex: the importance of patient-physician interaction. *Maturitas.* 2009;63:124–127.

5 Shindel AW, Parish SJ. Sexuality education in North American medical schools: Current status and future directions. *J Sex Med.* 2013;10:3–18.

6 Shindel AW. Sexuality education: a critical need. *J Sex Med.* 2015;12:1519–1521.

7 Coleman E, Elders J, Satcher D, *et al.* Summit on medical school education in sexual health: report of an expert consultation. *J Sex Med.* 2013;10: 924–938.

8 Obedin-Maliver J, Goldsmith ES, Stewart L, *et al.* Lesbian, gay, bisexual, and transgender-related content in undergraduate medical education. *JAMA*, 2011;306:971–977.

9 Brotto LA, Bitzer J, Laan E, *et al.* Women's sexual desire and arousal disorders. *J Sex Med.* 2010; 7, 586–614.

10 Bitzer J., Giraldi A, Pfaus J. Sexual desire and hypoactive sexual desire disorder in women. Introduction and overview. Standard operating procedure (SOP Part 1). *J Sex Med.* 2013;10:36–49.

11 Parish SJ, Rubio-Aurioles E. Education in sexual medicine: proceedings from the international consultation in sexual medicine, 2009. *J Sex Med.* 2010;7:3305–3314.

12 Bitzer J. Definition and diagnosis of sexual problems. In Wylie KR (ed.) *ABC of Sexual Health*, 3rd edn. Chichester, UK: John Wiley & Sons Ltd; 2015, pp.77–80.

13 Al-Azzawi F, Bitzer J, Brandenburg U, *et al.* Therapeutic options for postmenopausal female sexual dysfunction. *Climacteric.* 2010;13:103–120.

14 Bitzer J, Platano G, Tschudin S, Alder J. Sexual counseling in elderly couples. *J Sex Med.* 2008;5:2027–2043.

15 American Psychological Association. *Diagnostic and Statistical Manual of Mental Disorders, Fifth Edition: DSM-5.* Arlington, VA: American Psychological Association; 2013.

16 McCabe MP, Sharlip ID, Atalla E, *et al.* Definitions of sexual dysfunctions in women and men: A Consensus Statement From the Fourth International Consultation on Sexual Medicine 2015. *J Sex Med.* 2016;13:135–143.

17 Parish SJ, Goldstein AT, Goldstein SW, *et al.* Toward a more evidence-based nosology and nomenclature for female sexual dysfunctions – Part II. *J Sex Med.* 2016;13:1888–1906.

18 Bitzer J, Giraldi A, Pfaus J. A standardized diagnostic interview for hypoactive sexual desire disorder in women: standard operating procedure (SOP Part 2). *J Sex Med.* 2013;10:50–57.

19 Parish SJ, Hahn SR. Hypoactive sexual desire disorder: a review of epidemiology, biopsychology, diagnosis, and treatment. *Sex Med Rev.* 2016;4:103–120.

20 Goldstein I, Kim NN, Clayton AH, *et al.* Hypoactive sexual desire disorder: International Society for the Study of Women's Sexual Health (ISSWSH) Expert Consensus Panel Review. *Mayo Clin Proc.* 2017;92:114–128. doi: 10.1016/j. mayocp.2016.09.018.

21 Giraldi A, Rellini AH, Pfaus J, Laan E. Female sexual arousal disorders. *J Sex Med.* 2013;10:58–73.

**Part I**

**Hypoactive Sexual Desire Disorder**

# 3

# Nosology and Epidemiology of Hypoactive Sexual Desire Disorder

*Leonard R. Derogatis*

### Abstract

The chapter reviews the history and development of the diagnosis hypoactive sexual desire disorder (HSDD) and discusses its close ties to the evolution of the diagnostic system of the American Psychiatric Association (i.e. DSM-I to DSM-5). It reviews the principal criteria underlying the diagnosis and their underlying significance. The chapter also discusses the widespread dissatisfaction with the current DSM-5 system and the development, in response, of the new ISSWSH diagnostic system for female sexual dysfunctions. Diagnostic standards for the HSDD diagnosis in the ISSWSH system are described and elucidated as an alternative to the DSM-5 system. In addition, the chapter also provides a brief review of the current status of epidemiological research focused on the prevalence of HSDD as defined in contemporary nosological systems.

**Keywords:** *diagnosis; prevalence; nosology; nomenclature; FSD; HSDD*

## Nosology

Historically, the diagnoses of female sexual dysfunctions (FSD), including hypoactive sexual desire disorder (HSDD), have been made primarily based on clinical presentation and patient history rather than a formal nosology grounded in etiology, pathogenesis, and clinical phenomenology. The evolution of the diagnostic concept of HSDD is closely tied to the development of the American Psychiatric Association's Diagnostic (DSM) system [1–7]. This is, in large measure, due to the belief of experts in the postwar twentieth century medicine that female sexual dysfunctions have a primarily psychological etiology.

The modern diagnostic category of HSDD has existed for approximately 30 years, beginning with the DSM-III [3]. Antecedent diagnostic categories for low desire in the first two iterations of the DSM were labeled as "Psychophysiological autonomic and visceral disorders" and were consistent with the strong psychoanalytic influence holding sway at the time; etiology was attributed to repressed emotions. When Masters and Johnson [8] published their work in 1970, they did not identify nor emphasize disorders of sexual desire. However, Helen Singer Kaplan [9] and Harold Lief [10] writing independently in 1977 questioned the omission of this important dimension of sexual behavior, which led to modifications in the Masters and Johnson paradigm, and the inclusion of a category for desire disorders ("Inhibited sexual desire") in the DSM-III [3].

Desire disorder was initially labeled "Inhibited sexual desire" in the DSM-III [3], which was modified to "Sexual desire disorder" in the DSM-III-R [4]. Finally, in the

*Textbook of Female Sexual Function and Dysfunction: Diagnosis and Treatment*, First Edition. Edited by Irwin Goldstein, Anita H. Clayton, Andrew T. Goldstein, Noel N. Kim, and Sheryl A. Kingsberg.
© 2018 John Wiley & Sons Ltd. Published 2018 by John Wiley & Sons Ltd.

DSM-IV [5] the term "Hypoactive sexual desire disorder" was introduced. The most recent iterations of the DSM definitions of desire disorder are represented by the text revised version of the DSM-IV (i.e. DSM-IV-TR) [6] and the DSM-5 [7].

The DSM-IV-TR diagnosis requires the dual criteria of (A), the symptomatic presentation associated with desire disorder, and (B), "marked distress or interpersonal difficulty". The manifestation of the symptoms of low sexual desire are further specified as having to be "persistent or recurrent". Beyond these criteria the condition must be specified as occurring *lifelong* versus *acquired* and *situational* in nature versus *generalized*.

The DSM-5 definition of desire disorder fundamentally requires three criteria be met: Category (A) specifies the clinical phenomenology of the condition, somewhat more precisely than previous editions, and requires that defining clinical characteristics be present in a majority (e.g. 75%) of the encounters or episodes; a second (B) criterion requires the condition to have been present for at least six months; and third, the condition must cause "clinically significant distress in the individual". In addition, the patient is requested to make a judgment as to the severity level of the condition, choosing from "mild", "moderate", or "severe" as descriptors. These added criteria help to distinguish actual sexual dysfunctions from transient sexual difficulties and should help to further homogenize diagnostic groupings by reducing within-groups variation.

The most dramatic change in the DSM-5 involved eliminating HSDD as a distinct nosologic entity, replacing it with an amalgamation of the DSM-IV HSDD and DSM-IV female sexual arousal disorder (FSAD) diagnoses. The resulting compounded diagnosis has been termed female sexual interest/arousal disorder (FSIAD). This revised classification has proven to be highly controversial among experts in the area of sexual medicine, as there is little empirical support or confirmation for the new diagnostic category and the logics upon which the compounded diagnosis are based appear less than compelling [11, 12].

The resulting dissatisfaction with the DSM-5 nomenclature is one of the principal factors giving impetus to development of a new diagnostic system for female sexual dysfunctions, established under the auspices of two international expert panels, representing the ISSWSH Nomenclature Committee [13] and the International Consultation in Sexual Medicine [14]. In the new ISSWSH nomenclature, HSDD has been restored to an independent diagnostic category [11], as has arousal disorder.

In the ISSWSH nomenclature [11], the diagnostic criteria for desire disorder have been extended and simplified, and the diagnostic label of HSDD has been restored, an important decision in light of the very large body of empirical evidence that has been established under this label. In the new ISSWSH nomenclature, HSDD presents with any of the following characteristics for a minimum period of at least six months:

- Lack of motivation for sexual activity characterized by:
  - decreased or absent spontaneous desire (i.e. sexual thoughts or fantasies);
  - decreased or absent responsive desire to erotic cues or stimulation or inability to maintain desire or interest through sexual activity.
- Loss of desire to initiate or participate in sexual activity, including behavioral responses such as avoiding situations that could lead to sexual activity that is not secondary to sexual pain disorders.

The manifest characteristic(s) must be accompanied by clinically significant personal distress that includes frustration, grief, guilt, incompetence, loss, sadness or worry. In addition, the experience and impact of the symptoms of HSDD as a whole should be rated by the affected person as mild, moderate or severe.

Importantly, the new ISSWSH nosologic system is highly compatible with the International Statistical Classification of Diseases and Related Health Problems, 11th Revision (ICD-11) [15], which will be soon utilized worldwide. In ICD-11, HSDD is also represented by an independent diagnostic category, i.e. hypoactive sexual desire dysfunction.

## Epidemiology

By far the large majority of our epidemiological studies in FSD are *observational-descriptive* in nature, with very few *analytic* trials being reported. This state of affairs is due, in large measure, to the historical imprecision of the diagnostic systems used and the relative absence of standardized and well-articulated methods [16]. Imprecise diagnostic definitions lead to inaccurate estimates of occurrence rates and greatly impede the development of accurate rates for risk factors. As an example, Dunn [17] and her associates reviewed 28 studies of FSD and concluded, "...the heterogeneity of the studies ruled out the possibility of formally pooling the data" (p. 418). They further felt that the variation in methodology was so great across the studies that deriving a reliable pooled overall estimate of prevalence for these disorders was just not possible. Several years later, Hayes [18] and his colleagues in their review of prevalence studies concluded, "As measures of sexual dysfunction and time frames differ between studies, it is still not possible to determine reliable overall prevalence estimates of FSD" (p. 594). More recent studies have shown methodological improvements, but variations in nomenclature have continued to impede progress. Until a scientifically valid and rigorously defined nosology is achieved and adopted, our epidemiological estimates of prevalence for HSDD will continue to reflect wide variation.

An important convention that should be employed when considering the epidemiology of HSDD is to distinguish those studies which require the presence of clinically significant personal distress to make the diagnosis from those in which the distress criterion is absent. This is a very critical distinction, since the occurrence of low sexual desire among women is quite common; however, low sexual desire in combination with sexually-related personal distress has a much lower occurrence. Also, these two elements represent the core facets of contemporary definitions of HSDD, while earlier definitions focused more exclusively on the clinical details of low sexual desire. This distinction underlies the disjunction between contemporary epidemiological prevalence estimates and prevalence rates from earlier research, where personal distress was not considered. Findings in earlier studies report much higher rates of dysfunction, primarily because the criterion of personal distress was not included. For this reason, our brief review of the prevalence of HSDD given here will focus exclusively on those studies that used a distress criterion in their HSDD definition.

Probably the most comprehensive contemporary study of FSD prevalence was completed by Shifren and her associates [19]. Termed the PRESIDE study, they reported on a large survey of over 50,000 households in the United States, with 31,581 respondents, which probably represents the most complete study to date on the prevalence of FSD in the United States. Their results revealed 38.7% of American women reported problems with low sexual desire, with the highest prevalence reported in the ≥65 year old group (74.8%) and the lowest prevalence observed in the youngest age group (22.2%). The middle group (45–64%) revealed a prevalence of 38.9% for problems of low sexual desire. However, since older women reported significantly lower rates of personal distress than the younger groups (12.6% vs. approximately 25% in the two younger groups), the rates of diagnosed HSDD remained roughly equivalent, i.e. 10.08% overall. It has been theorized that the low rates of distress in older women, even in the face of a higher prevalence of sexual difficulties, might be the result of changes in partner status or the relatively diminished importance of sex in long-term relationships. It is also distinctly possible that many older women viewed the lessening of sexual desire with age as a natural phenomenon, and not a condition to be treated.

Probably the most closely comparable recent study to PRESIDE is the Women's

International Study of Health and Sexuality (WISHeS) [20]. In this study, both low sexual desire and distress were measured in a sample consisting of 1591 partnered women from the USA and 1998 partnered women from Europe, aged 20–70 years. Much as was observed in PRESIDE, rates of low sexual desire significantly increased across age groups, while rates of personal distress decreased significantly with age. This disordinal interaction resulted in a finding analogous to the PRESIDE study, that the prevalence of HSDD did not significantly change with age. The overall prevalence estimates ranged from a low of 7% for premenopausal women in the 20–49 year old group, to a high of 16% for surgically menopausal women, 20–49 years of age. Conclusions were similar, to the effect that low sexual desire is a common problem among women across age groups, and even when the additional criterion of personal distress is added to certify an HSDD diagnosis, it remains a prevalent problem.

There is also a fairly consistent pattern of associated conditions reported with the occurrence of HSDD. Women diagnosed with HSDD are significantly more likely to report being dissatisfied with their sex lives than women with normal desire and feel more dissatisfied with their relationships. These women also tend to have more chronic illnesses and poorer general health status. Effects between HSDD and these conditions appear to be bidirectional for the most part. In terms of specific health conditions, diabetes, ovary removal, urinary tract problems, and breast cancer appear to be more prevalent among women with HSDD [21].

A strong bidirectional cooccurrence between HSDD and clinical depression has also been repeatedly observed, such that each is considered a significant risk factor for the other condition. In a large meta-analysis, depressed patients had a 50–70% increased risk of developing a sexual dysfunction and patients with sexual dysfunction had 130–210% increased risk of developing depression [22]. Similarly, the French ELIXIR study [23] reported a prevalence rate of 65% for sexual dysfunction in their sample of depressed patients, and rates for all sexual dysfunctions twice those found in women free of these conditions. West [24] and her associates observed a rate of HSDD that was three times greater among depressed individuals in her cohort (20.6%) than the rate (6.9%) among the nondepressed. Depression and HSDD are frequently comorbid conditions, particularly in light of the fact that loss of sexual desire may be a symptom of a major depressive episode. In women and men with sexual dysfunction, the risk of developing depression was increased 170–210% [22]. It is very difficult to establish definitive directionality of effects in this relationship, except via temporal differences in date of onset. In two cross-sectional analyses, more than one-third of women with HSDD had comorbid depression or treatment: 34% in the HSDD Registry for Women [25] and 40% in the PRESIDE study [26].

The data all point to the conclusion that HSDD is a very prevalent problem among women, independent of age, with numerous concomitant and comorbid conditions that tend to complicate effective treatment planning and problem resolution.

## References

1 American Psychiatric Association. *The Diagnostic and Statistical Manual of Mental Disorders*. Washington, DC: American Psychiatric Association; 1952.

2 American Psychiatric Association. *DSM-II: Diagnostic and Statistical Manual of Mental Disorders*, 2nd edn. Washington, DC: American Psychiatric Association; 1968.

3 American Psychiatric Association. *DSM-III: Diagnostic and Statistical Manual of Mental Disorders*, 3rd edn. Washington, DC: American Psychiatric Association; 1980.

4 American Psychiatric Association. *DSM-III-R: Diagnostic and Statistical Manual of Mental Disorders*, 3rd edn revised. Washington, DC: American Psychiatric Association; 1987.

5 American Psychiatric Association. *DSM-IV: Diagnostic and Statistical Manual of Mental Disorders*, 4th edn. Washington, DC: American Psychiatric Association; 1994.

6 American Psychiatric Association. *DSM-IV-TR: Diagnostic and Statistical Manual of Mental Disorders*. 4th edn revised. Washington, DC: American Psychiatric Association; 2000.

7 American Psychiatric Association. *DSM-5: Diagnostic and Statistical Manual of Mental Disorders*, 5th edn. Washington, DC: American Psychiatric Association; 2013.

8 Masters WH and Johnson, VE. *Human Sexual Inadequacy*. New York: Bantam; 1970.

9 Kaplan HS. *The New Sex Therapy*. New York: Brunner/Mazel; 1974.

10 Lief HI. Inhibited sexual desire. *Medical Aspects of Human Sexuality*, 1977;7: 94–95.

11 Clayton AH, Derogatis LR, Rosen R, *et al.* Does clinical research data support sexual desire and arousal disorders as distinct diagnoses? *J Sex Med.* 2010;7(S3):143–144.

12 Derogatis LR, Clayton AH, Rosen R, *et al.* Do multiple convergent measures of female sexual dysfunction support sexual desire and arousal disorders as distinct diagnoses? *J Sex Med.* 2010;7(S3):142–143.

13 Parish SJ, Goldstein AT, Goldstein SW, *et al.* Toward a more evidence-based nosology and nomenclature for female sexual dysfunctions – Part II. *J Sex Med.* 2016;13:1888–1906.

14 McCabe MP, Sharlip ID, Atalla E, *et al.* Definitions of sexual dysfunction in women and men: a consensus statement from the Fourth International Congress on Sexual Medicine 2015. *J Sex Med.* 2016; 13:135–143.

15 Reed GM, Drescher J, Krueger RB, *et al.* Disorders related to sexuality and gender identity in the ICD-11: revising the ICD-10 classification based on current scientific evidence, best clinical practices, and human rights considerations. *World Psychiatry*, 2016; 15:205–221.

16 Derogatis LR, Sand M, Balon R, *et al.* Toward a more evidenced-based nosology and nomenclature for female sexual dysfunctions – Part 1. *J Sex Med.* 2016; 13:1881–1887.

17 Dunn KM, Jordan K, Croft PR, *et al.* Systematic review of sexual problems: epidemiology and methodology. *J Sex & Mar Ther.* 2002; 28:399–420.

18 Hayes RD, Bennett CM, Fairly CK, *et al.* What can prevalence studies tell us about female sexual difficulty and dysfunction. *J Sex Med.* 2006; 3:589–595.

19 Shifren JL, Monz BU, Russo PA, *et al.* Sexual problems and distress in United States women: prevalence and correlates. *Obstet Gynecol.* 2008; 112(5):970–978.

20 Dennerstein L, Koochaki P, Barton I, Graziottin A. Hypoactive sexual desire disorder in menopausal women: A survey of Western European women. *J Sex Med.* 2006; 3:212–222.

21 Derogatis LR, Burnett A. The epidemiology of sexual dysfunctions. *J Sex Med.* 2008; 5:289–300.

22 Atlantis E, Sullivan T. Bidirectional association between depression and sexual dysfunction: A systematic review and meta-analysis. *J Sex Med.* 2012; 9(6):1497–1507.

23 Bonierebale M, Lancon C, Tignol, J. The ELIXIR study: evaluation of sexual dysfunction in 4557 depressed patients in France. *Curr Med Res Opin.* 2003; 19:114–124.

24 West SL, D'Aloisio AA, Agans, RP, *et al.* Prevalence of low sexual desire and HSDD in a nationally representative sample of US women. *Arch Intern Med.* 2008. 168:1441–1448.

25 Clayton AH, Maserejian NN, Connor MK, *et al*. Depression in premenopausal women with HSDD: baseline findings from the HSDD Registry for Women. *Psychosom Med*. 2012; 74(3):305–311.

26 Johannes CB, Clayton AH, Odom DM, *et al*. Distressing sexual problems in United States women revisited: prevalence after accounting for depression. *J Clin Psychiatry*. 2009; 70(12):1698–1706.

4

# Central Nervous System Anatomy and Neurochemistry of Sexual Desire

*James G. Pfaus and Sherri L. Jones*

### Abstract

Sexual desire comprises objective physiological, subjective psychological, and behavioral aspects, and can be defined as a presence of desire for, and fantasy about, sexual activity. In animals and humans, desire can be inferred by measuring behaviors such as willingness to work for sexual reinforcers, or locomotor activity in anticipation of sexual activity. Inherent in all models of sexual behavior is the notion that the different components of sexual behavior require activation of different brain regions or networks for their coordination. That coordination requires tightly regulated feedback systems as well as molecular mechanisms that allow those systems to be amenable to steroid hormones and experience. In this chapter, we review central nervous system structures and the underlying neurochemistry involved in sexual excitation, inhibition, and disinhibition, drawn primarily from basic preclinical research in animals. We then discuss three potential treatments for female sexual desire or interest disorders that have undergone clinical trials.

**Keywords:** *dopamine; HSDD; melanocortin; neuroanatomy; neurochemistry; ovarian hormones; sexual desire; testosterone; solicitations; serotonin*

> Sexual desire is in the brain.
>
> Sexual desire is driven by the expectation of sexual pleasure.
>
> Excitatory and inhibitory systems in the brain integrate internal and external stimuli to generate desire as a final endpoint.

## Introduction

Sexual desire is a difficult concept to grasp, as it entails objective physiological, subjective psychological, and behavioral variables that reflect conscious recognition of its own state. This implies a dynamic regulation of desire in the brain. No agreed-upon definition of sexual desire exists except that inferred from the definition of hypoactive sexual desire disorder by the International Society for the Study of Women's Sexual Health (ISSWSH) [1], and

recommended for adoption into the ICD-11 [2], in which desire for, and fantasy about, engaging in sexual activity are chronically or recurrently deficient or absent. By converse logic, sexual desire would be the presence of desire for, and fantasy about, sexual activity. The Diagnostic and Statistical Manual of Mental Disorders 5 (DSM-5) of the American Psychiatric Association kept hypoactive sexual desire disorder but combined it for women with sexual arousal disorder into a new moniker called Female Sexual Interest and Arousal

*Textbook of Female Sexual Function and Dysfunction: Diagnosis and Treatment*, First Edition. Edited by Irwin Goldstein, Anita H. Clayton, Andrew T. Goldstein, Noel N. Kim, and Sheryl A. Kingsberg.
© 2018 John Wiley & Sons Ltd. Published 2018 by John Wiley & Sons Ltd.

Disorder [3], despite the fact that women can present with predominantly low desire, predominant arousal problems, or a combination of the two [4]. Indeed, desire can be viewed as distinct from arousal in animals and humans, with desire constituting a psychological interest in sex and behaviors that reflect such interest. Despite this separation of arousal and desire, it is likely that desire is informed or confirmed by the presence of autonomic or central arousal. In fact, many women and men regard sexual desire and arousal as parts of one another, despite being given distinct definitions [5]. Thus, desire as it is expressed physically in conscious, goal-directed behavior, most closely resembles the terms "lust", "libido", and "horny" [1].

Desire can be inferred in both animals and humans by their willingness to work for sexual reinforcers, or in behavior that reflects the anticipation of sexual activity [6]. In all species, sexual behavior is directed by a complex interplay between steroid hormone actions in the brain that give rise to sexual arousability, and experience with sexual reward or pleasure that gives rise to expectations of competent sexual activity, including sexual arousal, desire, and elements of copulatory performance [7]. Sexual experience allows animals to form instrumental and Pavlovian associations (i.e. associations formed between behaviors and devices such as levers or unrelated stimuli such as sound) that predict sexual outcomes and, thereby, direct the strength of sexual response. Although the study of animal sexual behavior by neuroendocrinologists has traditionally been concerned with mechanisms of copulatory response related to reproduction (e.g. lordosis in females and erections, mounts, intromissions, and ejaculations in males), more recent use of conditioning and preference paradigms, and a focus on environmental circumstances and experience, has revealed sexual behaviors in a variety of species that are driven by reward-related mechanisms in the brain that are analogous or homologous to human sexual

desire [7–10]. But from both a biological and psychological perspective, this makes logical sense: animals must be able to respond to hormonal and neurochemical changes that signal their own sexual arousal and desire, and be able to interact with external sexual incentives. Animals must be able to identify external stimuli that predict where potential sex partners can be found, and subsequently seek them out, solicit, court, or otherwise work to obtain them, distinguish sensory cues and behavioral patterns of potential partners from those that are not interested or receptive, and pursue desired sex partners once sexual contact has been made.

## The Sexual Brain

The brain organizes sexual stimulation into an overall interactive sense of sexual excitation and inhibition that integrates societal, psychological, and physiological factors (Figure 4.1). This is accomplished in evolutionarily-conserved sets of neurochemical pathways or "modules" that integrate endogenous sex "drive" (e.g. gonadal hormone status and energy metabolism) with autonomic arousal in the hypothalamus, the intensity of incentive sexual stimuli (unconditioned and conditioned stimuli that activate or "prime" attention and movement from distal to proximal to interactive) in the hypothalamus and limbic system, and the evaluation of sexual context and executive function as it relates to sexual excitation or inhibition overall [6]. In particular, cortical activation controls the coding of information into "gestalts" (e.g. sets of physical or interpersonal characteristics that individuals find conditionally attractive or unattractive; contexts that are suitable or unsuitable for sexual activity; etc., following from Pavlov [11]) and involves the activation of the medial prefrontal cortex and the descending inhibition of motor acts as part of executive function. Within each are excitatory and inhibitory neurochemical systems that control sexual response at any given

## Dual control model

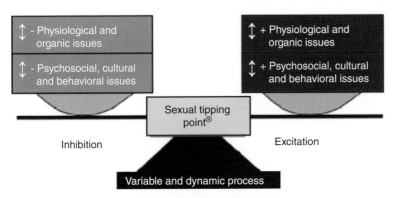

**Figure 4.1** Sexual tipping point model of sexual excitation and inhibition. Cultural, psychological, and physiological factors conspire to tip the balance either toward excitation or inhibition. Sexually functional individuals maintain a degree of lability in the balance, and an ability to have it tipped toward either excitation or inhibition. Persons with hypoactive sexual desire disorder are likely to have the balance weighed down by inhibition. This can occur because of hypofunctional excitation, hyperfunction inhibition, or a combination of the two. After Perelman [67]. (*See plate section for color representation of the figure*)

time. These systems are activated or suppressed by steroid hormones as well as by experience-driven changes in gene expression and neurochemical function [6]. It is through these systems that priming stimuli or drugs alter sexual response by changing the interpretation of stimuli and context.

Attentional and emotional components are encoded largely in limbic structures, notably in the nucleus accumbens, septum, and amygdala (Figure 4.2), that allow the animal to focus on pleasure (or punishment) related stimuli in the environment. The hippocampus provides spatial maps of the external world and episodic memory for important sexual encounters, and the paleocortex (e.g. anterior cingulate gyrus) regulates autonomic function along with anticipation of reward, decision making, and empathy [12, 13]. Along with limbic activation, hypothalamic structures, notably the medial preoptic area and ventromedial hypothalamus, activate sexual response in relation to hormonal status and metabolism, and in concert with regions, such as the paraventricular nucleus and supraoptic nucleus, coordinate autonomic activation with elements of sexual desire (e.g. solicitations, pursuit). Those structures

also participate in the generation of partner and mate preferences. The medial preoptic area is well suited as a central processor in the linking of metabolic need, hormonal status, and autonomic outflow, with the stimulation of mesolimbic dopamine neurons in the ventral tegmental area. The mesolimbic dopamine system projects to several important limbic and cortical structures, notably the nucleus accumbens, corticomedial amygdala, lateral and medial septum, and medial prefrontal cortex, and is critical for all animals' attention to incentive stimuli [14]; genitosensory, attentional, and emotional systems are engaged at the same time following the hormonal stimulation that occurs around ovulation, linking reward-related incentive motivation to reproduction.

Finally, as mentioned above, although sexual responses can include thoughts and fantasies (at least in humans), they are reflected in all animals as behavior. Coordinated purposeful behavior comes from the activity of both fine and gross motor acts that are derived from the coordinated activation of motor cortex and the basal ganglia, along with other motor structures in the midbrain and the cerebellum. In addition

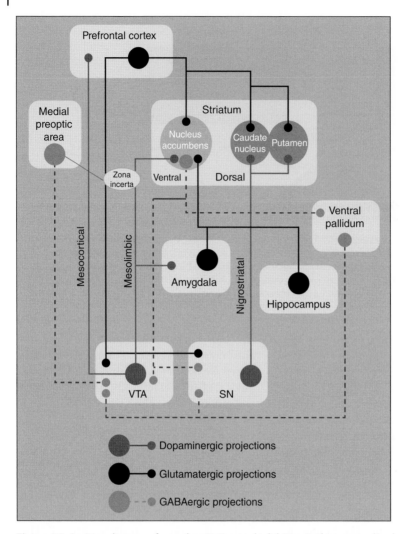

**Figure 4.2** A wiring diagram of sexual excitation and inhibition in the mammalian brain that reflects current understanding of neuroanatomical and neurochemical pathways. VTA: Ventral tegmental area; SN: substantia nigra. Modified from Kingsberg *et al.* [119]. (*See plate section for color representation of the figure*)

to coordinating body movements in space and time, these structures crystallize motor memory, a function that is critical for motor habit formation (the phenomenon whereby motor acts at the beginning of behavioral learning are choppy and uncoordinated, but become virtually automated with practice). Although the formation of motor habits in males with extensive sexual experience protects sexual behavior against treatments or situations that might disrupt it, including novel environments, stress, genital anesthesia, brain lesions, and even castration

or endogenous hypogonadism (reviewed in Pfaus *et al.* [7]), it is not yet known whether sexual experience provides females with similar protection.

## Structure of Female Sexual Behavior

For all animals, sexual behavior occurs as a sequence or "cascade" of behavioral events. Beach [15] recognized the heuristic value of separating sexual behavior into *appetitive* and *consummatory* phases. Essentially, this scheme followed from the work of early twentieth century ethologists and experimental psychologists [16, 17], who defined appetitive (or "preparatory") behaviors as those which bring an animal from distal to proximal and into contact with goal objects or incentives, like potential sex partners. In contrast, consummatory behaviors are performed once an animal is in direct contact with the incentive (i.e. to "consummate" the goal). Consummatory sexual behaviors tend to be species specific, sexually differentiated, and stereotyped, whereas appetitive behaviors are more flexible. This also makes sense, as survival often depends on behavioral flexibility, on an animal's ability to learn a variety of strategies to obtain goals in different environments or appetitive circumstances [7, 18]. As in animals, human sexual desire and subjective sexual arousal fit into an appetitive framework [7, 10, 19], whereas the more stereotyped patterns of copulatory behavior fit into a consummatory framework.

Perhaps the most well-known description of human sexual response is that of Masters and Johnson's "EPOR" (Excitation, Plateau, Orgasm, Resolution) model (Figure 4.3) [20]. This model, derived from Moll's original (1908) four-stage model [21], flows in time as a cascade of behavioral and neurophysiological events, starting with sexual excitement (blood flow to the genitals and other erogenous erectile tissues), then plateau (parasympathetic maintenance of genital

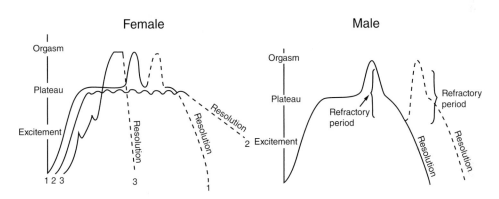

Modified by Kaplan (1974) and Georgiadis et al. (2012)

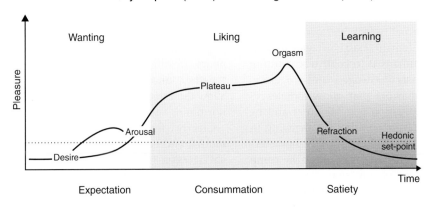

**Figure 4.3** The "EPOR" (Excitation, Plateau, Orgasm, Resolution) model of Masters and Johnson, with modifications by Kaplan [21] and Georgiadis *et al.* [24] to fit more current models of arousal, desire, and incentive motivation.

blood flow during sexual intercourse), culminating in orgasm (a defining moment of euphoria, ecstasy, and pleasure in which sympathetic systems move blood out of the genitals), followed by resolution (also called a refractory period during which inhibitory systems of the brain are activated to reduce the salience of external and somatosensory sexual stimuli). The EPOR model describes at least three distinct patterns for women that vary in the structure of the plateau, the intensity and number of orgasms, and the temporal offset of arousal during the resolution phase, although it does not differentiate the particular characteristics of the sexual stimuli used to achieve orgasm (e.g., external clitoral only, external and internal clitoral, cervical, blended clitoral and cervical, extragenital, etc.), nor was it based on an analysis of actual genital blood flow. Subsequently, Kaplan [22] added a phase of sexual desire, consisting of fantasies and thoughts about sexual activity, along with behavior aimed at obtaining sexual partners and/or sexual gratification. The phases can also be described in terms of wanting (desire), liking (arousal, plateau and orgasm), and inhibition (resolution) [23, 24].

Despite overarching theoretical models of human and animal sexual response that did not posit sex differences in the basic response structure, female sexual behavior has, until fairly recently, been considered "passive." This is due, in part, to a general social construction in Western society of female sexuality as something that is "done to," relative to more active male sexuality that "performs," and to the labeling of female sexual behavior in both animals and humans as "receptive", consisting largely in animals of estrogen- and progestin-dependent behaviors that allow females to accept male initiation (e.g. mounts) and be open to vaginal penetration by engaging in postural changes like lordosis, the characteristic arching of the back that raises the rump to allow penile intromission. Similarly, in humans, hormone- and context-dependent "responsive desire" has been viewed as allowing females to be responsive to a partner's active pursuits [25]. However, it is clear that women and some other primate females can have sexual intercourse anytime during the ovulatory cycle. This can even occur without hormone priming in hypogonadal individuals and, indeed, without prior desire or consent [26]. Although sexually receptive behaviors clearly exist in females of all species, they are far from passive when it comes to sex. Based on observations of a variety of species, Beach [15] proposed that female-initiated sexual behaviors can be partitioned into a cascade of essentially three temporal phases: *attractivity* (behaviors like approach or scent marking that lure males to the females), *proceptivity* (behaviors that precede receptive behaviors and focus the male on pursuing the female), and *receptivity* (behaviors like lordosis and lateral tail deflection in rats and hamsters, respectively, or sexual positions in humans that allow vaginal penetration). More recently, Basson [25] (Figure 4.4) described how "innate" sexual desire (potentially induced at ovulation, for example by the combined action of estrogens and androgens in the hypothalamus and limbic system), activates attention to incentive sexual stimuli, sexual arousal, and sexual receptive behaviors that, if positively reinforced, lead to a sensitization of attention and sexual arousal in the presence of salient and competent incentive sexual cues. Her model is easily applicable to all species and is similar to incentive models for sexual motivation produced by others [19, 27].

Inherent in all models of sexual behavior is the notion that the components are separable. This would require different brain regions or networks to control the components, feedback systems that link them together, and molecular mechanisms that allow their activation to be altered by steroid hormones and experience.

Clearly, females and males engage in mutual and complementary patterns of sexual activity; however, it is the females that initiate and control successful sexual interaction, including the initiation and temporal patterning of copulation. This occurs by a complex interaction of *appetitive*

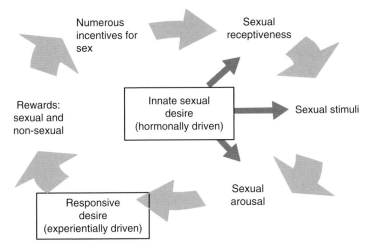

**Figure 4.4** Circular feedback model of sexual responsiveness by Basson. Note that experience with sexual reward in the model can increase the likelihood of response, whereas experience with sexual nonreward or punishment can diminish expectations of pleasure that reduce the functionality of the feedback system. From Basson [25].

*precopulatory behaviors* that attract and solicit sex from males. These behaviors are taken to reflect both innate and "receptive" sexual desire, and may well be informed by or sum with sexual arousal. Once copulation begins, females engage in *receptive behaviors* such as lordosis, *pacing behaviors* that control the rate of sexual stimulation received during sexual interaction and copulation, and *defensive behaviors* used either to pace the copulatory contact if females cannot otherwise do so, or to terminate the sexual interaction [27–29]. These behaviors serve to optimize the rate and strength of sexual stimulation received by females, which, in turn, initiates neuroendocrine reflexes associated with fertility and pregnancy.

## Sexual Behavior of Human Females

Like other primates, the sexual behaviors of women can be organized into specific patterns of sexual desire, arousal, orgasm, and sexual inhibition, all of which are exquisitely sensitive to context, social learning, and real experience [25]. However, despite the gen-eral view that sexual behavior in women is "freed" from the dependence on steroid hormones, women display a characteristic increase in self-reported sexual desire and arousal during ovulation (Figure 4.5) [30]. Across the ovarian cycle of women, steroid hormone levels fluctuate in a cyclical manner. Circulating levels of estrogens, progestins, and androgens rise around the time of ovulation, correlating with an increase in sexual interest, activity and fantasies [19, 27, 30–34]. Removal of cyclic steroid hormone release by long-term administration of estrogen-containing oral contraceptives often results in a decline in sexual desire, activity, and genital blood flow [31, 35–38]. It is unclear whether the blunting of the cyclical induction of sexual activity and fantasies is directly due to the removal of the cyclicity of the hormones acting on relevant tissues, or whether it is secondary to downstream effects of chronic administration of estrogens. Long-term exposure to estrogens has physiological effects that might disrupt sexual behavior. For example, estrogens upregulate steroid hormone binding globulin production by the liver, which are transport proteins that bind androgens with higher

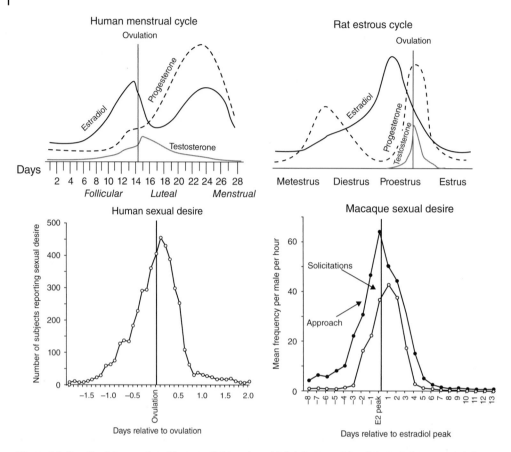

**Figure 4.5** Top: Ovulatory cycles of humans (left) and rats (right). Bottom: Sexual desire in humans and rhesus macaques. Note how measures of desire peak around the time of ovulation. Secondary peaks have been reported around the time of menstruation in humans. From Pfaus *et al.* [27], after Wallen [26], Stanislaw and Rice [30].

affinity than estrogens [39–41]. As such, the administration of an estrogen can lower circulating androgens such as testosterone. Given the importance of androgens for sexual desire in women, a reduction in circulating androgens by chronic use of oral contraceptives may be one reason why some women experience a decrease in sexual desire on the pill.

A decline in sexual desire and activity also occurs following surgical, natural, and chemically-induced menopause. Surgically menopausal women, induced by bilateral oophorectomy with or without hysterectomy, experience a sudden and drastic decline in sexual arousal and desire [42–44]. These symptoms can be restored following adequate hormone replacement regimens,

particularly with replacement of estrogens in combination with testosterone [42, 45–53]. For women with chemically-induced menopause (i.e. following chemotherapy or gonadotropin-releasing hormone agonists), those that experience chronic ovarian failure report higher levels of sexual desire problems than menstruating women with past chemotherapy treatment [54]. In postmenopausal (55–70 year olds) breast-cancer survivors, those treated with adjuvant hormone treatments report lower levels of sexual arousal and desire compared to age-matched controls [55]. Moreover, those treated with aromatase inhibitors report lower sexual interest compared to five years earlier than do those treated with estrogen receptor blockers or age-matched controls. As such, ample evidence suggests that fluctuating ovarian steroid hormone levels are important in normal sexual function in women, as they are in other species.

Despite a wealth of knowledge from animal studies, sexual desire in women is a matter of great controversy. Although sexual arousal and desire can be defined by subjective reports, only arousal has been defined objectively (as increased genital blood flow). There is not yet an objective measure of desire, thereby forcing it to be inferred from subjective self-report or intuitively observed behavior (e.g. flirtations). Desire appears to occur spontaneously in some women whereas in others it occurs in response to the right male(s) or females(s) making the right verbal and nonverbal gestures in the right contexts. As mentioned above, self-reported desire peaks during ovulation. This makes antecedent hormonal conditions – effects of estradiol, testosterone, and perhaps also progesterone, in the brain - likely motivational variables in its stimulation. Responsive desire, or the ability of the "right" stimuli to activate incentive motivational pathways in the brain and excite attention and behaviors that are indicative of desire, is also activated by steroid hormones. As mentioned above, desire is then expressed both as a spontaneous motivation and an attention toward competent sexual stimuli [19, 27]. In both cases, the emergent conscious awareness of sexual desire activates movement from distal to proximal to interactive, like the approach and solicitations of rats and macaques. Humans thus learn a baffling array of appetitive responses that work differently in different cultures and contexts, or differently within a single culture at different epochs, and indeed differently with different people. And cultures constrain women's responses, and indeed their own knowledge of their own sexuality, to appropriate times and places. The brain must balance these excitatory and inhibitory influences to achieve an optimal level for pleasure. And it must do this with hormonal influences weighing it toward excitation, especially during ovulation, and

experience directing attention and behavior toward individuals and stimuli previously associated with sexual reward.

The copulatory patterns of women are also fraught with problems of interpretation. Although more stereotyped than appetitive responses, consummatory patterns of copulation in humans are, nonetheless, extremely variable, even in cultures where certain positions (e.g. missionary) are proscribed. Some heterosexual positions (e.g. woman on top) can maximize her ability to get optimal external and internal clitoral stimulation, possibly along with direct stimulation of the cervix, from the male. Other positions may embellish other stimulus zones, and thus engage different motor patterns to maximize the stimulation achieved. And, of course, some women are extremely sensitive to external clitoral stimulation, and can only achieve orgasm in that way, whereas others achieve orgasms with blended internal and external clitoral stimulation. Interestingly, there is no human analogue to the lordosis reflex, although lordosis-like positions can be observed in women being mounted from behind. A lordosis-like arching of the back, however, is not a hormone-induced and/or facilitated spinal reflex; those do not exist in humans, a fact that continues to limit the human clinical application of the neuroendocrine work done on lordosis in animals. Being "receptive" to vaginal penetration in women involves a conscious decision to expose the vulva and open it to penetration. Experience with orgasm or other types of sexual pleasure and intimacy leads to expectancies of which positions "work", thus further constraining the sexual positions and patterns of both women and men.

## Ovarian Hormones Set the Stage

As mentioned above, the cyclic actions of estradiol, testosterone, and progesterone in females leads to changes in sexual response and increases in sexual arousal and desire around the time of ovulation in all vertebrate species, including humans [30, 56], although a smaller increase in arousal and desire has been reported around the time of menstruation [57]. Of the three steroids released from the ovaries of mammalian females, testosterone is at its highest level around the time of ovulation, whereas estradiol rises a few days earlier, peaking just before ovulation (Figure 4.5). Progesterone levels rise before, during, or after ovulation, depending on the species. This hormonal milieu during the periovulatory follicular phase alters the way in which visual sexual stimuli are processed in women [58–61], which presumably leads to a shift in the incentive value of the stimuli. Analogous findings have been reported in other primates, for example in approaches and solicitations made around the time of the mid-cycle estradiol peak in rhesus macaques [62], and in the appetitive and consummatory sexual behaviors that characterize the periovulatory period of female rats [63]. Steroid hormones drive sexual arousal and desire in response to competent incentive stimuli. In turn, experience with sexual reward (and inhibition) modulates the strength and trajectory of responses to incentive sexual cues. This is timed in most female mammals to the period around ovulation, thus stimulating females to engage in the most rewarding behaviors under the most reproductively-relevant circumstances (see *Pacing Behavior*). This contrasts with the relatively stable and continuous testicular androgen secretion in mammalian males (and its aromatization to neural estradiol in different regions of the brain) that maintains sexual arousability and responsiveness in a relatively continuous manner [64].

## How do We Study the Central Nervous System Regulation of Female Sexual Desire?

Although human sexual behavior is best studied in humans, it is often impossible to do so with experimental precision or at a level that allows any degree of finely-grained neural or molecular analysis. Recent advances in brain imaging and eye-tracking technology have allowed cortical and subcortical activation, and visual gaze, to be assessed in women viewing erotic visual stimuli, and some important paradigms have emerged to correlate aspects of subjective sexual arousal, desire, and orgasm to overall brain activation patterns (Figure 4.6) [23]. Such data reveal a great deal about the cognitive and limbic control of different aspects of female sexual behavior under different hormonally-modulated, pharmacological, or experiential conditions, and in ways that confirm data from females of other species. Nevertheless, these paradigms lag behind the scope of neuroanatomical, neuropharmacological, histochemical, and molecular methods that can be used with animal models.

Most of the research done on the neurobiology of female sexual desire comes from rodent subfamilies, like rats, mice, hamsters, gerbils, voles, and musk shrews, lagomorphs like rabbits and myomorphs like guinea pigs, less so from primates like rhesus and Japanese macaques, and even less so from humans. Understanding the behavioral structure of each species' appetitive and consummatory phases is vitally important for a sophisticated understanding of the neurobiological mechanisms that control it. In many studies, the female's receptive lordosis posture is taken as an index of her copulatory or "mating" behavior, rather than the full repertoire of appetitive and consummatory sexual responses. It is often the case in laboratory settings that females are tested in small chambers that do not allow them to approach or escape the male or, in the case of females that pace the copulatory contact, allow them to regulate the timing and intensity of that contact. When appetitive responses are taken together with lordosis, it becomes immediately apparent that there is extensive conservation of the neurochemical mechanisms that control sexual behavior, which generates homologies in the way that sexual stimulation is perceived by the brain and induces competent responses. Behavior is

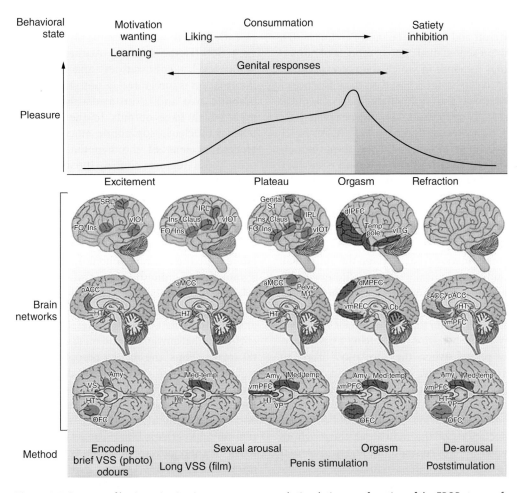

**Figure 4.6** Patterns of brain activation in response to sexual stimulation as a function of the EPOR stages of sexual response. From Georgiadis *et al.* [23]. (*See plate section for color representation of the figure*)

the ultimate arbiter and can never be supplanted by the processes that underlie it. For example, release of the neurotransmitter dopamine in mesolimbic terminals like the nucleus accumbens may be involved in all forms of appetitive motivation toward rewarding incentives like sex partners, but just observing dopamine released there does not allow the viewer to conclude that whatever the animal was doing is positively hedonic. Understanding the neurobiology of animal sexual behavior also allows the consideration of models of sexual function and dysfunction that are directly applicable in the preclinical testing of drugs or other treatments.

## Excitation, Inhibition, and Disinhibition of Sexual Responses

As mentioned previously, the notion of separate, but interactive, neural systems for behavioral excitation and inhibition goes back to the work of early neurophysiologists like Sechenov, Sherrington, and Pavlov, and more modern psychologists like Gray, who applied the idea to the study of fear and anxiety [65]. It has important implications for sexual behavior because it posits that behavior can commence either due to direct excitation or through a process of disinhibition.

This concept was advanced further by Bancroft and Janssen [66] and Perelman [67], who presented dual control models of human sexual response in which the net expression of sexual behavior is based on the influence of excitatory and inhibitory neurochemical mechanisms in the brain and periphery, set around a "sexual tipping point" (Figures 4.1 and 4.7). As in Gray's theory, these models stress the adaptive nature of both excitatory and inhibitory processes. For example, the adaptive nature of sexual excitement would drive individuals to seek out sex partners for reproductive or reward purposes. The adaptive nature of sexual inhibition would guard against situations that threaten the individual, including chronically stressful life events. It would also be important to keep the optimal expression of behavior constrained to the "right time," as in the case of females that display sexual behavior only during a periovulatory period, when they are most likely to become pregnant. Bancroft and Janssen viewed the propensity for sexual excitement or inhibition as an individual tendency based on the genetic makeup and/or behavioral expectations of the individual: those whose propensity for central inhibition of sexual response is too high have increased vulnerability to sexual dysfunction, whereas those whose inhibitory propensity is too low would be more likely to engage in hypersexual or high risk sexual behavior. Indeed, the study of sexual inhibition is also critical if we are to understand how certain events or drugs like alcohol, cocaine, or amphetamine, may induce sexual disinhibition and the propensity to engage in risky sexual behaviors [68].

## Excitation

Excitation can be viewed from autonomic arousal and genitosensory/erogenous stimulation as a "bottom-up" phenomenon, in which individual sensory modules come together at higher levels of processing. This occurs in the thalamus, and also in each domain of the hypothalamus, limbic system, and cortex, that make up the excitatory

sexual system of the brain [6]. These systems essentially tip the sexual tipping point toward excitation (Figure 4.8, left). At the hypothalamic level, genitosensory and olfactory information is integrated in both the medial preoptic area and ventromedial hypothalamus, which have outputs to the paraventricular nucleus, supraoptic nucleus, and arcuate nucleus of the hypothalamus. In turn, those regions control the release of oxytocin, vasopressin both in brain and from the posterior pituitary, and the release of melanocortins, opioids, and adrenocorticotropin hormone from the anterior pituitary. The medial preoptic area also sends lateral efferents to the ventral tegmental area, which stimulate dopamine neurons and dopamine release in mesolimbic and mesocortical terminals, such as the nucleus accumbens, anterior cingulate cortex, lateral septum, corticomedial amygdala, and medial prefrontal cortex. Thus, the medial preoptic area is well situated to "drive" the dopamine-mediated incentive motivational system in the presence of salient unconditional and conditional external sexual cues, and also to register and perhaps link those cues to genitosensory and autonomic input. In addition, noradrenergic inputs to the hypothalamus coming from the locus coeruleus are themselves stimulated by the reticular activating system, which is stimulated by general autonomic and somatic inputs from the spinal cord. For females, sensitivity to sexual arousal is enhanced during ovulation, and thus excitatory systems in the central nervous system appear to require steroid hormone priming.

Estradiol regulates a variety of neurotransmitter and second messenger systems in brain areas involved in sexual behavior [69, 70] (reviewed in Pfaus *et al.* [63]). Estradiol priming induces the synthesis of $\alpha_{1B}$-adrenergic receptors in the ventromedial hypothalamus and augments the release of dopamine in the striatum, nucleus accumbens, and medial preoptic area during copulation. Extracellular DOPAC, a dopamine metabolite, increases in the medial preoptic area in the afternoon to the early evening of

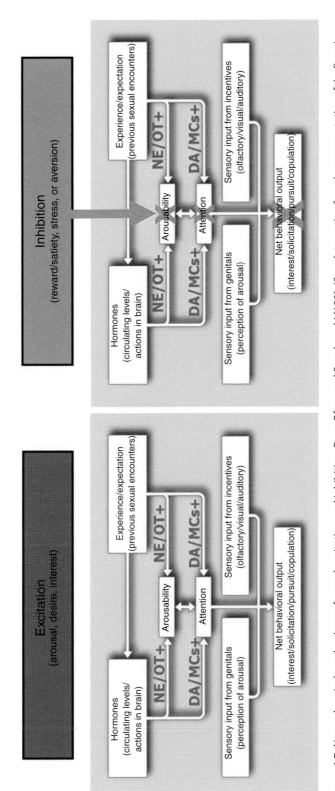

**Figure 4.7** Neurochemical mechanisms of sexual excitation and inhibition. From Pfaus and Scepkowski [120]. (*See plate section for color representation of the figure*)

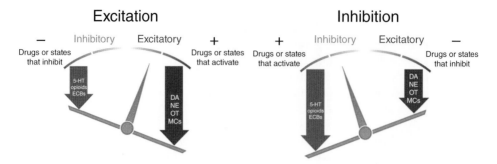

**Figure 4.8** Neurochemical mechanisms of sexual excitation within a tipping point model. Left: sexual excitation. Right: Sexual inhibition. From Pfaus [6]. (*See plate section for color representation of the figure*)

proestrus, around the time that sexual behavior is activated. Dopamine is also released within the medial preoptic area in ovariectomized female rats treated with estradiol benzoate and progesterone; however, this release is not detected in females treated with estradiol benzoate alone. Hormone dependent differences also occur with the application of dopamine agonists to the medial preoptic area, such that in females primed with estradiol benzoate alone, D2 receptor subtype agonists facilitate sexual behavior, whereas in estradiol benzoate + progesterone-primed females D1 receptor subtype activation facilitates sexual behavior. Tonic dopamine release activates D2 receptors, whereas phasic dopamine release stimulates D1 receptors. Thus, priming with estradiol benzoate alone may tonically activate D2 receptors, whereas subsequent P administration may stimulate phasic dopamine release within the medial preoptic area, and activate D1 receptors, to facilitate sexual behaviors. Estradiol also stimulates the synthesis of melanocortin type 4 receptors in the hypothalamus and synthesis of proopiomelanocortin in arcuate nucleus neurons, and stimulates the synthesis of cholinergic receptors and enkephalin within the ventromedial hypothalamus. Gamma-aminobutyric acid and glutamate activation are also stimulated by estradiol in these regions (see sections *Solicitations; Role of melanocortins; Glutamate in the ventrolateral portion of the ventromedial*

*hypothalamus; and Lordosis*). Although testosterone is important in the expression of sexually appetitive behaviors in EB-treated rats [71], and its facilitative effects have been well-documented in male rat sexual behavior [72], the neurobiological mechanisms in females have not been explored.

### Inhibition

Inhibitory synapses make up a large part of the central nervous system and local inhibitory networks can hone a response by eliminating competing responses that would interfere with it (e.g. as happens in the visual system with lateral inhibition by amacrine cells). Such inhibition can be observed when behavior comes in bouts or phases, and in a sexual response cycle would be consonant with the "R" phase, a period of postorgasmic refractoriness in which further sexual interest is diminished. Local inhibition can also play a role in the timing of behavior to make it occur only during optimal periods. Female desire and lordosis behavior in animals are obvious examples.

General behavioral inhibition, however, is typically viewed as a "top-down" phenomenon involving the cognitive process of "executive function" [73]. Animals always have to choose among different drives and motivations (e.g. between feeding and copulation), and, indeed, between several possibilities per motivational system, to achieve an optimal outcome. The medial prefrontal cortex organizes this by creating behavioral hierarchies based on expectancies, planned actions, and calculations. The medial prefrontal cortex (and likely other cortical areas) therefore, must inhibit a complex and ongoing interplay of motor tendencies to arrive at planned and sustained actions. People or rats with disrupted prefrontal function, either due to lesions or neurochemical imbalance, have great difficulty focusing attention on tasks, are unable to inhibit competing responses, and experience retroactive and proactive interference [73]. With regard to sexual behavior, such top-down inhibition can be activated as "morality" and would be based on a cultural value system that imposes "right" and "wrong" on certain behaviors, such that some that feel good are "right" and can be experienced without guilt, whereas others are "wrong" and carry the weight of guilt and/or rule of law against them. This type of inhibition gives rise to the classic "approach–avoidance" conflict, where the expectation of reward drives the desire, but the inhibition imposed by the real or perceived aversive consequences of engaging in sexual activity blunts the initiation of behavior. Such inhibition may well lie at the root of the inhibited sexual response experienced by women who are not taught to express their sexual desires without some form of guilt. Such inhibition would likely be reinforced if women experienced sexual nonreward during copulation, and such reinforced inhibition would likely overlay itself on desire components to suppress them directly. Some women may be more susceptible to this type of inhibition than others. Accordingly, the "prosexual" nature of drugs such as alcohol, cocaine, and methamphetamine, may be a function of their ability to disinhibit such suppressed sexual response [68].

Refractory inhibition that comes after orgasm involves the activation of at least three neurochemical systems: opioids that induce pleasure, euphoria, and ecstasy; endocannabinoids that induce sedation; and serotonin that induces satiety [6] (Figure 4.7, right). The reward states induced by clitoral stimulation, vaginocervical stimulation, or paced mating in rats appear to be independent of steroid hormone priming, although the priming is necessary to activate the excitatory systems that bring about the behavior in the first place [7, 74]. At present it is not known where such inhibition actually takes place. Indeed, the mPOA and VMH have receptors for all three transmitter systems, indeed for all three opioid systems. Activation of delta opioid receptors in the mPOA inhibit lordosis [75], whereas activation of mu opioid receptors in the VMH inhibits lordosis [76]. Inhibition also comes in the form of estrous termination [77].

## Disinhibition

As noted above, certain prosexual drugs can disinhibit sexual response, but only in individuals with sexual inhibition (reviewed in Pfaus *et al.* [68]). Male rats trained not to copulate with sexually nonreceptive females will attempt copulation with them under the influence of alcohol, amphetamine, cocaine, and methamphetamine. Alcohol and cocaine stimulate appetitive behaviors in females primed with estradiol alone. Intermittent amphetamine or methamphetamine administration sensitizes sexual approaches and solicitations in female rats and increases neuronal activation in the medial amygdala and ventromedial hypothalamus following copulation. However, methamphetamine treatment also makes female rats less selective in preference for particular males.

Disinhibition may also occur as a function of hormone priming. Systems that normally maintain inhibition over female sexual behavior during nonovulatory periods likely must be inhibited to allow the behavior to occur. This appears to be the case for some systems in the ventromedial hypothalamus that help to time the behavior and that help to bring about estrous termination (see *Glutamate in the ventrolateral portion of the ventromedial hypothalamus*). Thus, the brain is set up with modules that gather and interpret sensory input and generate competent motor outputs at optimal times. This allows reward systems to be activated when females engage in the right behaviors at the right times, and allows such behavior to optimize the reproductive outcomes. The fact that paced copulation is both rewarding to females and results in stronger copulatory stimulation from males, leading to a greater chance of successful impregnation, is a good example of the intricate timing systems that blend the two. Far more is known about the neural and neurochemical control of lordosis than appetitive sexual approach, solicitation, or pacing behaviors. These are outlined in the next sections.

## Sexual Approach Behaviors

Mesolimbic dopamine is involved in the sensitization and crystallization of incentive response [14], especially within terminals in the nucleus accumbens. Microdialysis studies have shown that dopamine in the nucleus accumbens increases during copulation in ovariectomized female rats or hamsters primed fully with estradiol benzoate and progesterone. In rats the increase is approximately 150% of baseline when females are presented with a gonadally intact, sexually vigorous male rat behind a screen, and increases to approximately 180% when the screen is removed and copulation ensues [78]. The temporal resolution of microdialysis (e.g. 10-min samples), however, does not permit specific behaviors to be correlated with the rise in dopamine, especially during copulation. However, the degree of release is positively correlated with the number of attempts made by the female to nose-poke through the wire-mesh divider. dopamine release increases more in the NAc and dorsal striatum in hormonally-primed females that must make an operant response to gain access to males compared to females that do not [79], suggesting that mesolimbic and striatal dopamine release helps orient the female

towards a sexually active male and make approach responses in anticipation of sexual stimulation and reward.

## Solicitations

The pioneering work of Wallen *et al.* [62], McClintock [29], and Erskine [28] refined Beach's [15] general category of "proceptive" behaviors in female macaques and rats into species-specific descriptions of sexual approach, solicitation, and pacing. In rats, solicitations could be defined as full (head-wise orientation to the male followed by a runaway) or partial (hops and darts, and perhaps also ear-wiggles) depending on how close in proximity the female was to the male and whether she had room to run away. Pacing could be operationalized as any behavior that imposed temporal control over the rate of mounts, intromissions, and ejaculations. Female mounting of sexually sluggish or naïve males was considered by Beach to be a "super-solicitation behavior" that would allow females to "show" the male what they wanted (reviewed in Pfaus *et al.* [63]).

Lesion studies show distinct effects on appetitive and consummatory behaviors. Excitotoxic lesions of the medial preoptic area abolished both full and partial solicitations, but enhanced lordosis in sexually-experienced ovariectomized rats primed with estradiol benzoate and progesterone [80]. Lesions of the medial prefrontal cortex also inhibited the temporal patterning of full solicitations [81], In contrast, lesions of the lateral septum or ventral tegmental area did not alter the frequency of hops and darts. However, lesions of the medial preoptic area, ventromedial hypothalamus, or medial amygdala, abolished the mounting of sexually sluggish males in ovariectomized rats primed with estradiol benzoate + progesterone, whereas crystalline implants of estradiol to the ventromedial hypothalamus, but not the medial preoptic area or medial amygdala, induced the behavior in ovariectomized rats.

## Role of Incertohypothalamic Dopamine

As with lesions of the medial preoptic area, systemic administration of dopamine antagonists such as haloperidol abolish solicitations but augment lordosis [82, 83]. This effect does not appear to be mediated by mesolimbic dopamine, as 6-hydroxydopamine lesions of ventral tegmental area dopamine neurons projecting to the nucleus accumbens did not alter solicitations in small chambers [84]. However, dopamine in the medial preoptic area plays a key role in the stimulation of solicitations, with D2 receptor activation facilitating solicitations in ovariectomized rats treated with estradiol benzoate alone, and D1 receptor activation facilitating solicitations in ovariectomized rats treated with estradiol benzoate and progesterone [85, 86]. Dopamine projections to the medial preoptic area originate in the zona incerta and dopamine turnover in the zona incerta increases with estradiol administration [87]. Extracellular DOPAC, a dopamine metabolite, increases in the medial preoptic area in the afternoon to the early evening of proestrus, around the time that sexual behavior is activated, and dopamine is also released within the medial preoptic area in ovariectomized rats treated with estradiol benzoate and progesterone, but not in rats treated with estradiol benzoate alone [88–91]. Infusions of SCH-23390, a D1 antagonist, to the medial preoptic area of ovariectomized rats primed with estradiol benzoate + progesterone significantly reduced solicitations selectively [86].

## Role of Melanocortins

Melanocortins like α-melanocyte stimulating hormone are derived from proopiomelanocortin, a precursor peptide made largely in the arcuate nucleus, from which is also derived the opioid β-endorphin and adrenocorticotropic hormone [92]. α-Melanocyte stimulating hormone synthesis is stimulated by estradiol [93] within arcuate nucleus neurons. Projections of those neurons terminate in the medial preoptic area and secrete α-melanocyte stimulating hormone. Two melanocortin receptors exist in the brain, MC3 and MC4, of which the latter is found in the medial preoptic area. Bremelanotide is a synthetic analogue of α-MSH and is the active metabolite of melanotan-II. Systemic administration of bremelanotide stimulates solicitations selectively in female rats primed with estradiol benzoate or estradiol benzoate + progesterone [94]. The precursor, melanotan-II, produces a weaker effect [95], although five consecutive days of melanotan-II administration produces an effect similar to bremelanotide in magnitude. The enhancement of solicitations by bremelanotide is duplicated by infusions to the lateral ventricles or medial preoptic area, but not the ventromedial hypothalamus [9]. Systemic bremelanotide also stimulates dopamine release in the medial preoptic area, but not nucleus accumbens or dorsal striatum of ovariectomized rats treated with estradiol benzoate and progesterone. Finally, the stimulation of solicitations by systemic bremelanotide can be reversed by a infusions of a selective MC4 antagonist (HS019) to the medial preoptic area, but not ventromedial hypothalamus [9]. It can also be reversed by infusions of the D1 antagonist SCH-23390 to the mPOA [9], suggesting that incertohypothalamic. Dopaminergic terminals in the medial preoptic area contain MC4 receptors that drive dopamine release, which, in turn, stimulates solicitations by acting on D1 receptors in this brain region. Thus, the integration between melanocortin and dopamine systems in the medial preoptic area is a critical component in the regulation of solicitations.

## Glutamate in the Ventrolateral Portion of the Ventromedial Hypothalamus

Full and partial solicitations are also under the control of the ventromedial hypothalamus. In a series of studies, Georgescu *et al.* [96, 97]

investigated the inhibitory role of glutamate neurons in the ventrolateral VMH on the sexual behavior of female rats. Both full and partial solicitations were inhibited dramatically by infusions of glutamate, and also by infusions of the selective ionotrophic receptor agonists AMPA and kainate to sexually experienced ovariectomized rats primed with estradiol benzoate and progesterone acutely, or repeatedly primed with estradiol benzoate alone and receiving AMPA infusions in place of copulation [98]. Conversely, infusions of the dual AMPA/kainate receptor antagonists CNQX and DNQX to the ventrolateral ventromedial hypothalamus of sexually experienced OVX rats primed with EB alone increased full and partial solicitations [97].

### Differential Effect of Opioid Receptors

Pfaus and Pfaff [99] reported that infusion of the delta opioid agonist DPDPE, but not the kappa opioid agonist U50-488h, or the mu opioid agonist DAMGO, to the lateral ventricles of sexually experienced ovariectomized rats primed with estradiol benzoate alone or estradiol benzoate and a low dose of progesterone (to induce moderate lordosis and low solicitations) increased solicitations in bilevel chambers significantly over control infusions. It is not known at present where in the brain this facilitation of solicitations may occur.

Taken together, these data suggest that the connections between the ventromedial hypothalamus and medial preoptic area are critical in the regulation of solicitations relative to lordosis. This is evident from the fact that medial preoptic area lesions suppress solicitations but augment lordosis, and is an example of the kind of mutually-exclusive behavioral patterns discussed by Konorski [100]. Females cannot hold a lordosis posture while making a forward-directed solicitation and vice versa. Mutually interactive inhibitory subsystems in the two regions likely regulate the timing of solicitations and lordosis.

## Pacing Behavior

The ability of female rats to pace the copulatory contact is critical for the timing of intromissions. This timing leads to distributed stimulation of the external glans clitoris, internal clitoris/G-spot, and cervix, stimulation that female rats find rewarding [88, 90, 91], and that facilitates pregnancy or the induction of pseudopregnancy and sets the reward state necessary for the induction of partner preference [101, 102]. Female rats pace at a faster rate early in the copulatory interaction, but with successive ejaculations the number of level changes per mount in bilevel chambers increases dramatically, thereby increasing male interintromission intervals. In unilevel pacing chambers, the latency to return to the male's side after mounts, intromissions, and ejaculations shows a progressive increase in time, which increases with successive ejaculatory series. Low, steady rates of pacing are induced in ovariectomized rats by estradiol benzoate and progesterone, whereas ovariectomized rats administered estradiol benzoate alone show higher rates of pacing and rejection responses. Fully primed female rats tested in small chambers that offer no escape from the male also display rejection responses (e.g., rearing and boxing postures [103]) at a higher rate than females tested in chambers where they can escape. It would appear that females use rejection responses to pace the copulatory contact if they cannot do so otherwise. However, in those conditions, copulation does not induce a reward state sufficient to induce conditioned place preference or conditioned partner preferences, and does not facilitate pregnancy or pseudopregnancy.

Very little work has been done examining the neural control of pacing. However, bilateral radiofrequency lesions of the lateral septum, but not the medial preoptic area, disrupted the pattern of female exits from the male side of a three-hole unilevel pacing chamber [104]. In general, females with lateral septal lesions did not leave the male side after mounts and took significantly more time than sham-lesioned females to leave the male side after intromissions or ejaculations. This suggests that activation of the lateral septum by copulatory stimulation is an important component of the regulation of pacing. It is not known whether such lesions would facilitate or inhibit the development of place or partner preferences. Guarraci *et al.* [105] found that cell body lesions of the medial preoptic area, but not medial amygdala or bed nucleus of the stria terminalis, increased the intromission and ejaculation contact-return latencies of females in pacing chambers, and increased the number of withdrawals from the male's side following intromisisons, suggesting that medial preoptic area activation is critically involved in keeping females with males, consistent with its role in solicitations. Interestingly, clitoral anesthesia induced by lidocaine injections also increased the number of exits and returns displayed by ovariectomized, estradiol benzoate and progesterone-primed rats in a four-hole unilevel pacing chamber, decreased the amount of time spent with males, and increased the ejaculation return latency [106]. This indicates that clitoral stimulation maintains low rates of pacing, which increase if the stimulation is blunted. As noted above, polysynaptic clitoral afferents project to the medial preoptic area and clitoral stimulation activates Fos in medial regions of the medial preoptic area of female rats. It is not yet known whether the reward induced by clitoral stimulation is eliminated by medial preoptic area lesions, although such lesions clearly disrupt conditioned place preference induced by vaginocervical stimulation [107].

## Lordosis

Lordosis is a hormonally modulated spinal reflex that characterizes sexual "receptivity" in females of most mammalian species (Figure 4.6). The arching of the back raises the rump that, in turn, allows the male's penis to penetrate the vagina. It also exposes the external clitoral glans to stimulation from the male's pelvis as he thrusts from behind. More is known about lordosis than any other behaviorally relevant spinal reflex with supraspinal control, except perhaps the control of penile erection [108] and the conditioned eye-blink response [109, 110]. We may consider the propensity for female rats to show lordosis, in a context where they have the choice to approach and withdraw from the male, as an analogy to Basson's concept of "sexual receptiveness," a form of responsive desire that indicates a willingness to engage in sexual behavior with a partner.

The seminal work of Pfaff [111, 112] merged electrophysiology with anatomy and pharmacology and behavioral neuroendocrinology with molecular biology to determine the modular supraspinal components of the lordosis reflex and its control by ovarian hormones acting on specific receptors in the brain (Figure 4.7). The action of steroids on those receptors alters the brain's neurochemistry though both direct and indirect genomic actions, which, in turn, activate excitatory sexual systems and inhibit inhibitory sexual systems. This activation/disinhibition alters the reaction of the female to incentive sexual stimuli, which leads her to being attracted to competent sexual cues. It engages approach behaviors and solicitation of sex from the male and, upon simple palpation of the flanks and perineum, the female no longer reacts with violent intense rejection but rather with ear wiggles and sexual receptivity. Thus, the behavioral reflex is linked by the mechanics of gene transcription and translation in critical hypothalamic circuits to the timing of ovulation so that the two can co-occur.

Coordinating physiological responses with behavior requires timing. Hormone priming essentially sets up a timing system for lordosis onset and offset. Although some of the neurochemical systems involved in onset are part of the excitatory system, others are actually inhibitory and keep lordosis from occurring too soon. Likewise, activation of the excitatory neurochemical systems keeps the potential for lordosis on long after the female has taken herself out of the mating game. In general, the hypothalamic targets of estradiol include neurosecretory neurons, such as gonadotropin-releasing hormone and dopamine neurons, that affect both pituitary secretion and sexual behavior, and local circuitry neurons, such as proopi-omelanocortin, gamma-aminobutyric acid, and glutamate.

### Activation of Excitatory Systems

Estradiol and progesterone activate gene expression for a number of neurochemical systems in the hypothalamus, most notably in the medial preoptic area and ventromedial hypothalamus, which stimulate lordosis. This includes an upregulation of specific neurotransmitter receptors by estradiol (e.g. progestin receptors, oxytocin receptors, adrenergic $\alpha_1$ receptors, muscarinic receptors, melaocortin 3 and 4 receptors, and delta opioid receptors, gonadotropin-releasing hormone receptors, GABA-A receptors, and D1 dopamine receptors – reviewed in Pfaus et al. [63]). This changes how the circuit between the two regions operates. Enzymes are also upregulated in this system, including nitric oxide synthase, prostaglandin-D synthase, and dopamine $\beta$-hydroxylase (that metabolizes dopamine to noradrenaline), leading to an upregulation of the end products. Nitric oxide, in particular, is a critical and ubiquitous player in neurotransmitter release, so its upregulation is important in helping to set the stage for the upregulated neurochemical systems to play a functional role in the generation of the behavior. Pharmacological studies help to confirm the role played by these neurochemical substrates.

### Inhibition of Inhibitory Systems

Tonic inhibitory systems exist for lordosis in the medial preoptic area and ventromedial hypothalamus that must be overridden to activate lordosis. This action then constrains lordosis to the periovulatory period. Local actions of both mu and delta opioids, and glutamate, appear to keep lordosis constrained until such time as those systems are either inhibited directly or the action of excitatory neurochemical systems overcomes the inhibitory tone. Serotonin is the most intensely studied transmitter in this category and, as might be expected, projections from the raphe to the ventromedial hypothalamus inhibit female sexual behavior, as do projections to the prefrontal cortex that induce top-down inhibition. Treatment of ovariectomized rats with behaviorally effective doses of estradiol plus progesterone significantly reduces the turnover of serotonin in the ventromedial hypothalamus in a manner that correlates with changes in lordosis behavior. Decreased serotonin in parallel with increased sexual behavior is also seen across the estrous cycle. This inhibitory effect of serotonin on female sexual behavior is associated with an inhibitory effect on ventromedial hypothalamus neuronal activity, although the affected cell types have not been described. The serotonin receptor subtype 2C has been localized to the ventromedial hypothalamus. Acute systemic treatment with the selective serotonin reuptake inhibitor fluoxetine disrupts estrous cyclicity and reduces lordosis and the amount of time ovariectomized rats primed with estradiol benzoate and progesterone spend with males.

In summary, neurobiological studies in rodent models show that lesions to specific regions can have distinct effects on components of sexual response. The connections between the ventromedial hypothalamus and medial preoptic area appear to be critical to this dissociation, and numerous neuropeptide and neurotransmitter systems can be acting to excite, inhibit, or disinhibit at any one time. Just as the initiation of female sexual desire can be complex, disordered sexual desire likely requires targeting of multiple neurobiological mechanisms in an individualized approach.

# Relevance of Animals to Humans

An important example of how basic preclinical research in animals translates into clinical treatments comes from the study of the neurochemistry of sexual desire. At least three potential treatments for disorders of sexual desire or interest in women have undergone clinical trials (Figure 4.9), including the serotonergic mixed 5-HT$_{1A}$ agonist/5-HT$_{2A}$ antagonist flibanserin (approved by the Food and Drug Administration in the United States as Addyi®), the melanocortin agonist bremelanotide, and a combined pill containing testosterone and a phosphodiesterase 5 inhibitor called Lybrido®. Chronic flibanserin increased solicitations and reduced rejection responses in ovariectomized rats primed with estradiol benzoate or estradiol benzoate and progesterone [113]. Microdialysis samples from the medial prefrontal cortex, nucleus accumbens, and medial preoptic area showed that acute flibanserin increased basal levels of norepinephrine in all areas, along with dopamine in the medial prefrontal cortex and medial preoptic area, but not

the nucleus accumbens. Acute flibanserin also decreased serotonin levels in all areas. However, chronic flibanserin increased dopamine and norepinephrine significantly in the medial prefrontal cortex, but did not alter serotonin, glutamate, or gamma-aminobutyric acid relative to chronically injected controls. Likewise, acute bremelanotide increased solicitations selectively in preclinical models using ovariectomized rats primed with low doses of estradiol benzoate, or low estradiol benzoate and progesterone, and increased dopamine release selectively in the medial preoptic area. Finally, acute treatment of ovariectomized rats primed with low estradiol benzoate with testosterone and a phosphodiesterase 5 inhibitor increased solicitations and hops and darts. All three drugs have shown significant efficacy in increasing self-reported sexual desire in pre- and postmenopausal women diagnosed with hypoactive desire disorder [9, 114–118]. The ability of these three drugs to stimulate solicitations in a rat model of hypoactive sexual desire predicts their functional application in women with hypoactive sexual desire and interest. This suggests

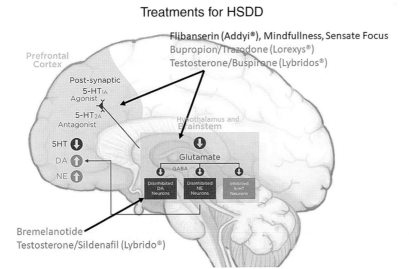

**Figure 4.9** Treatments for sexual desire disorders and their potential mechanisms of action in the brain. From Pfaus [121]. (*See plate section for color representation of the figure*)

strongly that the neurochemical systems underlying appetitive sexual behaviors that reflect sexual desire are conserved between at least rats and humans, and that transla-tional work on the neural and hormonal systems that mediate sexual responses in women can be derived from basic and preclinical research in other species.

# References

1 Parish SJ *et al.* Toward a more evidence-based nosology and nomenclature for female sexual dysfunctions – Part II. *J Sex Med*, **13**, 1888–1906 (2016).

2 Reed GM *et al.* Disorders related to sexuality and gender identity in the ICD-11: revising the ICD-10 classification based on current scientific evidence, best clinical practices, and human rights considerations. *World Psychiatry*, **15**, 205–221 (2016).

3 American Psychiatric Association. *Diagnostic and Statistical Manual of Mental Disorders (DSM-5®)*. American Psychiatric Association (2013). doi:10.5555/appi. books.9780890425596.x00pre

4 Sarin S, Amsel R, Binik YM. A streetcar named 'derousal'? A psychophysiological examination of the desire–arousal distinction in sexually functional and dysfunctional women. *J Sex Res*, **53**, 711–729 (2015).

5 Toledano R, Pfaus JG. The sexual arousal and desire inventory (SADI): a multidimensional scale to assess subjective sexual arousal and desire. *J Sex Med*, **3**, 853–877 (2006).

6 Pfaus JG. Pathways of sexual desire. *J Sex Med*, **6**, 1506–1533 (2009).

7 Pfaus JG. *et al.* Who, what, where, when (and maybe even why)? How the experience of sexual reward connects sexual desire, preference, and performance. *Arch Sex Behav*, **41**, 31–62 (2012).

8 Agmo A, Ellingsen E. Relevance of non-human animal studies to the understanding of human sexuality. *Scand J Psychol*, **44**, 293–301 (2003).

9 Pfaus JG, Giuliano F, Gelez H. Bremelanotide: an overview of preclinical CNS effects on female sexual function. *J Sex Med*, **4** (Suppl 4), 269–279 (2007).

10 Pfaus JG, Kippin TE, Coria-Avila GA. What can animal models tell us about human sexual response? *Annu Rev Sex Res*, **14**, 1–63 (2003).

11 Pavlov IP. *Conditioned Reflexes*. Courier Dover Publications (1927).

12 Bush G. Dorsal anterior cingulate cortex: A role in reward-based decision making. *Proc Natl Acad Sci USA*, **99**, 523–528 (2001).

13 Carter CS *et al.* Anterior cingulate cortex, error detection, and the online monitoring of performance. *Science* **280**, 747–749 (1998).

14 Robinson TE, Berridge KC. The neural basis of drug craving: an incentive-sensitization theory of addiction. *Brain Res Brain Res Rev*, **18**, 247–291 (1993).

15 Beach FA. Sexual attractivity, proceptivity, and receptivity in female mammals. *Horm Behav*, **7**, 105–138 (1976).

16 Craig W. Appetites and aversions as constituents of instincts. *The Biological Bulletin* (1918).

17 Woodworth RS. *Dynamic Psychology*. Columbia University Press (1918).

18 Mackintosh NJ. *The psychology of animal learning*. Academic Press (1974).

19 Toates F. An integrative theoretical framework for understanding sexual motivation, arousal, and behavior. *J Sex Res*, **46**, 168–193 (2009).

20 Masters WH, Johnson VE. *Human sexual response*. Boston, MA: Little (1966).

21 Moll, A. *The Sexual Life of the Child*. Macmillan (1908), pp. 1–17.

22 Kaplan HS. *The New Sex Therapy*. Brunel/Mazel (1974).

23 Georgiadis JR, Kringelbach ML, Pfaus JG. Sex for fun: a synthesis of human and animal neurobiology. *Nat Rev Urol*, **9**, 486–498 (2012).

24 Georgiadis JR, Kringelbach ML. The human sexual response cycle: Brain imaging evidence linking sex to other pleasures. *Prog Neurobiol*, **98**, 49–81 (2012).

25 Basson R. Women's sexual dysfunction: revised and expanded definitions. *CMAJ*, **172**, 1327–1333 (2005).

26 Wallen K. *The evolution of female sexual desire*. 57–79 (University of Chicago Press, 1995).

27 Pfaus JG. Revisiting the concept of sexual motivation. *Annu Rev Sex Res*, **10**, 120–156 (1999).

28 Erskine MS. Solicitation behavior in the estrous female rat: a review. *Horm Behav*, **23**, 473–502 (1989).

29 McClintock M. Group mating in the domestic rat as a context for sexual selection: Consequences for the analysis of sexual behavior and neuroendocrine responses. *Adv Study Behav*, **14**, 2–50 (1984).

30 Stanislaw H, Rice FJ. Correlation between sexual desire and menstrual cycle characteristics. *Arch Sex Behav*, **17**(6), 499–508 (1988).

31 Adams DB, Gold AR, Burt AD. Rise in female-initiated sexual activity at ovulation and its suppression by oral contraceptives. *N Engl J Med*, **299**, 1145–1150 (1978).

32 Dennerstein L *et al.* The relationship between the menstrual cycle and female sexual interest in women with PMS complaints and volunteers. *Psychoneuroendocrinology*, **19**, 293–304 (1994).

33 Harvey SM. Female sexual behavior: fluctuations during the menstrual cycle. *J Psychosom Res*, **31**, 101–110 (1987).

34 Van Goozen SH, Wiegant VM, Endert E, *et al.* Psychoendocrinological assessment of the menstrual cycle: the relationship between hormones, sexuality, and mood. *Arch Sex Behav*, **26**, 359–382 (1997).

35 Cechetto DF, Shoemaker JK. Functional neuroanatomy of autonomic regulation. *Neuroimage*, **47**, 795–803 (2009).

36 Iversen S, Iversen L, Saper CB. The autonomic nervous system and the hypothalamus. In Kandel ER, Schwartz JH, Jessell TM (eds) *Principles of Neural Science*, 4th edn. New York: McGraw Hill (2000), pp. 960–981.

37 Graham CA, Sherwin BB. The relationship between mood and sexuality in women using an oral contraceptive as a treatment for premenstrual symptoms. *Psychoneuroendocrinology*, **18**, 273–281 (1993).

38 Warner P, Bancroft J. Mood, sexuality, oral contraceptives and the menstrual cycle. *J Psychosom Res*, **32**, 417–427 (1988).

39 Selye H. Confusion and controversy in the stress field. *J Human Stress*, **1**, 37–44 (1975).

40 Bancroft J. Sexual effects of androgens in women: some theoretical considerations. *Fertil Steril*, **77**, 55–59 (2002).

41 Mathur RS, Landgrebe SC, Moody LO, *et al.* The effect of estrogen treatment on plasma concentrations of steroid hormones, gonadotropins, prolactin and sex hormone-binding globulin in post-menopausal women. *Maturitas*, 7, 129–133 (1985).

42 Shifren JL *et al.* Transdermal testosterone treatment in women with impaired sexual function after oophorectomy. *N Engl J Med*, **343**, 682–688 (2000).

43 Leiblum SR, Koochaki PE, Rodenberg CA, *et al.* Hypoactive sexual desire disorder in postmenopausal women: US results from the Women's International Study of Health and Sexuality (WISHeS). *Menopause*, **13**, 46–56 (2006).

44 Dennerstein L, Koochaki P, Barton I, Graziottin A. Hypoactive sexual desire disorder in menopausal women: A survey of western European women. *J Sex Med*, **3**, 212–222 (2006).

45 Braunstein GD. Androgen insufficiency in women. *Growth Horm IGF Res*, **16**, 109–117 (2006).

46 Braunstein GD *et al.* Safety and efficacy of a testosterone patch for the treatment of hypoactive sexual desire disorder in surgically menopausal women: a randomized, placebo-controlled trial. *Arch Intern Med*, **165**, 1582–1589 (2005).

47 Burger HG *et al.* The management of persistent menopausal symptoms with oestradiol-testosterone implants: clinical, lipid and hormonal results. *Maturitas,***6**, 351–358 (1984).

48 Burger H, Hailes J, Nelson J, Menelaus M. Effect of combined implants of oestradiol and testosterone on libido in postmenopausal women. *Br Med J (Clin Res Ed)*, **294**, 936–937 (1987).

49 Davis SR, Braunstein GD. Efficacy and safety of testosterone in the management of hypoactive sexual desire disorder in postmenopausal women. *J Sex Med*, **9**, 1134–1148 (2012).

50 Nachtigall L *et al.* Safety and tolerability of testosterone patch therapy for up to 4 years in surgically menopausal women receiving oral or transdermal oestrogen. *Gynecol Endocrinol*, **27**, 39–48 (2011).

51 Panay N *et al.* Testosterone treatment of HSDD in naturally menopausal women: the ADORE study. *Climacteric*, **13**, 121–131 (2010).

52 Sherwin BB, Gelfand MM, and Brender W. Androgen enhances sexual motivation in females: a prospective, crossover study of sex steroid administration in the surgical menopause. *Psychosom Med*, **47**, 339–351 (1985).

53 Sherwin BB. Randomized clinical trials of combined estrogen-androgen preparations: effects on sexual functioning. *Fertil Steril*, 77(Suppl 4), S49–54 (2002).

54 Ochsenkühn R *et al.* Menopausal status in breast cancer patients with past chemotherapy determines long-term hypoactive sexual desire disorder. *J Sex Med*, **8**, 1486–1494 (2011).

55 Baumgart J, Nilsson K, Evers AS, *et al.* Sexual dysfunction in women on adjuvant endocrine therapy after breast cancer. *Menopause*, 1–7 (2012). doi: 10.1097/gme.0b013e31826560da

56 Slob AK, Ernste M, Werff ten Bosch JJ. *Menstrual cycle phase and sexual arousability in women. Arch Sex Behav*, **20**, 567–577 (1991).

57 Singer I, Singer J. Periodicity of sexual desire in relation to time of ovulation in women. *J Biosoc Sci*, **4**, 471–481 (1972).

58 Gizewski ER *et al.* There are differences in cerebral activation between females in distinct menstrual phases during viewing of erotic stimuli: A fMRI study. *Exp brain Res*, **174**, 101–108 (2006).

59 Krug R, Plihal W, Fehm HL, Born J. Selective influence of the menstrual cycle on perception of stimuli with reproductive significance: An event-related potential study. *Psychophysiology*, **37**, 111–122 (2000).

60 Mass R., Hölldorfer M, Moll B, *et al.* Why we haven't died out yet: Changes in women's mimic reactions to visual erotic stimuli during their menstrual cycles. *Horm Behav*, **55**, 267–271 (2009).

61 Rupp HA *et al.* Neural activation in the orbitofrontal cortex in response to male faces increases during the follicular phase. *Horm Behav*, **56**, 66–72 (2009).

62 Wallen K, Winston LA, Caventa S, *et al.* Periovulatory changes in female sexual behavior and patterns of ovarian steroid secretion in group-living rhesus monkeys. *Horm Behav*, **18**, 431–450 (1984).

63 Pfaus JG, Jones SL, Flanagan-Cato LM, Blaustein JD. Female sexual behavior. In Plant T and Zeleznik A (eds) *Knobil and Neill's Physiology of Reproduction*, 4th edn. Elsevier (2014), pp. 2287–2370.

64 Hull E, Dominguez JM, Muschamp JW. *Neurochemistry of Male Sexual Behavior.* Springer Verlag (2007).

65 Gray JA. *The Psychology of Fear and Stress.* Cambridge University Press (1987).

66 Bancroft J, Janssen E. The dual control model of male sexual response: a theoretical approach to centrally mediated erectile dysfunction. *Neurosci Biobehav Rev*, **24**, 571–579 (2000).

67 Perelman MA. The sexual tipping point: a mind/body model for sexual medicine. *J Sex Med*, **6**, 629–632 (2009).

68 Pfaus JG *et al.* Inhibitory and disinhibitory effects of psychomotor stimulants and

depressants on the sexual behavior of male and female rats. *Horm Behav*, **58**, 163–176 (2010).

69 Fink G, Sumner BE, Rosie R, *et al.* Estrogen control of central neurotransmission: effect on mood, mental state, and memory. *Cell Mol Neurobiol*, **16**, 325–344 (1996).

70 Kow L-M, Mobbs CV, Pfaff DW. Roles of second-messenger systems and neuronal activity in the regulation of lordosis by neurotransmitters, neuropeptides, and estrogen: a review. *Neurosci Biobehav Rev*, **18**, 251–268 (1994).

71 Jones SL, Ismail N, Pfaus JG. Facilitation of sexual behavior in ovariectomized rats by estradiol and testosterone: A preclinical model of androgen effects on female sexual desire. *Psychoneuroendocrinology*, **79**, 122–133 (2017).

72 Hull EM, Dominguez JM. Getting his act together: roles of glutamate, nitric oxide, and dopamine in the medial preoptic area. *Brain Res*, **1126**, 66–75 (2006).

73 Robbins TW. Shifting and stopping: fronto-striatal substrates, neurochemical modulation and clinical implications. *Philos Trans R Soc Lond B Biol Sci*, **362**, 917–932 (2007).

74 Parada M, Vargas EB, Kyres M, *et al.* The role of ovarian hormones in sexual reward states of the female rat. *Horm Behav*, **62**, 442–447 (2012).

75 Sinchak K, Mills RH, Eckersell CB, Micevych PE. Medial preoptic area delta-opioid receptors inhibit lordosis. *Behav Brain Res*, **155**, 301–306 (2004).

76 Acosta-Martinez M, Etgen AM. Activation of mu-opioid receptors inhibits lordosis behavior in estrogen and progesterone-primed female rats. *Horm Behav*, **41**, 88–100 (2002).

77 Pfaus JG, Smith WJ, Byrne N, Stephens G. Appetitive and consummatory sexual behaviors of female rats in bilevel chambers II. *Patterns of estrus termination following vaginocervical stimulation. Horm Behav*, **37**, 96–107 (2000).

78 Pfaus JG, Damsma G, Wenkstern D, Fibiger HC. Sexual activity increases dopamine transmission in the nucleus accumbens and striatum of female rats. *Brain Res*, **693**, 21–30 (1995).

79 Jenkins WJ, Becker JB. Dynamic increases in dopamine during paced copulation in the female rat. *Eur J Neurosci*, **18**, 1997–2001 (2003).

80 Hoshina Y, Takeo T, Nakano K, *et al.* Axon-sparing lesion of the preoptic area enhances receptivity and diminishes proceptivity among components of female rat sexual behavior. *Behav Brain Res*, **61**, 197–204 (1994).

81 Afonso VM, Sison M, Lovic V, Fleming AS. Medial prefrontal cortex lesions in the female rat affect sexual and maternal behavior and their sequential organization. *Behav Neurosci*, **121**, 515–526 (2007).

82 Grierson JP, James MD, Pearson JR, Wilson CA. The effect of selective D1 and D2 dopaminergic agents on sexual receptivity in the female rat. *Neuropharmacology*, **27**, 181–189 (1988).

83 Ismail N *et al.* Conditioned ejaculatory preference in male rats paired with haloperidol-treated females. *Physiol Behav*, **100**, 116–121 (2010).

84 Hansen S, Harthon C, Waslin E, *et al.* Mesotelencephalic dopamine system and reproductive behavior in the female rat: Effects of ventral tegmental 6-hydroxydopamine lesions on maternal and sexual responsiveness. *Behav Neurosci*, **105**, 588–598 (1991).

85 Graham MD, Pfaus JG. Differential regulation of female sexual behaviour by dopamine agonists in the medial preoptic area. *Pharmacol Biochem Behav*, **97**, 284–292 (2010).

86 Graham MD, Pfaus JG. Differential effects of dopamine antagonists infused to the medial preoptic area on the sexual behavior of female rats primed with estrogen and progesterone. *Pharmacol Biochem Behav*, **102**, 532–539 (2012).

87 Wilson CA, Thody AJ, Hole DR, *et al.* Interaction of estradiol, alpha-melanocyte-stimulating hormone, and dopamine in the regulation of sexual receptivity in the female rat. *Neuroendocrinology*, **54**, 14–22 (1991).

88 Parada M, Chamas L, Censi S, *et al.* Clitoral stimulation induces conditioned place preference and Fos activation in the rat. *Horm Behav*, **57**, 112–118 (2010).

89 Matuszewich L, Lorrain DS, Hull EM. Dopamine release in the medial preoptic area of female rats in response to hormonal manipulation and sexual activity. *Behav Neurosci*, **114**, 772–778 (2000).

90 Paredes RG, Alonso A. Sexual behavior regulated (paced) by the female induces conditioned place preference. *Behav Neurosci*, **111**, 123–128 (1997).

91 Paredes RG, Vazquez B. What do female rats like about sex? *Paced mating. Behav Brain Res*, **105**, 117–127 (1999).

92 Cooper PE, Martin JB. Neuroendocrinology and brain peptides. *Ann Neurol*, **8**, 551–557 (1980).

93 Khorram O, Bedran de Castro JC, *McCann SM. The effect of the estrous cycle and estrogen on the release of immunoreactive* α-melanocyte-stimulating hormone. *Peptides*, **6**, 503–508 (1985).

94 Pfaus JG, Shadiack A, Van Soest T, *et al.* Selective facilitation of sexual solicitation in the female rat by a melanocortin receptor agonist. *Proc Natl Acad Sci USA*, **101**, 10201–10204 (2004).

95 Rössler A-S *et al.* The melanocortin agonist, melanotan II, enhances proceptive sexual behaviors in the female rat. *Pharmacol Biochem Behav*, **85**, 514–521 (2006).

96 Georgescu M, Pfaus JG. Role of glutamate receptors in the ventromedial hypothalamus in the regulation of female rat sexual behaviors: I. Behavioral effects of glutamate and its selective receptor agonists AMPA, NMDA and kainate. *Pharmacol Biochem Behav*, **83**, 322–332 (2006).

97 Georgescu M, Pfaus JG. Role of glutamate receptors in the ventromedial hypothalamus in the regulation of female rat sexual behaviors. II. Behavioral effects of selective glutamate receptor antagonists AP-5, CNQX, and DNQX. *Pharmacol Biochem Behav*, **83**, 333–341 (2006).

98 Jones SL, Farisello L, Mayer-Heft N, Pfaus JG. Repeated administration of estradiol promotes mechanisms of sexual excitation and inhibition: Glutamate signaling in the ventromedial hypothalamus attenuates excitation. *Behav Brain Res*, **291**, 118–129 (2015).

99 Pfaus JG, Pfaff DW. Mu-, delta-, and kappa-opioid receptor agonists selectively modulate sexual behaviors in the female rat: differential dependence on progesterone. *Horm Behav*, **26**, 457–473 (1992).

100 Konorski J. *Integrative Activity of the Brain*. Chicago University Press (1967).

101 Coria-Avila GA, Ouimet AJ, Pacheco P, *et al*. Olfactory conditioned partner preference in the female rat. *Behav Neurosci.* **119**, 716–725 (2005).

102 Coria-Avila GA. *et al*. Conditioned partner preference in female rats for strain of male. *Physiol Behav*, **88**, 529–537 (2006).

103 Barnett SA. *The Rat: A Study in Behaviour*. Chicago, IL: Aldine Publishing Company (1963).

104 Xiao K, Kondo Y, Sakuma Y. Differential regulation of female rat olfactory preference and copulatory pacing by the lateral septum and medial preoptic area. *Neuroendocrinology*, **81**, 56–62 (2005).

105 Guarraci FA, Megroz AB, Clark AS. Paced mating behavior in the female rat following lesions of three regions responsive to vaginocervical stimulation. *Brain Res*, **999**, 40–52 (2004).

106 Parada M, Jafari N, and Pfaus JG. Sexual experience blocks the ability of clitoral stimulation to induce a conditioned place preference in the rat. *Physiol Behav*, **119**, 97–102 (2013).

107 Meerts SH, Clark AS. Lesions of the medial preoptic area interfere with the display of a conditioned place preference for vaginocervical stimulation in rats. *Behav Neurosci*, **123**, 752–757 (2009).

108 McKenna KE. Central nervous system pathways involved in the control of penile erection. *Annu Rev Sex Res*, **10**, 157–183 (1999).

109 Bracha V *et al.* The cerebellum and eye-blink conditioning: learning versus network performance hypotheses. *Neuroscience* **162**, 787–796 (2009).

110 Thompson RF, Steinmetz JE. The role of the cerebellum in classical conditioning of discrete behavioral responses. *Neuroscience*, **162**, 732–755 (2009).

111 Pfaff DW. *Estrogens and brain function: Neural analysis of a hormone-controlled mammalian reproductive behavior.* Springer Verlag (1980).

112 Pfaff DW. *Drive: Neurobiological and Molecular Mechanisms of Sexual Motivation.* MIT Press (1999).

113 Gelez H, Greggain-Mohr J, Pfaus JG, *et al.* Flibanserin treatment increases appetitive sexual motivation in the female rat. *J Sex Med*, **10**, 1231–1239 (2013).

114 Clayton AH, Dennerstein L, Pyke R, Sand M. Flibanserin: a potential treatment for Hypoactive Sexual Desire Disorder in premenopausal women. *Womens Health (Lond)*, **6**, 639–653 (2010).

115 Diamond LE. *et al.* An effect on the subjective sexual response in premenopausal women with sexual arousal disorder by bremelanotide (PT-141), a melanocortin receptor agonist. *J Sex Med*, **3**, 628–638 (2006).

116 Katz M *et al.* Efficacy of flibanserin in women with hypoactive sexual desire disorder: results from the BEGONIA trial. *J Sex Med*, **10**, 1807–1815 (2013).

117 Perelman MA. Clinical application of CNS-acting agents in FSD. *J Sex Med*, **4**(Suppl 4), 280–290 (2007).

118 van der Made F *et al.* The influence of testosterone combined with a PDE5-inhibitor on cognitive, affective, and physiological sexual functioning in women suffering from sexual dysfunction. *J Sex Med*, **6**, 777–790 (2009).

119 Kingsberg SA, Clayton AH, Pfaus JG. The female sexual response: Current models, neurological underpinnings, and agents currently available or under investigation for the treatment of hypoactive sexual desire disorder. *CNS Drugs*, **29**, 915–933 (2015).

120 Pfaus JG, Scepkowski LA. The biologic basis for libido. *Curr Sex Health Rep*, **2**, 95–100 (2005).

121 Pfaus JG. Treatment for hypoactive sexual desire. *Cell*, **163**, 533 (2015).

# 5

# Psychological Management of Hypoactive Sexual Desire Disorder

*Sheryl A. Kingsberg and Stanley E. Althof*

### Abstract

Hypoactive sexual desire disorder (HSDD) is best understood using a biopsychosocial model to capture the interaction of physiologic, psychologic and sociocultural influences. This model also enables a comprehensive approach to treatment that is rooted in the psychological, interpersonal, cultural and biological domains. The decision regarding which modality is appropriate is individualized and based upon the specifics of any patient's presenting problem. Psychotherapy focuses primarily on the psychological and sociocultural factors contributing to distressing low desire and seeks to ameliorate some of the impact of HSDD on the woman and her relationship. Sex therapy generally consists of psychoeducation, couple exercises including sensate focus, and individual and group psychotherapeutic approaches including cognitive behavioral therapy and mindfulness cognitive behavioral therapy.

**Keywords:**   *hypoactive sexual desire disorder (HSDD); psychotherapy; sex therapy; biopsychosocial*

---

Desire is best understood as being under the influence of biological, psychological and interpersonal factors.

Regardless of the precipitating causes of hypoactive sexual desire disorder, biologic, psychologic, and interpersonal changes will occur over time, thus impacting the woman's sexual desire and the couple's sexual equilibrium.

Combining medical and psychotherapeutic interventions is the natural extension of the biopsychosocial model.

---

## Introduction

The biopsychosocial model (Figure 5.1), which has been used broadly in medicine and psychiatry for decades, captures the ever changing influences of biological, psychological, and cultural societal concerns [1]. It is a dynamic rather than static model that captures a snapshot of the woman at only one point in time. Regardless of the precipitating causes of hypoactive sexual desire disorder, biological, psychological, and interpersonal changes will occur over time, thus impacting the woman's sexual desire and the couple's sexual equilibrium.

Some of the influences in the biological sphere may include: the woman taking an antidepressant that negatively affects her libido and orgasmic ability, neurotransmitter imbalance such as that experienced with major depression, or the hormonal changes associated with menopause. Undesirable impacts from the psychological and interpersonal sphere may include a history of sexual

*Textbook of Female Sexual Function and Dysfunction: Diagnosis and Treatment*, First Edition. Edited by Irwin Goldstein, Anita H. Clayton, Andrew T. Goldstein, Noel N. Kim, and Sheryl A. Kingsberg.

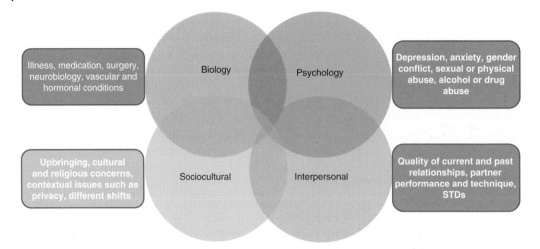

**Figure 5.1** Biopsychosocial model of sexual response. (*See plate section for color representation of the figure*)

or physical abuse that makes feeling sexual desire unsafe, symptoms of depression, the partner's infidelity, ghosts of previously distressing relationships, the partner's sexual dysfunction, psychiatric or substance abuse problems, or the threat of abandonment. Cultural concerns may include religious prohibitions or teachings that sex is dirty and should not be enjoyable. Given the multitude of potential etiologic factors impacting desire, the use of a more comprehensive global assessment of sexual issues may provide a more accurate understanding of what initiates and maintains hypoactive sexual desire disorder.

Additionally, the biopsychosocial model enables a comprehensive approach to treatment rooted in the psychological, interpersonal, cultural and biological domains [2, 3]. The model also explains the failure of treatments for biological problems that ignore relevant psychological contributions and psychological treatments that disregard the biomedical factors.

In addition to the biopsychosocial model, another organizing principle of evaluation is the division of etiological variables into predisposing, precipitating, maintaining, and contextual factors [2, 3]. Predisposing factors may make the woman susceptible to

hypoactive sexual desire disorder. These may include body image issues, childhood genital surgeries, attachment concerns, restrictive upbringing, troubled family relationships, inadequate sexual information, and traumatic early sexual experiences. Precipitating factors are ones that trigger the onset of hypoactive sexual desire disorder and may include a new medication, surgery, discovery of infidelity, struggles with infertility, trauma, psychological impact of an illness or its treatment (e.g. mastectomy) and/or relationship distress. Maintaining factors, which reinforce the persistence of the symptom, include performance anxiety, guilt, psychiatric disorder, relationship discord, loss of attraction between partners, fear of intimacy, impaired self-image, restricted foreplay, sexual myths, and poor communication. Finally, contextual factors may include the current stresses from attempting to conceive, fatigue from full time employment, child rearing, and caring for the home.

The biopsychosocial model follows a logical progression examining all relevant biomedical and psychological aspects that may account for the condition of hypoactive sexual desire disorder and other related sexual problems, such as arousal disorder, anorgasmia, and pain. Such an evaluation is a collaborative endeavor between the clinician and patient that offers the patient the advantage of shared decision making. The clinical synthesis derived from this process serves as a pragmatic road map for treating all of the biopsychosocial variables identified that precipitate or maintain the symptom of hypoactive sexual desire disorder.

The focus here is on the psychological, interpersonal and cultural/contextual contributions to hypoactive sexual desire disorder, as other chapters will present the biological in greater detail.

## Psychotherapy/Sex Therapy for Hypoactive Sexual Desire Disorder

Historically, women with sexual dysfunctions were treated using psychoanalytic methods. Other than anecdotal case reports, no large scale, systematic trials or data were available. Psychoanalysts initially viewed women's sexual desire as "pale imitations of the more robust sexual drive in men." [4].

In the 1960s and 1970s, Masters and Johnson revolutionized the treatment of sexual problems by working with couples to overcome the psychological and behavioral obstacles that may impede natural function [5, 6]. They developed a highly structured two-week treatment model employing male and female cotherapy teams. The multiple facets of their treatment included physical examination, history taking, individual and couples' psychotherapy, and prescription of behavioral tasks, such as sensate focus. Based on their clinical judgment, Masters and Johnson reported both an end of treatment outcome and a five-year follow-up outcome. They reported astounding success rates of 72–98% for female sexual dysfunctions and only a 5% relapse rate after five years.

A core component of Masters and Johnson's work and sex therapy in general is the prescription of sensate focus, a graded series of nondemand sensual touching exercises [5, 6]. In a couple-based approach, the objectives of sensate focus therapy are to reduce avoidance of sensual touching or sexual activity and related anxiety, improve sexual communication between partners, and improve intimacy by re-introducing sexual activity in a gradual way. Exercises might begin with non-genital touching, and assuming successful achievement of each successive series of exercises, move to genital touching, and ultimately intercourse [7].

Modern sex therapy is an extension of Masters and Johnson's work that uses specific techniques to address problems of sexual desire, arousal, orgasm, and pain. Generally, sex therapy is a short-term (approximately three months) treatment conducted in an individual, couples, or group setting [8]. The decision regarding which modality is appropriate is based upon the specifics of any patient's presenting problem. Sex therapy generally consists of psychoeducation, couple exercises including sensate focus, and counseling.

Cognitive behavioral therapy approaches gained prominence in the early 1980s. Cognitive behavioral therapy focuses on identifying and altering behaviors (e.g. avoidance of sexual activity) and cognitions (e.g. unrealistic expectations) that contribute to low sexual desire in women [9, 10]. Because cognitive distraction during sexual activity is prevalent among women with hypoactive sexual desire disorder, the application of cognitive challenging strategies (i.e. identifying, challenging, and replacing irrational thoughts) is a mainstay of cognitive behavioral sex therapy. Education is also an important component of cognitive behavioral therapy and can help the woman/couple understand how adequate erotic stimulation and physical stimulation contribute to their sexual desire and arousal.

Mindfulness techniques were incorporated into a cognitive behavioral framework by Brotto *et al.* [11, 12]. Mindfulness is derived from Buddhist meditation practices and focuses on being present and nonjudgmental awareness of bodily sensations or perceptions. Mindfulness cognitive behavioral therapy can be especially helpful for women who have a disconnect between genital and subjective arousal (a positive mental engagement/focus in response to a sexual stimulus) [13].

## Psychotherapy/Sex Therapy Outcomes

The majority of the psychotherapy outcome studies are notoriously flawed, with few using control groups or validated outcome measures. Outcome studies demonstrate sex therapy to be moderately effective at improving sexual desire, especially when compliance with the recommended exercises is high. Overall the noncontrolled efficacy rates for the treatments in these studies range between 52 and 74% [14]. A 2013 systematic analysis found an effect size of 1.03 on the outcome of symptom severity and of 0.86 for sexual satisfaction, suggesting a high level of efficacy [15].

For women with low relationship satisfaction, improving sexual function alone may not be sufficient to alleviate their sexual distress. Therefore, focusing on improving the intimate relationship would be an important first step for a woman with low sexual desire and concomitant low relationship quality. However, couple/marital therapy alone, without adjunct sex therapy, may not be sufficient to improve women's sexual desire [16].

## Integrating Psychotherapy in Multimodal Treatments for Hypoactive Sexual Desire Disorder

Combining medical and psychotherapeutic interventions is the natural extension of the biopsychosocial model. In men with erectile dysfunction and premature ejaculation, combination therapy harnesses the power of both treatments to quickly reverse symptoms, enhance efficacy, increase treatment and relational satisfaction, and decrease patient discontinuation [8, 17–21].

To date, there are no studies on combination therapy for female sexual dysfunction. However, combining current pharmacologic treatments with psychosocial interventions is likely to enhance the positive effects of pharmacotherapy. It also offers support to women with the distressing problem of hypoactive sexual desire disorder and may confer positive benefit to their relationship as well.

## Conclusion

A biopsychosocial model informs both etiology and treatment. However, it should also be noted that one size does not fit all. Some women will benefit more from psychotherapeutic options, some from pharmacologic options, and some from an integrated multimodal approach. A thorough evaluation of underlying psychological, interpersonal, and cultural causes may lead to the most optimal approach.

## References

1 Althof S, Leiblum S, Chevret-Meason, *et al.* Psychological and interpersonal dimensions of sexual function or dysfunction. *J Sex Med.* 2005;**26**:793–800.

2 Bitzer J, Giraldi A, Pfaus J. Sexual desire and hypoactive sexual desire disorder in women. Introduction and overview. Standard operating procedure (SOP Part 1). *J Sex Med.* 2013;**10**:36–49.

3 Bitzer J, Giraldi A, Pfaus J. A standardized diagnostic interview for hypoactive sexual desire disorder in women: standard operating procedure (SOP Part 2). *J Sex Med.* 2013;**10**:50–57.

4 Lief H, Friedman R. History of psychologic treatments. In: Goldstein I, Meston C, Davis S, and Traish A (eds) *Women's Sexual Function and Dysfunction.* London: Taylor and Francis; 2006, pp. 427–433.

5 Masters WH, Johnson VE. *Human Sexual Response.* Boston, MA: Little, Brown & Company; 1966.

6 Masters WH, Johnson VE. *Human Sexual Inadequacy.* Boston, MA: Little, Brown & Company; 1970.

7 Kaplan H. *The New Sex Therapy.* New York: Bruner Mazel; 1974.

8 Althof S. Sex therapy and combined (sex and medical) therapy. *J Sex Med.* 2011;**8**:1827–1828.

9 Carvalho J, Nobre P. Sexual desire in women: an integrative approach regarding psychological, medical, and relationship dimensions. *J Sex Med.* 2010;7:1807–1815.

10 Nobre P. Determinants of sexual desire problems in women: Testing a cognitive-emotional model. *J Sex Marital Ther.* 2009;**35**:360–77.

11 Brotto LA. Evidence-based treatments for low sexual desire in women. *Front Neuroendocrinol.* 2017;**45**:11–17.

12 Brotto LA, Basson R. Group mindfulness-based therapy significantly improves sexual desire in women. *Behav Res Ther.* 2014;**57**:43–54.

13 Brotto LA, Chivers ML, Millman RD, Albert A. Mindfulness-based sex therapy improves genital-subjective arousal concordance in women with sexual desire/arousal difficulties. *Arch Sex Behav.* 2016;**45**:907–921.

14 Kingsberg S, Althof S, Simon J, *et al.* Female sexual dysfunction-medical and psychological treatments. *J Sex Med.* 2017;**14**(12):1463–1491.

15 Günzler C, Berner MM. Efficacy of psychosocial interventions in men and women withsexual dysfunctions – a systematic review of controlled clinical trials. *J Sex Med.* 2012;**9**:3108–3125.

16 McCabe M. Editorial comment on "Psychological treatment trials for hypoactive sexual desire disorder: A sexual medicine critique and perspective." *J Sex Med.* 2015;**12**:2459–2460.

17 Althof S. New roles for mental health clinicians in the treatment of erectile dysfunction. *J Sex Educ Ther.* 1998;**23**:229–231.

18 Althof S. Sex therapy in the age of pharmacotherapy. *Annu Rev Sex Res.* 2006:116–132.

19 Comio L, Massenio P, La Rocca R, *et al.* The combination of dapoxetine and behavioral treatment provides better results than dapoxetine alone in the management of patients with lifelong premature ejaculation. *J Sex Med.* 2015;**12**:1609–1615.

20 Perelman M. Combination therapy: Integration of sex therapy and pharmacotherapy. In: Balon R and Taylor Segraves R (eds) *Handbook of Sexual Dysfunction.* New York: Marcel Dekker; 2005, pp. 13–41.

21 Perelman M. A new combination treatment for premature ejaculation: A sex therapist's perspective. *J Sex Med.* 2011;**3**:1004–1012.

# 6

# Pathophysiology and Medical Management of Hypoactive Sexual Desire Disorder

*Anita H. Clayton and Linda Vignozzi*

## Abstract

Human sexual behavior is stimulated by numerous hormonal, cerebral (neurotransmitter) and social factors. Therefore, several physical and medical factors as well as some medications have been associated with low sexual desire. Validated questionnaires such as the Decreased Sexual Desire Screener (DSDS) are extremely useful tools to establish the diagnosis of hypoactive sexual desire disorder and to identify potential causes or exacerbating factors for reduced desire. Therefore, the first line intervention for women with reduced sexual desire is to address any modifiable risk factor, following the process of care. Other important medical treatment options consist of either the use of central nervous system (CNS) agents or hormonal therapy. Indeed, sex hormones such as androgens have been recognized as important determinants of female sexual function, therefore representing an important therapeutic strategy to positively modulate sexual desire.

**Keywords:** *female sexual desire; hormones; neurotransmitters; hypoactive sexual desire disorder; HSDD; hypoandrogenism; depression; SSRI; antidepressants; testosterone; flibanserin*

---

Sex hormones, in particular testosterone, are important determinants of female sexual desire. Other hormones (i.e. thyroid hormones, prolactin) have been reported to modulate sexual desire.

Psychiatric conditions (depression) are frequently comorbid with hypoactive sexual desire disorder with a bidirectional risk relationship; some medical conditions, such as metabolic/endocrine and neurological disorders have been reported to modulate sexual desire

An evidence-based flowchart for management of hypoactive sexual desire disorder includes:

- diagnosis (using validated questionnaire or interview);
- evaluation for the presence of organic diseases that may be contributing to acquired, generalized hypoactive sexual desire disorder;
- modification of any medical, sexual, psychological, and social factors that may potentially cause or worsen hypoactive sexual desire disorder (intervention includes psychotherapy);
- treatment (use of central nervous system agents or hormonal therapy).

---

## Neurobiological Endocrinology

### Sex Steroid Hormones

In the human species, instinctive behaviors, such as sexual behavior, are stimulated by numerous hormonal, cerebral (neurotransmitter), and social factors. In particular, in females relevant changes in behavior occur not only across the reproductive life but have also been hypothesized to occur across the menstrual cycle; the famous Duke of Mantua's aria from Giuseppe Verdi's opera Rigoletto (*"La donna è mobile, qual piuma al*

*Textbook of Female Sexual Function and Dysfunction: Diagnosis and Treatment*, First Edition. Edited by Irwin Goldstein, Anita H. Clayton, Andrew T. Goldstein, Noel N. Kim, and Sheryl A. Kingsberg.

*vento, muta d'accento, e di pensiero*", "Woman is flighty like a feather in the wind, she changes in voice and in thought"; 1851), depicts as one illustration the provocative concept that women's behavior may be considered mobile ("inconstant") and rapidly changing over time. From a more scientific perspective, a wide amount of research has recently addressed the potentially adaptive changes in human female mating (including sexual behaviors) across the menstrual cycle [1–7].

Fluctuations in female sex steroids across the reproductive cycle seem to orchestrate these shifts in sexual behavior. However, adding layers to this complexity, three kinds of difficulty accompany any attempt to ascertain the precise function of hormones in the sexual behavior of women: (i) their changes at the individual level according to development (puberty, menopause) and the men-

strual cycle; (ii) their variations in response to other hormones or neurotransmitters; (iii) their secondary variations in response to psychological modifications, which may be individual, interindividual within the couple, and psychosocial.

## Steroid Biosynthesis and Metabolism

A simplified scheme of steroid biosynthesis is shown in Figure 6.1. The three main classes of steroid hormones are glucocorticoids, mineralocorticoids, both synthesized by the adrenal cortex, and sex steroids (progestogens, androgens, and estrogens), synthesized by the adrenal cortex and the gonads.

Cholesterol is the major substrate of the biosynthesis of steroids, representing the basic molecular structure of all steroid

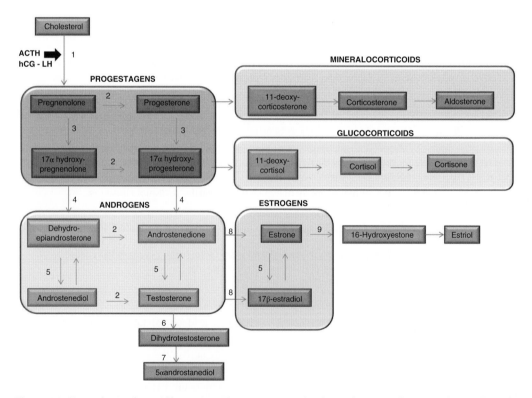

**Figure 6.1** Biosynthesis of steroid hormones. The enzymes involved in androgen and estrogen biosynthesis or metabolism are indicated by numbers. 1 = 20,22-desmolase; 2 = 3β-hydroxysteroid dehydrogenase-isomerase; 3 = 17α-hydroxylase; 4 = 17,20-desmolase; 5 = 17β-hydroxysteroid dehydrogenase; 6 = 5α-reductase; 7 = 3β-ketoreductase; 8 = aromatase; 9 = 16α-hydroxylase.

hormones. Cholesterol can be synthesized by steroidogenic cells but is mainly up taken from circulating lipoproteins. Micellar lipoproteins are complex macromolecules constituted by a central fraction, made by triglycerides and cholesterol esters, surrounded by a hydrophilic layer of phospholipids, free cholesterol, and multiple proteins (apolipoproteins). The lipoproteins are classified according to their hydrated density into five major classes: chylomicrons, very low density, intermediate density, low density, and high density lipoproteins. Low density lipoprotein-cholesterol is currently thought to bind to the membrane receptors on the steroidogenic cells and to be internalized. Its protein content is degraded and cholesterol content transferred to intracellular compartments, from where it is transported back to the liver as high density lipoprotein. Cholesterol is cleaved to form pregnenolone, which is converted to the biologically active progesterone. Subsequent hydroxylation of progesterone at three different positions (C21, C11, C18) leads to the formation of aldosterone, the most potent mineralocorticoid. Pregnenolone and progesterone are both hydroxylated at the C17 position to form the relative 17α-hydroxyl-derivatives, which are the key precursors for the biosynthesis of either cortisol or androgens. Androgens, dehydroepiandrosterone and Δ4-androstenedione, a moderately active androgen, are reduced to testosterone, the most potent secreted androgen. Hence dehydroepiandrosterone, a steroid with weak androgenic activity, is actually the precursor for the most potent androgens. Androgens are metabolized at several sites. When testosterone enters a cell, it is converted to a more potent steroid, which exerts its action in autocrine/paracrine manner or on cells of other tissues. Testosterone is metabolized to dihydrotestosterone, and then to 5α-androstane-3α, 17β-diol (5α-androstane-diol), with androgenic activity 2.5 and 1.5 times greater than testosterone, respectively. The Δ4-androgens are also the essential precursors of estrogens. Estrone and 17β-estradiol are derived from Δ4-androstenedione and testosterone, respectively, through the loss of the C19-carbon residue and desaturation or aromatization of the A-ring. These steps involve aromatase, a complex microsomal enzyme. Estriol, the weakest natural estrogen, is mainly a metabolic product of estrone and estradiol.

## Plasma Transport of Sex Steroids

Unconjugated steroid hormones are relatively insoluble in aqueous solutions and, thus, circulate in blood bound to plasma proteins, mainly to albumin and to specific binding proteins. Albumin binds all unconjugated steroids with very high capacity but low affinity. Specific binding proteins that bind steroids with high affinity but lower capacity are also involved: androgens and, to a lesser extent, estrogens are specifically bound by sex hormone binding globulin. The plasma concentrations of sex hormone binding globulin are increased by estrogens and an excess of thyroid hormones, and decreased by androgens, synthetic progestins (derivatives of the 19-nor-testosterone precursor), and insulin. Sex hormone binding globulin decreases throughout puberty, more in males than in females. As a result, a sex difference is observed in adulthood, mean sex hormone binding globulin levels being about three times higher in men ($14.7 \pm 4.4\,\mu g/l$) than in women ($5.3 \pm 1.5\,\mu g/l$). In contrast, sex hormone binding globulin markedly increases during pregnancy (about 10-fold). Only a small percentage of the circulating sex steroids is present in the "free" (unbound) form. In the blood of adult women (follicular phase), only 1% of testosterone is free, 66% is bound to sex hormone binding globulin, 30% bound to albumin, and the rest to other plasma proteins. These proportions are respectively, 0.5%, 78%, 20%, and 1.5% for dihydrotestosterone, and 2%, 37%, 60% and 1% for estradiol. Vermeulen has shown that the rate of testosterone metabolism correlates with its free plus albumin-bound fraction.

An automatic calculator to evaluate free testosterone level is available at http://www.issam.ch/freetesto.htm [8].

### Secretion and Production of Sex Steroids

Steroids are not stored in the synthesizing cell, therefore if not used as substrate for a specific step in steroidogenesis, steroids are secreted and released in the blood stream. Steroid secreting glands are the main source of steroids. However, peripheral conversions between androgens and from androgens to estrogens do occur in several tissues (liver, brain, skin, fat, and target cells). The blood *production rate* of a hormone is the sum of the quantity secreted and the amount formed by peripheral conversion. Table 6.1 lists the production rate of sex steroids.

### Origin of Sex Steroids

The ovary and the adrenal glands are the two main organs producing sex steroids. Their relative contribution varies for each hormone, according to the phase of the menstrual cycle (Table 6.1). The menstrual cycle is usually divided into three periods: follicular, ovulatory, and luteal phases.

All cellular structures of the ovary produce steroids but in different amounts according to the secreting cells and/or the menstrual cycle phases. The interstitial cells have the principal function to synthesize and secrete androgens, such as Δ4-androstenedione and testosterone. In contrast, progesterone is mainly produced by luteinized granulosa cells. Aromatization of Δ4-androstenedione to estrone and of testosterone to estradiol takes place in the follicle and corpus luteum but is mainly the task of granulosa cells. During the menstrual cycle, developing follicles produce estrogens that dominate the follicular phase, the corpus luteum produces progesterone and estrogens in the luteal phase, and interstitial stroma cells produce androgens.

The adrenal glands produce a significant amount of progestogens and androgens. Adrenal androgens are mainly synthesized in the *zona reticularis* of the adrenal cortex. The relative contribution of the adrenal to the plasma pool of Δ4-androstenedione varies between 30 and 45% according to the phase of the menstrual cycle. In contrast, dehydroepiandrosterone, the most abundant androgen secreted, is mainly of adrenal origin (Table 6.1). Secretion of estrogens, mainly estrone, normally occurs in small amounts in the zona reticularis; in

**Table 6.1** Blood production rate and relative contribution (%) of glandular secretions and peripheral conversion to blood production of sex steroids in young adult women.

| Hormone | Production rate (mg/24 h) | % from adrenals | % from ovary | % from conversion |
|---|---|---|---|---|
| **Progesterone** | | | | |
| (follicular) | 0.8–2.5 | 50–70 | 10–25 | 20–55 |
| (luteal) | 15–50 | 5 | 90 | 1 |
| (pregnant) | 230–310 | (mostly from placental origin) | (mostly from placental origin) | (mostly from placental origin) |
| **Testosterone** | 0.25–0.3 | 15–20 | 25–30 | 50–60 |
| **Δ4-androstenedione** | 2–5 | 30–45 | 45–60 | 10 |
| **DHEA** | 7–15 | 60–70 | 10–25 | 15 |
| **Estrone** | 0.6–0.8 | 1–2 | 60–70 | 30–40 |
| **17β-estradiol** | 0.01–0.1 | 0 | 85–90 | 10–15 |

DHEA = dehydroepiandrosterone

contrast, adrenal glands do not secrete estradiol at any stage of life.

In children, ovarian secretions are insignificant or nonexistent. In contrast, the adrenal contribution to all sex hormones is prominent. From about seven years of age, adrenal production of dehydroepiandrosterone rises abruptly and progressively, in parallel to the relative development and enlargement of the zona reticularis within the adrenal cortex. This process continues throughout puberty. This change in the pattern of adrenal secretion (referred to as "adrenarche") precedes by 2–3 years the onset of puberty. In postmenopausal women, the main source of estrogens is extra-gonadal, such as fat, liver and specific nuclei in the hypothalamus. In this period of life, the adrenals are the major source of Δ4-androstenedione; its conversion into estrone accounts for virtually all the estrone produced. The postmenopausal ovary continues to produce androgens (testosterone and Δ4-androstenedione).

## Sex Hormone Levels

In normally menstruating women, the gradual or day-to-day changes in the plasma levels of sex steroids reflect the changing secretory activities of the various ovarian cells. A typical profile is illustrated in Figure 6.2.

During the first half of the follicular phase (early follicular phase), the ovarian secretion of estrogens, androgens, and progestins is relatively stable. The second half of the follicular phase (late follicular phase), beginning about 7–8 days before the preovulatory luteinizing hormone surge, is characterized by a rise in estrogen levels. Estradiol rises slowly at first and then reaches a maximum several hours before the luteinizing hormone mid-cycle peak. The estrone level rises in parallel, but less. Increases in plasma levels of Δ4-androstenedione and testosterone precede the mid-cycle luteinizing hormone surge by several days, reaching their maximum on the day of the luteinizing hormone peak. Shortly before the luteinizing hormone peak and

prior to ovulation, estradiol levels drop and plasma progesterone begins to rise. Follicular rupture occurs 16–24 hours after the luteinizing hormone peak. The most important feature of the luteal phase is the marked increase in progesterone levels, which reach their maximum about eight days after the luteinizing hormone peak. In the absence of ovulation, sex hormone levels resemble those observed in the early follicular phase. In postmenopausal women, sex steroids are at significantly lower levels. Mean (±SD) values observed at different periods of reproductive life are listed in Table 6.2.

## Regulation of the Hypothalamus–Pituitary–Ovary Axis

Schematically, steroid secretion by the ovary is regulated by two polypeptides hormones, luteinizing hormone and follicle-stimulating hormone, which are produced by the gonadotropic cells of the anterior pituitary gland. From a neurobiological perspective, the gonadotropin releasing hormone secretory system anatomically develops relatively early in life, when activation of the gonadotropin releasing hormone secretory system may be important for masculinization of the brain and attainment of subsequent sexual behavior. In female primates, these early periods of gonadotropin releasing hormone secretion seem to occur at low levels throughout the juvenile period [9]. Therefore, the synthetic capacity of gonadotropin releasing hormone is present even before puberty in that gonadotropin releasing hormone expression reaches adult levels. After the first year of postnatal life, the hypothalamic–pituitary–gonadal axis is quiescent until reactivation occurs to prompt pubertal onset. Puberty onset is a function of the central control of gonadotropin releasing hormone secretion, reflecting the integration of multiple internal and external cues acting upon a genetically determined process. A plethora of different pathways involving neuropeptides and systemically produced steroids can *directly*

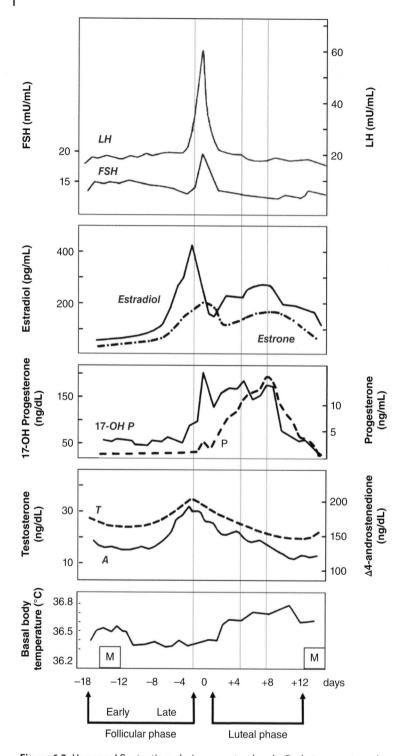

**Figure 6.2** Hormonal fluctuations during menstrual cycle. Body temperature change is also shown.

**Table 6.2** Blood levels of the main sex steroids at different periods of reproductive life.

| Hormone | Follicular phase Early | Late | Mid-luteal phase | Postmenopausal | Pregnancy 3rd trimester |
|---|---|---|---|---|---|
| **Progesterone (ng/dl)** | 56 ± 10 | 56 ± 10 | 1350 ± 490 | 25 ± 8 | 12 361 ± 3394 |
| **Testosterone (ng/dl)** | 22 ± 5 | 37 ± 9 | 35 ± 6 | 25 ± 12 | 67 ± 46 |
| **Δ4-androstenedione (ng/dl)** | 77 ± 28 | 220 ± 45 | 149 ± 43 | 75 ± 20 | 166 ± 111 |
| **DHEA (ng/dl)** | 515 ± 107 | 515 ± 107 | 515 ± 107 | 220 ± 80 | 363 ± 233 |
| **Estrone (pg/ml)** | 49 ± 8 | 75 ± 220 | 84 ± 8 | 29 ± 15 | 541 ± 278 |
| **17β-estradiol (pg/ml)** | 68 ± 14 | 180 ± 500 | 123 ± 11 | 12 ± 4 | 16 640 ± 2375 |

DHEA = dehydroepiandrosterone

modulate gonadotropin releasing hormone release. Kisspeptin-1 and its receptor is one of the major regulatory system of gonadotropin releasing hormone neurons [10, 11]. Genetic studies demonstrated that disabling mutations and targeted deletions of the G-protein-coupled receptor of kisspeptin-1 (previously called GPR54) in humans and mice resulted in sexual infantilism and hypogonadotropic hypogonadism [12, 13]. Kisspeptin neurons in the hypothalamic arcuate nucleus act on gonadotropin releasing hormone nerve terminals in the median eminence and regulate basal pulsatile gonadotropin releasing hormone/luteinizing hormone release [14, 15]. Kisspeptin-1 is highly expressed in cells residing in the anteroventral periventricular nucleus, the medial amygdala, and the arcuate nucleus. Interestingly, similar to other neurons present in the arcuate nucleus, kisspeptin-1 neurons are dependent on energy status and are able to respond to metabolic cues [16–18].

Interindividual variability in the timing of puberty indicates that the onset of puberty is not only a function of chronological age. A multitude of information about metabolic fuels, energy stores and somatic development and social environment impact upon the gonadotropin releasing hormone secretory network. Gonadotropin releasing hormone is synthesized by a limited group of 2000 neurons of the anterior hypothalamus projecting dorsally in the hypothalamic medial basal area, where gonadotropin releasing hormone is secreted into the hypothalamic–hypophyseal portal system. The pulsatile gonadotropin releasing hormone release is an inherent function of gonadotropin releasing hormone neurons, acting directly on the pituitary gonadotrope cells to maintain gonadotropins (luteinizing hormone and follicle-stimulating hormone) secretion. During puberty, the amplitude of luteinizing hormone and follicle-stimulating hormone release increases progressively and stimulates the ovaries to produce the gonadal sex steroids (testosterone and estradiol). The reactivation of gonadotropin releasing hormone release up to the first signs of physical maturation is referred to as "gonadarche". As stated above, an independent endocrine process of maturation of the adrenal glands, known as "adrenarche", contributes to sex steroid secretion that occurs during puberty. Adrenal androgens, including dehydroepiandrosterone, dehydroepiandrosterone sulfate, and androstenedione progressively increase after birth and continue during adolescence and into young adulthood [19].

## Factors Modulating Secretion of Gonadotropin Releasing Hormone and Gonadotropins

Gonadotropin releasing hormone release into the portal blood is characterized by intermittent pulses superimposed on a lower level of continuous secretion. Gonadotropin releasing hormone pulse characteristics are major determinants of gonadotropin pulsatile secretion, which varies both in amplitude and frequency according to the phase of the menstrual cycle. Luteinizing hormone pulses occur every 1–2 hours in the early follicular phase with increasing amplitude until preovulation. In the preovulatory period there is an increase in both amplitude and frequency. During the luteal phase, there is a remarkable reduction in luteinizing hormone pulsatility to once every four hours, while the amplitude is about twice as high as in the follicular phase. The frequency of gonadotropin releasing hormone secretion is determined by the firing rate of the neurons, while the amplitude is determined by stimuli acting either at the cell body or at the nerve terminals. Sex steroids acting on kisspeptin-1 system in the arcuate nucleus exert negative feedback. Indeed, while gonadotropin releasing hormone neurons do not express estrogen receptor alpha, a high percentage of kisspeptin-expressing cells express steroid receptors. Therefore, kisspeptin-1 neurons are considered as the main steroid-sensitive neurons mediating the feedback effects of sex steroids on gonadotropin releasing hormone secretion. However, estrogens also stimulate kisspeptin-1 signalling in the anteroventral periventricular nucleus of the hypothalamus, thus stimulating gonadotropin releasing hormone release. Estradiol robustly stimulates the expression of kisspeptin-1 in the anteroventral periventricular nucleus of the female rat and mouse [20, 21]. These and other observations led to the hypothesis that kisspeptin neurons in the anteroventral periventricular nucleus mediate the positive feedback effect of estradiol. These differential effects exerted in the arcuate nucleus and anteroperiventricular nucleus are the neurobiological basis of the negative and positive feedback, respectively, of estrogens on gonadotropins during the menstrual cycle. Therefore, circulating concentrations of estrogens define the levels of kisspeptin-1 mRNA expression in the female brain in a site-specific manner.

Other stimuli influencing gonadotropin releasing hormone release are:

*Opioid peptides*: β-endorphin and enkephalins inhibit the release of luteinizing hormone and to a lesser extent that of follicle-stimulating hormone. On the other hand, naloxone (an opiate receptor antagonist) increases luteinizing hormone levels; this effect was positively correlated with the previous endogenous levels of estradiol. Indeed, β-endorphin levels in hypophyseal portal blood are reduced after ovariectomy and restored by estrogen supplementation [22]. Therefore, it seems that estrogens may have a positive feedback on the release of opioid peptides.

*Neurotransmitters*: various monoaminergic brain neurotransmitters control gonadotropin releasing hormone neuronal activity and, thus, the amplitude of gonadotropin releasing hormone secretion. Noradrenaline has a facilitatory action on the gonadotropin releasing hormone neurons. Dopamine is considered an inhibitor of gonadotropin releasing hormone secretion and its action is enhanced by estrogens. Direct serotonin input from serotonin neurons located in raphe nuclei to preoptic gonadotropin releasing hormone neurons has been demonstrated in rodents. Treatment of immortalized mouse gonadotropin releasing hormone neurons with a nonselective serotonin receptor agonist causes a transient increase in gonadotropin releasing hormone release followed by reduction of pulsatile gonadotropin releasing hormone secretion [23].

*Prolactin*: this hormone exerts short-loop feedback on the release of gonadotropins. Prolactin acts as a neurotransmitter and may influence the turnover of catecholamines in the brain. It could also reduce luteinizing hormone/follicle-stimulating hormone levels by raising of hypothalamic dopamine and, in high concentration, reduce the pulsatile release [24].

## Effects of Sex Hormones Variation on Brain, Sexual Function and Behavior

### Early Development

A wealth of evidence indicates that androgens play a critical role in organizing gender identity, sexual orientation, and other behavioral traits in humans, specifically through binding to androgen receptors in the brain [25]. In contrast, animal models in rodents demonstrated that androgens aromatization into estrogens and binding of estrogen to estrogen receptors is necessary for brain masculinization [26, 27]. This interspecies discrepancy is most probably due to the fact that alpha-fetoprotein binds estrogen and prevents it from entering and masculinizing the brain in rodents [26, 27], but not in humans, where it shows a very low affinity for estrogen [28]. If masculinization of the brain was also estrogen-mediated in humans as in rodents, then unbound estrogens would cross the blood–brain barrier and masculinize the human female brain. In addition, women with complete androgen insensitivity syndrome, despite producing normal-to-high male levels of testosterone [29], show female gender identity [30], sexual attraction to men [31], and feminine brain architecture and behavior [32]. Additionally, human males with aromatase deficiency typically present as normal males, despite the absence of aromatization in the brain or elsewhere [33]. This suggests that androgens and a functional androgen receptor are actually necessary for masculinizing the human brain and behavior. In a case-control double-blind study involving data from the US/Denmark Prenatal Development Project, prenatal exposure to progesterone was associated with higher rates of bisexuality, regardless of sex [34]. In contrast, estrogen receptor stimulation seems to exert a limited role.

### Puberty

The next crucial life history transition is puberty. Both gonadarche and adrenarche are relevant contributors to brain and behavioral development that occur during puberty. Indeed, puberty is not only loosely anchored to marked internal and external physical changes and secondary sexual characteristics and fertility, but also to the profound changes in drives, motivations, psychology, and social life. The attainment of complex social and behavioral capacities mold the perceptions, motivations, and behavioral repertoire necessary for reproductive success. Steroid hormones are key determinants in the development and organization of brain during the adolescent transition from childhood to adulthood, when sociosexual maturity is attained. The specific behaviors that are organized by gonadal hormones are gender-dimorphic. However, research on the role of ovarian hormones in the organization of female sociosexual behaviors lags far behind that in males.

The complex interplay of luteinizing hormone, follicle-stimulating hormone, and steroidal hormones is hypothesized to facilitate sexual behavior in adolescence, emerging perceptual sensitivity for facial cues related to sexual interest, and the development of adult mating preferences [35]. Adolescence is characterized by an emerging "receptivity" (interest in sexual objects), which does not necessarily equate with "proceptivity" (the urge to seek and initiate sexual activity) [36]. Hormonal changes of puberty have been suggested to induce sexual dimorphism in neuroanatomical development across adolescence [37, 38]. Interestingly, the amygdala and hippocampus are the brain structures where a high density of estradiol and androgen receptors are found [35]. Therefore, these two brain regions are expected to be selectively influenced by sex hormones during adolescence.[35]. Goddings and colleagues found pubertal related amygdala growth for both sexes [39]. Indeed, pubertal sex hormones testosterone and estradiol, independent of age, drive sex differences in gray matter, white matter, amygdala and caudate volumes across adolescence. Changes in testosterone levels are associated with the development of total white matter, right amygdala, and bilateral caudate volumes in boys, whereas estradiol was related to the development of total white matter, right amygdala, and total gray matter volume in girls. Therefore, individuals with higher estradiol levels displayed increases in amygdala volumes across adolescence. Interestingly, in animal models, a similar gender dimorphism was found in the amygdala in male rats compared to females during puberty [40]. Estrogen has been found to increase dendritic spine density in the medial amygdala in female rats. Animal [41] and human [42] models have also demonstrated estradiol to reduce myelination during puberty in females. In summary, these results indicate that estradiol and testosterone may drive sexually dimorphic changes in the amygdala during pubertal development in both human and animal models.

This plasticity in brain volumes, driven by sex hormones, may have important implications for gender-related differences in behavior and mental health. It has been hypothesized that these changes seen across puberty in brain volumes of total white matter, cortex, and amygdala may account for different affective processing in girls and boys. However, further research is necessary to definitively elucidate the actions of sex hormones on microstructural development during adolescence. Indeed, the amygdala tightly connects with cortical regions to regulate emotion and can respond to cues of motivational significance (both fears and desires), even when occur outside awareness. Even though the amygdala is well known for its rapid response to signals for danger [43], it has been recently demonstrated to respond also to rapid "unseen" sexual as well as drug stimuli, thus indicating its importance in the processing of signals for reward [44, 45]. Interestingly, a decrease in amygdala responsiveness to arousing stimuli has been described in women with postpartum decrease in sexual interest [46]. This brain's rapid response to sexual reward cues may stem from the brain's capacity to initiate sexual desire in an instant, also outside awareness, and without heavy regulatory influence from frontal regions [47]. Therefore, the ability of testosterone and estradiol to trigger amygdala development and activation is a paramount feature in the understanding of how sex steroids may modulate appetitive sexual motivation within and outside awareness. The mesolimbic dopamine system is probably the best known neurobiological pathway able to enhance "wanting," and to process romantic love. Several neurobiological studies conclude that love is characterized by significantly increased activation of specific brain regions such as the ventral tegmental area, medial insula, anterior cingulate cortex, hippocampus, nucleus accumbens, caudate nucleus, and hypothalamus, which also mediate reward, motivation, and emotion regulation [48].

### Adulthood

There is compelling experimental evidence that brain structural alteration does occur also in adulthood. A recent study demonstrated that women's brains might modify slightly every month, in synchronization with menstrual cycles. Thirty women underwent magnetic resonance imaging and levels of estrogen in the blood were measured. Both grey and white matter in the brain increased as estrogen levels rose, causing the hippocampus to increase in volume, which, in turn, may affect women's behavior [49]. This important study is the first to link subtle hormonal variations during the menstrual cycle to a rapid, remarkable microstructural change in the hippocampus (within days). These data are consistent with evidence from other studies reporting the influence of the menstrual cycle on the human brain [50, 51]. At the time of ovulation, gray matter volume significantly increases by about 1.8% [52]. Studies comparing regional brain variations in women during different phases of the menstrual cycle reported larger gray matter volumes in the right fusiform/parahippocampal gyrus during the early follicular phase, i.e. between onset of menstruation to five days before ovulation [53], as well as increased gray matter volume in the right anterior hippocampus and decreased gray matter in the right dorsal basal ganglia (globus pallidus/putamen) in the high-estrogen, late-follicular phase, i.e. days 10–12 after onset of menses [50]. Perturbations in adult hippocampal neurogenesis plays an important role in the pathophysiology of various disease states, including depression [54, 55]. In summary, brain structure in adulthood is dramatically plastic and influenced by hormonal fluctuations [54, 56, 57]. Progressive age-related brain atrophy was observed in postmenopausal women and in women receiving antiestrogens [58, 59], thus suggesting a neuroprotective role for estrogens [60]. A recent study evaluated the time course of regional brain activity induced by visual sexual stimulation in premenopausal and menopausal women, and assessed the effect of menopause on the brain areas associated with sexual arousal in menopausal women using functional magnetic resonance imaging [61]. The brain areas with significantly higher activation in premenopausal women versus menopausal women included the thalamus, amygdala, and anterior cingulate cortex. This reduced brain activity of the thalamus, amygdala, and anterior cingulate cortex in menopausal women might be the neurobiological correlate of a menopause-related decrease in sexual arousal [61]. Structural and functional investigations have also revealed significant changes within the brain in women using hormonal contraceptives. A significant increase in gray matter volume in the pre- and postcentral gyri, parahippocampal gyrus, fusiform gyrus, and the superior, middle and inferior temporal gyri was observed in women taking hormonal contraceptives [53]. In particular, the precentral gyrus is a brain area with a high density of estrogen receptors [62] and has greater relative volume in women than in men [63]. In men, activation of the precentral gyrus has already been related to measures of penile turgidity under erotic vs. nonerotic visual stimulation [64]. Together with the cingulate cortex, precentral gyrus activation has been identified as one of the brain regions linked to behavioral inhibition and self-related anticipation of a sexual action [65]. Women taking oral contraceptives also show less activity in several prefrontal regions and fail to show the attenuation of activity in the amygdala observed in naturally cycling women [66]. Overall there is growing evidence that several brain areas, including the amygdala and hippocampus, are influenced by sex hormones, but future investigations are needed to identify the amygdala and hippocampus dependent behaviors influenced by sex hormones.

### Role of Estrogens and Progesterone

Both estrogen and progesterone activate classical genomic receptors as well as nonclassical membrane-associated receptors. The classical nuclear estrogen receptors (ERα and ERβ) [57, 60] and progesterone receptors [67] are highly expressed in brain areas involved in emotion and cognition, such as the amygdala and hippocampus. However, sex steroids can bind to multiple neuronal receptors, including serotonin, dopamine, and $GABA_A$ receptors [68, 69]. In addition to genomic actions, both estrogen and progesterone exert acute effects on synaptic physiology through the activation of multiple intracellular pathways to downstream membrane receptors [70]. The G protein-coupled estrogen receptor (GPER1, also known as GPR30) has been identified as one of the main estrogen-sensitive receptors responsible for the rapid nongenomic actions of estrogen. G protein-coupled estrogen receptor is highly expressed at the level of the synapse and rapidly regulates hippocampal dendritic morphology and synaptic plasticity. Therefore, some the neuroprotective actions of estrogens might be linked to G protein-coupled estrogen receptor activation [70].

A woman's lifespan is characterized by relevant periods of hormonal change, beginning with rising estrogen levels during puberty, high estrogen levels during pregnancy, and rapid falls postpartum, declining levels during peri-menopause, and extremely low levels in postmenopause [71]. Intriguingly, these major transitions in sex hormone levels seem to be associated with a parallel incidence of mood disorder. [72]. In addition to these major shifts in hormonal levels, mild changes in endogenous sex hormones, as occur during the monthly cycle, have also been associated with changes in mood [73] and sexual behavior [74]. In the pathology of premenstrual dysphoric disorder [74], an imbalance of the normal functioning of the serotonergic and dopaminergic system has been hypothesized. As previously reported, typically four main pathways are described for the dopaminergic system that are deeply involved in sexual desire (Chapter 4). Conflicting findings of estrogen effects on dopaminergic neurotransmission have been documented [72]; however, most of the studies report an overall facilitating effect on dopaminergic neurotransmission [75–78]. An estrogenic priming seems also to be necessary for progesterone-modulating effects on dopaminergic transmission [79]. However, further studies are needed before translating these preclinical findings to the human brain, behavior, and potential pathology. Nevertheless, recent studies support an interaction between estrogen and dopamine on cognitive domains, such as decision making [77], fear extinction [78], and memory bias [80]. In particular, estradiol is hypothesized to direct decision making toward more accessible, even if smaller, rewards [77], and to mediate memory bias through the interaction with dopamine in the dorsal striatum [80]. An interaction between estrogen and dopamine in prefrontal cortex function has also been suggested to play an important role during a working memory task [76]. The serotonin system plays a multitude of roles, most importantly balancing mood. Serotonergic neurons are highly expressed in the dorsal and medial raphe nuclei of the midbrain with ascending fibers projecting to the frontal cortex, striatum, thalamus, amygdala, hypothalamus, and hippocampus. In particular, two important serotonin-mediated physio-

logical functions, sexual behavior and the stress response, are tightly modulated by sex steroid hormones. Estrogen has been reported to heterogeneously modulate serotonin function via the regulation of neurotransmitter synthesis, degradation and binding to receptors [72]. In particular, acute estrogen administration has been reported to have opposite effects on the serotonin system as compared to a more chronic treatment-regimen. Therefore, the effect of estrogen on serotonin cannot be exclusively classified as stimulatory or inhibitory.

Also, progesterone has been reported to regulate serotonergic neurotransmission [72, 81]. Chronic progesterone treatment seems to decrease $5\text{-HT}_{1A}$ receptor expression in rats [82]. Progesterone is rapidly metabolized in the brain to 5α-pregnandione or 5β-pregnandione through a 5α- or 5β-reductase, respectively. Both pregnandiones can be reduced further in ring A, resulting in the formation of 3α- or 3β-pregnanolones. These reduced forms of progestins stimulate lordosis (sexual receptivity in female rats) when injected into the ventromedial hypothalamic nucleus and preoptic area in rodents [83]. Interestingly, in brain areas involved in progesterone regulation of female sexual behavior, such as the hypothalamus and preoptic area progesterone receptors, are upregulated by estrogens [83]. Facilitation of lordosis has been demonstrated in ovariectomized estrogen primed rats after implantation of 5α-, 3β-pregnenolone in the medial preoptic area. Intrahypothalamic total progesterone levels show a good correlation with the capacity of progesterone to stimulate lordosis in rats [83].

Interestingly, both estrogen and progesterone have been demonstrated to influence selective serotonin reuptake inhibitor treatment response [84]. In particular, estrogen blocks serotonin clearance, thus resulting in enhancement of serotonin function. This effect appears to be a consequence of estrogen receptor-β and/or G protein-coupled estrogen receptor stimulation. In humans, a recent study found an association between antidepressant efficacy and polymorphism of the serotonin transporter gene in premenopausal women only, but not in postmenopausal women [85]. These findings suggest that hormonal status is crucial for antidepressant efficacy, postmenopausal women gaining less benefit from antidepressant treatments compared to women of reproductive age [86, 87].

In conclusion, the interaction between ovarian hormone levels, age and genotype appear to modulate serotonin function in females. Interestingly, basic and clinical studies over the past three decades have consistently demonstrated that the serotonergic system is intimately involved in the pathogenesis of depression [88, 89]. Changes in serotonin neurotransmission have been repeatedly associated with the therapeutic response to antidepressant and mood stabilizing medication. Almost all currently employed treatments for depression, including the tricyclic antidepressants, the selective serotonin reuptake inhibitors, the monoamine oxidase inhibitors, and lithium, exert their antidepressant effects through a direct or indirect increase in serotonergic neurotransmission. Thus, the side effects of almost all these drugs include a reduction of sexual desire [90].

### Role of Androgens

It has been proposed that androgens have important effects in modulating sexual desire in women. The vaginal response to erotic stimuli is increased in women with high testosterone levels [91]. Additionally, a significant incidence of masturbatory activity corresponds with the midcycle peak of androgens [92]. Other data highlight the potential excitatory role of androgens on the reward system in humans [93, 94]. Several studies in adult rodents have demonstrated that testosterone administration induced conditioned place preference in rodents [95–97]. In another animal model, administration of a cocktail consisting of testosterone cypionate, nandrolone decanoate, and boldenone undecylenate, increased the rate of self-administration and enhanced the sensitivity

to amphetamine challenge [98]. Such effects were blunted by dopaminergic antagonists [99], suggesting that dopaminergic pathways mediate the behavioral outcomes induced by androgens. As stated previously, sexual desire and female-initiated sexual behavior change across the menstrual cycle, with a peak during the fertile phase [100–102]. Such variation across the cycle is not observed in women using oral contraceptives [101], which suppress ovulatory fluctuations of all sex steroids. In fact, not only estradiol but also testosterone peak near ovulation (Table 6.2) [71]; thus, testosterone is another good candidate for the cyclic shift in sexual desire. The evidence that androgens are important modulators of women's sexual function stems mainly from studies of testosterone therapy given to postmenopausal women with hypoactive sexual desire disorder (see later paragraph on "Treatment"). Some pioneering studies first suggested that testosterone positively regulates sexual desire not only in men but also in women. For example [103], low estradiol and testosterone levels during lactation were associated with low libido. Similarly, in a small observational study [104], antiandrogen therapy was found to negatively affect libido in women. In a representative sample of 1021 Australian women (ages 18–75), low androgens levels increased the risk of low sexual desire, arousal, and responsiveness [105]. In particular, in young women (<44 years old), low sexual desire, sexual arousal, or sexual responsiveness was significantly associated with a low dehydroepiandrosterone sulfate value [105]. Most recently, the association between androgens and sexual desire was investigated in 560 healthy Danish women 19–65 years old. Free testosterone and androstenedione were significantly linked with sexual desire both in women 19–24 years old and in women 25–44 years old [106]. In the Study of Women's Health Across the Nation, testosterone and dehydroepiandrosterone sulfate were both positively associated with masturbation frequency and desire across the menopausal transition [107].

In addition, oophorectomy, with a relevant reduction of not only estrogens but also androgens produced by the ovaries, is associated with decreased sexual desire and frequency of sexual fantasies [108]. Androgen treatment increased the intensity of sexual desire in oophorectomized women who were randomized to receive one of three different sex steroid replacement regimens: estrogen–androgen combined, an estrogen-alone drug, an androgen-alone drug, or a placebo [108]. Accordingly, combined supplementation with estradiol and androgen in oophorectomized women promoted sexual desire, sexual arousal, and increased numbers of fantasies vs. estradiol alone [109]. In addition, in a double-blind, placebo-controlled trial involving 533 oophorectomized women (ages 20 to over 65) with concurrent hypoactive sexual desire disorder, testosterone treatment significantly ameliorated both sexual desire and satisfying sexual activity [110]. The effects of exogenous estradiol vs estradiol plus testosterone were studied in six surgically menopausal women and five premenopausal women using functional magnetic resonance imaging patterns of brain activation in response to a sexual stimulus. Six weeks of estradiol was associated with global increases in the brain for erotic and neutral stimuli. Estradiol plus testosterone was associated with higher activation in the limbic system, which reached a level similar to that observed in premenopausal women [111]. These data suggest a positive effect of testosterone on sexual desire in women with reduced or absent ovarian androgen production.

However, the role of sex steroids on libido, and in particular whether the effect of testosterone is mediated by aromatization to _ estradiol, has been recently elucidated. A randomized controlled trial was conducted in 76 postmenopausal women using transdermal estradiol plus a 0.5% transdermal testosterone gel 400 ml/d who were randomly assigned to the aromatase inhibitor letrozole 2.5 mg/d or placebo for 16 weeks [112]. At 16 weeks, the two treatment groups reached similar serum testosterone levels and a similar significant increase in sexual function from baseline [112]. This study clearly suggested that the effect of testosterone on sexual function is not mediated by aromatization to estrogens in adequately estrogenized postmenopausal women.

With ageing, the mean circulating levels of total and free testosterone decrease progressively from the early reproductive years [113]; adrenal production of the androgen precursors, androstenedione and dehydroepiandrosterone, also decreases linearly with ageS [113, 114]. Therefore, an overall age-related decrease in testosterone is observed. Several pathophysiologic conditions are considered as common causes of low testosterone in women (Box 6.1).

In conclusion, androgens are important determinants of female sexual function. Low levels of total and free testosterone, $\Delta 4$ androstenedione, and dehydroepiandrosterone sulfate are linked to lower sexual desire. However, there is no threshold for any of these androgens that can be used to diagnose women with low sexual function or candidates for testosterone therapy.

---

**Box 6.1 Conditions associated to low testosterone in women.**

- Aging
- Panhypopituitarism
- Hyperprolactinemia
- Hypothalamic amenorrhea (i.e. anorexia nervosa)
- Primary ovarian insufficiency (all causes): bilateral oophorectomy; chemotherapy or radiation to pelvis or chemical ovarian suppression (e.g. gonadotropin releasing hormone analogs)
- Adrenal insufficiency
- Antiandrogen therapy (e.g. spironolactone, cyproterone acetate)
- Oral estrogen
- Glucocorticoid therapy

## Role of Kisspeptin in Female Sexual Desire

Kisspeptin is a crucial reproductive hormone that potently activates the reproductive axis, acting in the hypothalamus to stimulate downstream secretion of reproductive hormones [14, 115]. However, the expression of kisspeptin-1 and its cognate receptor (KISS1R) is not limited to the hypothalamus. As stated before, kisspeptin-1 neurons are also present in limbic brain structures in rodents and humans, including the medial amygdala. However, the role of kisspeptin-1 in these areas is far from clear. The limbic system has established roles in emotional and reproductive behavior and is considered the anatomical framework uniting sex, emotion, and reproduction in humans (for more details see Chapter 4). A recent randomized, double-blinded, cross-over, placebo-controlled study demonstrated that intravenous infusion of kisspeptin-1 (1 nmol/kg/h) in 29 healthy young men enhanced activity in key limbic and paralimbic structures when viewing sexual images [116]. These structures included the anterior and posterior cingulate as well as the left amygdala. Interestingly, sexual aversion decreased as a function of kisspeptin-1's enhancement of several structures of the sexual-processing network (including the cingulate, putamen, and globus pallidus), suggesting a role for kisspeptin-1 in sexual disinhibition [116]. Moreover, kisspeptin-1 stimulated key structures of the mesolimbic reward and fronto-striatal-amygdala-midbrain systems (including the hippocampus, amygdala, and cingulate) more in subjects with lower baseline sexual desire and reward trait [116]. In addition, kisspeptin also enhanced the response to bonding images activating regions similar to those activated with sexual images (i.e. the amygdala and the anterior and posterior cingulate), with additional activation of the thalamus and globus pallidus. Collectively, these data suggest that kisspeptin enhances limbic responses to sexual and bonding stimuli; the activation of these sexual arousal structures correlates with increased reward measures as well as with reduced sexual aversion [116].

## Role of Oxytocin in Female Sexual Desire

Oxytocin is a small neuropeptide synthesized in the supraoptic and paraventricular nucleus of the hypothalamus and secreted into the systemic circulation by nerve terminals in the posterior pituitary gland. Oxytocin is critically involved in female reproduction, facilitating pair bonding and affiliative behaviors in vertebrates from toads to humans [117]. The functions of oxytocin in uterine contractility and the breastfeeding are also well known. Oxytocin is released simultaneously by the brain of mother and her infant during suckling. It appears that oxytocin is essential for the onset of normal maternal behavior, as well as for the building of the mother/infant bond in all the animal species studied such far. However, oxytocin has also been implicated as having an important role in sexual responsiveness, arousal, and orgasm. Both sexual partners secrete oxytocin simultaneously during sexual intercourse. This parallel release of oxytocin reinforces the sexual arousal of both partners and is associated with affiliative, nonaggressive behavior, favoring the formation of pair bonding. The role of oxytocin in female sexual function and, especially, in desire is complex and not completely elucidated. However, animal studies provide a wealth of information about the biological function of oxytocin [117]. In rat studies, oxytocin administration has been found to increase lordosis (sexual receptivity in female rats), with the effect appearing dependent on sex steroids. However, oxytocin knockouts display normal mating behavior but do not experience bonding [117, 118]. Estradiol increases the expression of oxytocin and its receptors in the ventromedial hypothalamus of the rat [119], and a group of oxytocin receptor positive cells has been identified in the medial prefrontal cortex of female mice. In a small study enrolling 30 healthy premenopausal women, serum oxytocin levels were reduced in the luteal phase and were correlated with lower scores on the lubrication scale of the Female Sexual Function Index [120].

## Role of Prolactin in Female Sexual Desire

Prolactin is a hormone secreted by lactotrophs in the anterior pituitary. It enhances the turnover of dopamine in brain areas involved in the regulation of sexual behavior (i.e. nigrostriatal and mesolimbic tracts). In particular, in the tuberoinfundibular tract chronic increases of prolactin levels (hyperprolactinemia) induced dopamine release, thus leading to suppression of gonadotropin-releasing hormone with subsequent hypogonadotropic hypogonadism. Central hypogonadism may be the main underlying mechanism of hyperprolactinemia-associated low sexual desire. However, a direct effect of increased prolactin on sexual desire has been also hypothesized. In fact, prolactin receptors were found in the diencephalic incerto-hypothalamic dopaminergic system, which is tightly connected with the medial preoptic area, the most important area for the control of motivational and consummatory aspects of sexual behavior [121]. In contrast to other areas, in the incerto-hypothalamic dopaminergic system, prolactin did not release dopamine, suggesting a direct, inhibitory role of prolactin on sexual motivation. An extensive list of causes of hyperprolactinemia has been reported elsewhere [122].

## Role of Thyroid Hormones in Female Sexual Desire

In primary hypothyroidism, elevated hypothalamic thyrotropin releasing hormone stimulates prolactin secretion, with subsequent high prolactin levels. Although hypothyroidism is usually considered a possible cause of hyperprolactinemia, it is accompanied by normal serum prolactin levels in the majority of patients (roughly 60%). Therefore, additional mechanisms for decreased sexual desire in hypothyroidism should be taken into account. Hypothyroidism is often associated with depressive disorders, although the mechanism for this is unclear. Thyroid hormones are critically involved in the development of the central nervous system. However, an important role of thyroid hormones in the mature mammalian brain has been recently recognized [123]. In particular, in human cortical brain tissue thyroid hormones are present in high (nanomolar) concentrations. In peripheral tissues, where thyroxine is converted to triiodothyronine, thyroxine concentrations usually far exceed levels of triiodothyronine, the thyroid hormone with the highest biological activity. In contrast, in the brain thyroxine and triiodothyronine concentrations are in an equimolar range [124]. Their relative receptors are also prevalent in the mature brain. Indeed, nuclear receptors for triiodothyronine, the thyroid hormone with the highest biological activity, are widely distributed in adult rat brain, with the highest density in the amygdala and hippocampus. Thyroid hormones appear to play an important role in regulating central noradrenergic function and it has been suggested that thyroid dysfunction may be linked with abnormalities in central noradrenergic neurotransmission. An interaction of thyroid hormones with serotonin neurotransmission has been also documented [125]. Some evidence in humans with thyroid dysfunction suggests that hypothyroid status is associated with a reduced serotonin responsiveness. Furthermore, this appears to be reversible with thyroid replacement therapy [126, 127]. However, given the small number of studies in humans, and a limited sample size, definitive conclusions cannot be established. In contrast, results from studies in animals yielded stronger evidence that thyroid status has a relevant impact on serotonergic neurotransmission in the adult brain [128]. Thyroid hormone may enhance cortical serotonergic neurotransmission via two distinct mechanisms: (i) by disinhibiting cortical and hippocampal serotonin release through a reduction of the $5\text{-}HT_{1A}$ autoreceptors sensitivity in the raphe area; and (ii) by increasing cortical serotonin neurotransmission through an increase of cortical $5\text{-}HT_2$ receptor sensitivity [125, 128].

Hyperthyroidism has been also associated with reduced desire. Thyroid hormones influence androgen activity by altering the production of sex hormone-binding globulin by hepatocytes [129]. It has been hypothesized that these responses are mediated directly by thyroid hormone receptors acting at the level of the human sex hormone binding globulin gene. Thyroid hormones exert their effects at the gene level via thyroid hormone receptors, which generally bind as a heterodimer with the retinoid X receptor to thyroid hormone response elements within target gene promoters. However, a typical thyroid hormone response element has not been documented within the human sex hormone binding globulin promoter region [130]. It has been suggested that the thyroid hormone-induced increase in sex hormone binding globulin gene expression is mediated indirectly through the release of hepatocyte nuclear factor-4α [130]. Therefore, a change in the metabolic state of the liver after thyroxine treatment could in turn influence hepatocyte nuclear factor-4α expression, leading to increased sex hormone binding globulin expression. Suppression of the thyroxine-induced hepatocyte nuclear factor-4α levels in hapathocytes completely blocked the thyroxine-induced increase in sex hormone binding globulin promoter region activity [131]. In conclusion, a decreased free testosterone concentration due to a marked increase in sex hormone binding globulin might be the underlying mechanism for hypoactive sexual desire disorder in hyperthyroid women.

### Role of Metabolic Disease

Both obesity and metabolic syndrome have been recently associated with increased vascular resistance in the clitoris and impaired sexual arousal, suggesting that these cardiometabolic risk factors may have a greater direct negative impact at the genital level than at a central one [132, 133]. However, these metabolic diseases have also been associated with reduced sexual desire. Therefore, a reduced libido in patients affected by diabetes mellitus or metabolic syndrome may be, at least in part, related to reduced sexual arousal during intercourse.

# Pathophysiology

Several physical and medical factors as well as some medications have been associated with low sexual desire (Box 6.2).

---

**Box 6.2 Conditions and medications associated with low sexual desire.**

- Surgically induced menopause and other conditions associated to low androgen levels
- Hyperprolactinemia
- Thyroid disorders
- Diabetes mellitus/Obesity/Metabolic syndrome
- Depression
- Low urinary tract symptoms
- Neurological diseases
- Medications (antidepressant, antipsychotic, oral contraceptives, antiandrogens)

---

### Surgically Induced Menopause and Other Conditions Associated with Low Androgen Levels

Women who have undergone oophorectomy have been reported to have a higher risk of developing adverse health consequences, such as shorter life expectancy, with a 13% increase in all-cause mortality, coronary heart disease (23%), lung cancer (29%), and colorectal cancer (49%) [134]. It has been established that surgical menopause may lead to distressing and abrupt symptoms, especially sexual dysfunction, compared with women who undergo natural menopause [135, 136], with surgical menopause roughly doubling the risk of having low sexual desire than natural menopause [137]. Sexual desire scores are highly correlated with sexual arousal, orgasm, and sexual pleasure, demonstrating that low sexual desire is frequently associated with impaired functioning in other aspects of the sexual response. As described before, the ovary is one of the main sources of androgens in women. Most studies indicate that surgical menopause is associated with lower total and free testosterone levels than natural menopause [138–143]. Therefore, the reduction in androgen levels due to ovariectomy is the most plausible cause of increased risk for hypoactive sexual desire disorder in surgical menopause. Compared with the naturally postmenopausal ovary, which continues low-level secretion of testosterone, surgically induced menopause is associated with an abrupt cessation of steroid production [142]. This sudden and complete loss of all ovarian steroids is also associated with more severe menopausal symptoms (hot flashes, vaginal dryness, dyspareunia, and mood changes) as compared to naturally menopause [142]. However, women who had surgical menopause and took hormone therapy experienced significantly less severe symptoms, but hormone replacement therapy did not completely counteract vaginal dryness, pain with intercourse, and loss of interest in sex [142]. According to a Cochrane review, hormone replacement therapy had a small-to-moderate benefit when treating sexual dysfunction in perimenopausal and postmenopausal women [144]. Additionally, women who undergo surgical menopause show poorer psychosocial outcomes than those who undergo natural menopause [145], with younger women experiencing more depressive symptoms and lower psychosocial functioning than older women undergoing the same procedure [146].

Apart from surgical menopause, some other clinical conditions have been recognized to be associated with a reduction in androgens levels and with reduction of sexual desire (Box 6.1) [147]. A reduced level of testosterone was reported in women with premature ovarian insufficiency as compared to age-matched healthy counterparts [148–150]. In particular, in subjects with Turner syndrome, reduced circulating levels of several androgens (testosterone and Δ4-androstenedione) are roughly 40% lower than in age-controls and are also associated with reduced sexual desire [151].

Anorexia nervosa, is a psychiatric disorder complicated by severe hypogonadism leading to bone loss, cognitive impairment, and a high prevalence of mood and anxiety disorders, including major depressive disorder [152]. More importantly, a clear association between sexual problems, including low sexual desire, and eating disorder psychopathology has been identified [153].

Hypopituitarism often consists of hypogonadotropic hypogonadism and/or secondary adrenal insufficiency, thereby impairing the two major sources (ovary and adrenal gland) of androgen production. Reduced concentrations of total testosterone, free testosterone, and androstenedione have been demonstrated in women presenting with hypopituitarism [154]. In women with adrenal insufficiency (either secondary or primary), but not in women with hypogonadism, a relevant reduction of dehydroepidandrosterone sulfate is also described.

## Hyperprolactinemia

As stated before hyperprolactinemia is associated with hypogonadotropic hypogonadism, reduced ovarian production of sex steroids, and low sexual desire [155–157]. In a small study of 63 women with morphologically verified hypothalamic-pituitary disorders and hyperprolactinemia, decreased sexual desire was present in more than 30% of cases [156].

## Hypothyroidism/Hyperthyroidism

There is a paucity of data regarding thyroid disorders and female sexuality. However, hypothyroidism in women is another endocrine condition previously associated with decreased libido. Three case-control studies reported decreased sexual desire either in women with overt [158–160] or subclinical [158, 161] hypothyroidism. On the other hand, hyperthyroidism has also been associated with reduced sexual desire [160, 162], most probably linked to an increase of sex hormone binding globulin levels with a parallel reduction in free testosterone.

## Diabetes Mellitus

Female sexual dysfunction and urinary incontinence have been indicated as two of the major problems, negatively affecting quality of life among women with diabetes [163, 164]. A recent meta-analysis demonstrated that having any type of diabetes almost doubled the risk of sexual dysfunction [164]. Several of the studies in type 1 and 2 diabetes specifically reported a reduction of libido. In particular, in the long-term Epidemiology of Diabetes Interventions and Complications study, 57% of women with type 1 diabetes suffered from decreased sexual desire [165]. However, female sexual dysfunction associated with diabetes mellitus is likely to be multifactorial, with peripheral macrovascular/microvascular and neurogenic complications proposed [132, 133]. In particular, decreased capillary engorgement in response to erotic stimuli was found using vaginal photoplethysmography in women with diabetes as compared with healthy control subjects without diabetes [166]. A small study enrolling 30 women with diabetes and 20 control subjects, demonstrated that reduced (vibratory) sensation at multiple genital and extragenital sites was associated with diabetes mellitus [167]. Diabetes has been reported to greatly impact vaginal physiology, being associated with alterations of the vaginal lamina propria vascular network, nitrergic signaling, and androgen receptor expression [168]. In conclusion, diabetic end-organ complications may play a role in decreasing women's sexual arousal, with a subsequent reduction of sexual desire.

## Metabolic Syndrome

Data for metabolic syndrome and hypoactive sexual desire disorder are conflicting. Among 376 postmenopausal, community-dwelling women from the Rancho Bernardo Study (aged ≥40 years, mean baseline age = 73 years), women with metabolic syndrome showed significantly lower sexual activity and lower sexual desire compared with women without metabolic syndrome [169]. The number of metabolic syndrome criteria was strongly associated with reduced sexual activity and reduced sexual desire and satisfaction, suggesting a cumulative association of cardiovascular risk factors with sexuality. Among metabolic syndrome components, elevated triglyceride levels were the most tightly associated with low sexual desire [169]. Three other smaller case-control studies did not find any significant association between metabolic syndrome and sexual desire domain [170–172]. Therefore, available evidence suggests that metabolic syndrome might be associated with hypoactive sexual desire disorder, but further studies are needed.

## Obesity

In population-based studies, sexual desire was found to decrease as a function of obesity and increasing body mass index [173, 174]. However, this evidence was not confirmed in three clinical samples of women seeking or undergoing weight loss treatment [175–177]. These prior studies supporting an association between body mass index and sexual dysfunction observed lower sexual functioning at higher levels of body mass index. In one sample [178], more than half of women seeking bariatric surgery reported reduced sexual desire. It is important to note that women seeking weight loss surgery showed a significantly greater impairment in sexual functioning than obese women who do not [175]. Women seeking surgery for weight loss may thus experience more severe physiological or psychological distress that accounts for differences in sexual function. An intimate relationship between binge eating and sexual functioning has been also described in obese subjects [177]. The perceived lack of control over eating, which determines a sense of shame [179], was thus hypothesized to worsen sexual functioning. Alternatively, the reduced satisfaction in sexual life may lead to lifestyle changes, with increased calorie intake [180]. Observational studies have consistently demonstrated a trend towards an improvement of sexual desire after weight loss [181, 182]. More importantly, it was reported that change in reported sexual desire was associated with deviation from each woman's individual body mass index trajectory. In particular, greater-than-expected weight gain seems to be responsible for concurrent decrease in desire, whilst an increase in desire occurred in patients showing greater-than-expected weight loss. Weight loss after intensive lifestyle intervention was not significantly associated with resolution of female sexual dysfunction [183]. In contrast, a complete resolution of female sexual dysfunction for a majority of patients six months postbariatric surgery has been reported [181]. Improved body image, increased self-esteem, and perceived sexual attractiveness may be the most important determinant factors leading to improved sexual desire following intervention for weight loss [178, 181].

## Depression

As reported in the previous chapters, depression is an important risk factor for low sexual desire. In particular, in the Hypoactive Sexual Desire Disorder Registry Study, about 30% of women with acquired, generalized hypoactive sexual desire disorder presented concurrent symptoms or diagnosis of depression [184]. Adding a layer of complexity, most antidepressants are associated with decreased desire [185, 186]; therefore, use of antidepressant medication may actually substitute one causative factor of hypoactive sexual desire disorder for another. During the assessment phase, every patient with low sexual desire should thus be screened for depression, as depression and decreased sexual desire have demonstrated a strong bidirectional association [187].

## Urinary Tract Symptoms

Urinary tract symptoms in women are extremely common. According to the literature, 11–73% of women suffer from some urinary tract symptoms throughout their lifespan [188]. The most distressing urinary

dysfunctions in women include [189]: (i) overactive bladder, currently defined as a syndrome characterized by urinary urgency, associated with increased daytime frequency and nocturia; (ii) urgency urinary incontinence, defined as a loss of urine associated with urgency to void; (iii) stress urinary incontinence, which is the involuntary leakage of urine during maneuvers involving sudden increased intra-abdominal pressure; and (iv) mixed urinary incontinence, with concurrent stress urinary incontinence and urgency urinary incontinence. In general, lower urinary tract symptoms negatively affect quality of life and are commonly associated with female sexual dysfunction [190, 191]. Women with urinary incontinence and/or lower urinary tract symptoms were more likely to suffer from sexual dysfunction [190], mainly sexual pain disorder (44%) and hypoactive sexual desire (34%) than the general female population. Similarly, other studies reported that stress urinary incontinence and low urinary tract symptoms might negatively affect sexual desire [192]. The pathogenic mechanisms underlying this association are unclear. A contribution of serotonin on lower urinary tract function has been recognized. A wide variety of serotonin receptor subtypes are present in bladder urothelium, smooth muscle, autonomic excitatory nerve terminals, and central pathways controlling the micturition reflex [193–195]. Serotonin has both physiological and pathological functions in the lower urinary tract. Recently, serum serotonin has shown an independent negative correlation with lower urinary tract symptoms and with urinary incontinence. In the current National Institute for Health and Care Excellence guidelines, duloxetine, a serotonin-noradrenaline reuptake inhibitor, has been recommended as treatment for women with lower urinary tract symptoms who are not surgical candidates or those who prefer drugs to surgery [196]. Moreover, it may be that women with urinary incontinence avoid sexual intimacy because of fear of involuntary leakage of urine during intercourse or orgasm.

## Neurological Diseases

Various chronic neurological diseases show a negative influence on sexual desire in women. Examples include multiple sclerosis [197] and spinal cord injury [198]. Based on the available data, we conclude that some neurological diseases appear to be associated with decreased sexual desire, but data are limited.

## Medications

Among medications, special attention should be paid to antidepressant treatments (as discussed before), antipsychotics, and other drugs increasing prolactin levels [199]. In addition, a focused medical history should also ascertain the use of combined oral contraceptives [200], as well as antiandrogen drugs. The estrogen/progestin combination contraceptive pills inhibit the mid-cycle peak of gonadotropin releasing hormone from the hypothalamus, thus suppressing pituitary luteinizing hormone and follicle-stimulating hormone, and inhibiting ovulation [201]. Women taking oral contraceptives do not ovulate, do not experience physiological fluctuations in sex hormones (estradiol, progesterone, and testosterone), and therefore, do not experience cyclic peaks in sexual behaviors [200]. These hormones are not completely suppressed by oral contraceptives and the levels of endogenous sex steroids in the peripheral blood are maintained at level similar to that detected in the early follicular phase of the menstrual cycle [201]. However, even though all types of oral contraceptives decrease levels of total and free testosterone, the greatest effect on the increase of sex hormone binding globulin is seen with higher ethinyl estradiol dose and with a third or fourth generation progestins [202]. This relevant hormonal reduction might be responsible for lower levels of sexual desire reported in some oral contraceptive users [200]. A recent placebo-controlled, double-blind, randomized trial demonstrated that desire was significantly reduced by levonorgestrel-containing oral contraceptives in comparison to placebo [203]. Interestingly, duration of oral contraceptive use was found to be one of the most important predictors of a woman's subjective response to sexual stimuli. Similarly, antidepressant medications may also lower desire. Antiandrogen drugs are usually used in women with hirsutism [204]. Spironolactone and cyproterone acetate, the antiandrogens most commonly used in the treatment of hirsutism, possess intrinsic hormonal activity and interfere with steroidogenesis. Cyproterone acetate also shows significant antigonadotropic effects. Side effects of these drugs include frequent menstrual irregularity. Other antiandrogen drugs, such as flutamide and finasteride, can be also used in women with hirsutism. Flutamide is a nonsteroidal compound with pure antiandrogen activity that acts to block the androgen receptor site. However, some data suggest that flutamide might also reduce the synthesis of androgens and/or increase their metabolism to inactive molecules. Liver toxicity is a rare but potentially severe side effect of flutamide. Finasteride is a very potent inhibitor of the type 2 isoenzyme of 5α-reductase, the enzyme responsible for conversion of testosterone to the active metabolite dihydrotestosterone [204]. As increased 5α-reductase activity is considered a pathogenic mechanism of hirsutism, selective enzyme inhibition has been proposed as a rational medical approach to this condition as well.

Some antidepressants, such as selective serotonergic reuptake inhibitors, are well known to induce sexual side effects. As stated, selective serotonin reuptake inhibitors may inhibit gonadotropin releasing hormone, thus reducing testosterone levels. Recently the US Food and Drug Administration stated that antidepressant-related sexual dysfunction is an important entity that should be adequately assessed during clinical trials with the use of available instruments and described in product labels.

## Substances of Abuse

Numerous substances of abuse, including alcohol, tobacco, and opioids, are correlated with sexual dysfunction in women. Endogenous opioids exert an important action on the physiological sexual functioning through effects at specific opioid receptors and control of the release of gonadotropin releasing hormone and, thus, follicle-stimulating hormone and luteinizing hormone, with subsequent development of hypogonadotropic hypogonadism. Opioids use also exerts a negative influence on adrenal androgen. Studies show that long-term use of alcohol leads to inhibition of the hypothalamic-pituitary-gonadal axis and reduces the release of gonadotropins from the pituitary. Therefore, in both opioid and alcohol abusers, a reduction of androgen levels and libido have been observed [205].

## Diagnosis

Low or decreased sexual desire that causes personal distress is the core feature of hypoactive sexual desire disorder as defined by the Diagnostic and Statistical Manual, Fourth Edition, Revised (DSM-IV-TR) [206]. Hypoactive sexual desire disorder is a relatively common but often undiagnosed condition. As for other sexual dysfunctions, hypoactive sexual desire disorder may be defined according to the duration as lifelong (no previous history of normal functioning) or acquired (prior normal functioning) and according to whether it occurs only in limited circumstances (situational) or in all sexual experiences (generalized). The DSM-5 merged desire and arousal into the single diagnosis, female sexual interest-arousal disorder, but this new clinical entity has not been validated nor studied in any clinical trial. In conclusion, for the purpose of this chapter, we use the DSM-IV definition of hypoactive sexual desire disorder.

## Screening Tools

The Decreased Sexual Desire Screener [207] is a validated self-administered questionnaire that that can help clinicians in establishing the presence and severity of hypoactive sexual desire disorder (Box 6.3). The Decreased Sexual Desire Screener is an extremely useful tool to be also used by clinicians without expertise in sexual medicine. The first four yes/no questions make an accurate diagnosis of an acquired, distressing, reduction in sexual desire. The fifth question lists potential causes or exacerbating factors for reduced desire. Patients who do not endorse all of the first four questions are unlikely to have hypoactive sexual desire disorder.

---

**Box 6.3  Decreased Sexual Desire Screener.**

| | | | |
|---|---|---|---|
| 1) | In the past, was your level of sexual desire or interest good and satisfying to you? | YES | NO |
| 2) | Has there been a decrease in your level of sexual desire or interest? | YES | NO |
| 3) | Are you bothered by your decreased level of sexual desire or interest? | YES | NO |
| 4) | Would you like your level of sexual desire or interest to increase? | YES | NO |
| 5) | Please circle all the factors that you feel may be contributing to your current decrease in sexual desire or interest: | | |
| | A)  An operation, depression, injuries, or other medical condition | YES | NO |
| | B)  Medications, drugs, or alcohol you are currently taking | YES | NO |
| | C)  Pregnancy, recent childbirth, menopausal symptoms | YES | NO |
| | D)  Other sexual issues you may have (pain, decreased arousal, orgasm) | YES | NO |
| | E)  Your partner's sexual problems | YES | NO |
| | F)  Dissatisfaction with your relationship or partner | YES | NO |
| | G)  Stress or fatigue | YES | NO |

Other screening tools for female sexual dysfunction may be used, even though they are more dimensional and less specific to reduced sexual desire. The Female Sexual Function Index is a well-validated, 19-item self-report instrument that evaluates different dimensions of sexual function, including desire, arousal, lubrication, orgasm, satisfaction, and pain. It is useful to reliably differentiate between sexually dysfunctional and healthy women (with a cut-off score <26.5 indicating sexual dysfunction) and to measure treatment efficacy (www. fsfiquestionnaire.com) [208]. The Female Sexual Distressed Scale – Revised version [209] is a validated questionnaire consisting of 13 items scoring distress, dissatisfaction, and other negative feelings related to sexual dysfunctions, including low desire.

In general, patients with sexual dysfunctions expect clinicians to inquire about their general health. During assessment, the medical history should be focused to ascertain the presence or suspicion of organic diseases that may be contributing to acquired, generalized hypoactive sexual desire disorder. A list of medical conditions associated with hypoactive sexual desire disorder has been described previously (Box 6.2). In particular, depression should be carefully evaluated. Depressive illness can be easily identified with some questions evaluating the presence of depressed mood or anhedonia during the previous two weeks or the current use of antidepressant medications. However, according to the recent US Preventive Services Task Force Recommendation Statement, an accurate depression screening instrument is the Patient Health Questionnaire [210]. Although a general physical examination of patients who experience hypoactive sexual desire disorder is often unremarkable and it has a low diagnostic yield, a focused physical examination, including a pelvic examination, may facilitate important reassurance for the patient that she is anatomically normal or identify genital arousal or pain disorders.

There are no specific investigations to confirm or exclude acquired, generalized hypoactive sexual desire disorder, and additional laboratory (e.g., thyroid stimulating hormone, prolactin), or imaging investigations are only occasionally required based upon the patient's medical history and examination. In particular, if hyperprolactinemia is suspected, a prolactin blood test will be done. The initial determination of prolactin can be performed at any time of the day but it should absolutely avoid excessive venipuncture stress [199]. A single determination is usually sufficient to establish the diagnosis, but when in doubt 2–3 samples separated by at least 15–20 minutes should be drawn after obtaining venous access. Normal values of prolactin in women are generally lower than 25 µg/l. A prolactin level greater than 250 µg/l usually indicates the presence of a prolactinoma, whereas prolactin level greater than 500 µg/l is diagnostic of a macroprolactinoma [199]. However, it should be underscored that selected drugs, including antipsychotic medications and metoclopramide, may cause prolactin levels increase above 200 µg/l. In addition, in patients with asymptomatic hyperprolactinemia (without galactorrhoea, menstrual irregularity, infertility), assessment for macroprolactin is mandatory. The term *macroprolactinemia* indicates the situation in which a preponderance of the circulating prolactin consists of the larger molecules (such as a dimer, "big prolactin," and a much larger polymeric form, "big-big prolactin") [199]. Larger prolactin forms (macroprolactin) are characterized by a lower/absent bioactivity, and thus macroprolactinemia should be suspected when typical symptoms of hyperprolactinemia are absent. Polyethylene glycol precipitation is an inexpensive way to evaluate the presence of macroprolactin in the serum [199].

As mentioned before, both hypothyroidism and hyperthyroidism have been associated with reduced sexual desire. Therefore, if a disorder of thyroid function is suspected, a blood thyroid-stimulating hormone will be measured. Diagnosis of hypothyroidism is based on symptoms [211] and the results of a blood thyroid stimulating hormone level. Hypothyroidism commonly manifests as a slowing in physical and mental activity but may be asymptomatic. An elevated thyroid stimulating hormone requires measurement of the level of the thyroid hormone thyroxine. A low level of thyroxine and high level of thyroid stimulating hormone indicate overt hypothyroidism. Normal blood levels of triiodothyronine and thyroxine but a higher than normal level of thyroid stimulating hormone is a condition called subclinical hypothyroidism, which usually is without outward signs or symptoms. In contrast, hyperthyroidism is a condition in which the thyroid gland produces a high level of thyroid hormones and thyroid stimulating hormone is usually suppressed. Commonly reported symptoms of hyperthyroidism are palpitations, fatigue, tremor, anxiety, sleep disturbance, weight loss, heat intolerance, and sweating. Frequent physical findings are tachycardia, tremor of the extremities, and weight loss. In conclusion, thyroid stimulating hormone should be measured when a woman with hypoactive sexual desire disorder also presents clinical suspicion of hypothyroidism [211] or hyperthyroidism [212].

Although several studies indicate that androgen levels are positively associated with sexual interest and arousal in women (see previously), there is no cut-off level for any androgen that distinguishes women with/ without normal sexual function. Hence, measurement of androgens is not recommended to diagnose low sexual desire or any other female sexual dysfunction. Testosterone and sex hormone binding globulin levels are only required if considering testosterone therapy. However, since several conditions (Box 6.1) have been associated with reduced testosterone level, their presence should be carefully evaluated during the assessment phase.

# Therapeutic Strategies for Hypoactive Sexual Desire Disorder

## Modification of neuroendocrine factors contributing to low sexual desire

Following the ISSWSH process of care, [213] when the presence of acquired, generalized hypoactive sexual desire disorder is diagnosed, it is particularly crucial to take a focused medical, sexual, psychological, and social and drug history to identify any factors that may be potentially reversible. Indeed, etiology of hypoactive sexual desire disorder is often complex and multivariate, and several pathophysiological factors (see the section "Pathophysiology") may cause hypoactive sexual desire disorder by either decreasing sexually excitatory processes or increasing inhibitory ones. Therefore, the first line intervention for women with hypoactive sexual desire disorder is to remove any modifiable risk factor that has been identified during the assessment phase.

### Treatment of Hyperprolactinemia
Therapeutic strategy for hyperprolactinemia must be driven by the underlying etiology [199]. In symptomatic patients with suspected drug-induced hyperprolactinemia, discontinuation of the medication for 4–5 drug half-lives or substitution of an alternative drug, followed by re-measurement of serum prolactin is recommended. If the drug cannot be discontinued and the onset of the hyperprolactinemia is not temporally coincident with drug initiation, a pituitary magnetic resonance image should be obtained to exclude the presence of pituitary or hypothalamic mass. In contrast, in patients with asymptomatic medication-induced hyperprolactinemia, a treatment with dopamine agonists is not recommended, but the use of estrogen in patients with long-term hypogonadism is suggested. In symptomatic hyperprolactinemia due to prolactinoma, treatment with dopamine agonists is currently the gold standard therapy to lower prolactin levels, decrease tumor size,

and restore gonadal function [199]. Among dopamine agonists, cabergoline is the treatment of choice because it has higher efficacy in normalizing prolactin levels and restoring normal sexual function, as well as a higher frequency of pituitary tumor shrinkage. Cabergoline generally only needs to be administered either once or twice per week due to its extremely long half-life (weekly dose of 0.5–2.0 mg) [199]. In contrast, asymptomatic patients due to microprolactinomas should not be treated with dopamine agonists. Pituitary surgery, usually by the transsphenoidal approach, is generally reserved for prolactinoma resistant to maximal tolerable doses of dopamine agonists. In 70–90% of patients with hypoactive sexual desire disorder, dopamine agonists lower prolactin levels to normalize both hypoactive sexual desire and gonadal function.

### Treatment of Hypothyroidism/ Hyperthyroidism

Standard treatment for hypothyroidism involves daily use of the synthetic thyroid hormone levothyroxin. [211]. This oral medication restores adequate hormone levels, reversing the signs and symptoms of hypothyroidism. In contrast, several treatments for hyperthyroidism exist. The treatment choice is driven by patient's age, physical condition, underlying cause, and the severity of the hyperthyroidism. First-line treatment usually involves antithyroid medications, including propylthiouracil and methimazol, which gradually reduce symptoms of hyperthyroidism. Symptoms usually begin to improve in 6–12 weeks but treatment with antithyroid medications typically continues at least a year and often longer [214]. However, it is actually not known whether restoring a euthyroid state can improve low sexual desire in hypothyroid or hyperthyroid patients.

### Treatment of Conditions Related to Low Testosterone Level

As stated previously, another condition associated with low androgens levels is adrenal insufficiency, either primary or secondary. In women presenting with adrenal insufficiency, four months of treatment with dehydroepiandrosterone (50 mg/d) resulted in an increased frequency of sexual thoughts, interest, and satisfaction, as well as improved well-being and decreased depression and anxiety [215]. In contrast, many other subsequent studies did not confirm these results. In 2009, a meta-analysis demonstrated that dehydroepiandrosterone therapy in adrenal insufficiency showed a low-to-moderate improvement in health-related quality of life and depressive symptoms, but it had no effects on sexual well-being [216]. Accordingly, a recent guideline of the Endocrine Society recommends against the routine prescription of dehydroepiandrosterone for the treatment of women with low androgen levels due to hypopituitarism, adrenal insufficiency, surgical menopause, pharmacological glucocorticoid administration, or other conditions associated with low androgen levels, because there are limited data supporting clinical improvement with therapy [217]. Thus, available evidence does not support the use of dehydroepiandrosterone in women with or without adrenal insufficiency. Data on other low testosterone conditions like Turner syndrome, anorexia nervosa, and hypopituitarism are inadequate to support the use of testosterone.

### Treatment of Depression or Antidepressant-Induced Low Sexual Desire

Bupropion has selectivity for inhibition of the dopamine and norepinephrine reuptake transporters. It alleviates sexual symptoms caused by other antidepressant medication, hence providing a potential off-label approach in the treatment of hypoactive sexual desire disorder. A recent placebo-controlled functional magnetic resonance imaging study on healthy subjects receiving paroxetine or bupropion demonstrated that brain regions related to the processing of emotional and autonomic components of erotic stimulation showed reduced responsiveness under paroxetine but not with bupropion [218]. A recent systematic review and meta-analysis on the effectiveness of bupropion as an antidepressant identified 51 studies, dividing into four categories: bupropion as monotherapy for depression; bupropion prescribed with another antidepressant; bupropion in "other" populations (e.g. bipolar depression, elderly populations); and the evaluation of the side effects of bupropion. More methodologically robust trials demonstrated the superiority of bupropion over placebo, and most head-to-head trials showed an equivalent efficacy with other antidepressants. Moreover, most of the studies on the co-administration of bupropion with another antidepressant showed an additional effect [219]. Therefore, it is recommended as an alternative antidepressant treatment without adverse effects concerning sexual arousal and libido.

Some other newer antidepressants have also been associated with less sexual dysfunction. Agomelatine, a stable analog of melatonin, is a melatonin receptor agonist and a $5\text{-HT}_{2C}$ receptor antagonist. A recent meta-analysis demonstrated that agomelatine is an effective antidepressant with similar efficacy to standard antidepressants [220]. However, it shows similar rates of sexual dysfunction compared with placebo and lower rates compared with serotoninergic antidepressants [221].

Desvenlafaxine, the major metabolite of venlafaxine, has recently been associated with greater orgasmic dysfunction in healthy men, but not in a group of healthy women. There were no differences in other sexual areas (libido and arousal) in comparison with placebo [222]. An additional randomized controlled trial in a depressed population treated with desvenlafaxine 50–100 mg/d or placebo, sexual function was comparable between desvenlafaxine and placebo [223].

Vortioxetine, a new multimodal-serotonin antidepressant, displays robust procognitive properties in addition to antidepressant effects [224]. In addition to its blockade of serotonin transporter reuptake, it is an antagonist at $5\text{-HT}_{1D}$, $5\text{-HT}_3$, and $5\text{-HT}_7$ receptors, agonist at $5\text{-HT}_{1A}$ receptors, and partial agonist at $5\text{-HT}_{1B}$ receptors. This combined effect increases extracellular concentrations of serotonin, dopamine, and noradrenaline [225], and might be responsible for the less frequent sexual side effects. In a recent randomized, double-blind trial, treatment-emergent sexual dysfunctions were not significantly different between vortioxetine (15–20 mg/d) and placebo-treated groups [226]. Similar results were demonstrated in double-blind, placebo-controlled trial with vortioxetine (10–15 mg/d) in depressed patients [226]. Finally, vortioxetine has been recently found to improve escitalopram-associated sexual dysfunction in patients with well-treated major depressive disorder [227].

Vilazodone, a selective serotonin reuptake inhibitor with partial agonist activity at the $5\text{-HT}_{1A}$ receptor, approved for the treatment of major depressive disorder, has few sexual side effects [228]. Three studies showed that treatment with vilazodone 40 mg/d was associated with improved sexual function from baseline and limited adverse impact on sexual function relative to placebo [228]. In a recent phase IV study [229], the efficacy, safety, and tolerability of vilazodone (20 and 40 mg/d) versus placebo were evaluated in patients with major depressive disorder; citalopram was used as an active control. Across treatment groups, baseline sexual function improved in women and men, major depressive disorder responders, and patients with baseline sexual dysfunction [229].

Finally, management strategies for antidepressant-related sexual dysfunction include a progressive reduction of dosage, drug substitution, holiday weekends and the use of antidotes [230]. Controlled and open-label studies demonstrated the efficacy of bupropion to reverse antidepressant-associated sexual dysfunction [231].

Sexual dysfunction is a frequent long-term side effect of treatment with antipsychotics [232]. A decrease in dopamine activity and D2-receptor blockade removes the inhibitory effect of dopamine on prolactin secretion, thus inducing hyperprolactinemia, which might be the main potential determining factor of antipsychotic-associated loss of libido [232]. Several antipsychotics induce hyperprolactinemia, such as haloperidol, risperidone, paliperidone, and amisulpride, and are more likely to be associated with low libido. Additionally, a meta-analysis [233] demonstrated that significant differences exist across different antipsychotics with quetiapine, ziprasidone, perphenazine, and aripiprazole being less or not related to sexual dysfunction (16–27%), while olanzapine, risperidone, haloperidol, and clozapine were associated with higher sexual dysfunction rates (40–60%).

## Treatments for Hypoactive Sexual Desire Disorder

Apart from psychological interventions discussed in the previous chapter, important treatment options for women with hypoactive sexual desire disorder consist of either the use of central nervous system agents or hormonal therapy, following the process of care [213].

### Central Nervous System Agents

*Flibanserin*, the only Food and Drug Administration (FDA) approved drug for acquired (at least to the time of writing this chapter), generalized hypoactive sexual desire disorder in premenopausal women, is a serotonin 1A receptor agonist and a serotonin 2A receptor antagonist thought to increase dopamine and norepinephrine and decrease serotonin activity in the brain. The effectiveness of the 100 mg bedtime dose of flibanserin was evaluated in three 24-week randomized, double-blind, placebo-controlled trials involving over 3500 premenopausal women (mean age 36 years) with acquired, generalized hypoactive sexual desire disorder. In these three pivital phase 3 studies (Violet, Daisy, Begonia) [234–236], flibanserin increased satisfying sexual events and sexual desire as measured by the Female Sexual Function Index, with a reduction in distress indicated by the Female Sexual Distress Scale – Revised Item 13, compared to placebo. The most commonly reported adverse effects of flibanserin treatment were drowsiness (11.8%), vertigo (10.5%), and fatigue (10.3%) [234–236], which are generally mild and transient. Bedtime dosing mitigates these adverse effects. In contrast, these risks increase when the drug is taken during the daytime, with concomitant use of cytochrome P-450 3A4 inhibitors (i.e. some antiretroviral drugs, antihypertensive drugs, antibiotics, and fluconazole, which increases systemic exposure to flibanserin by a factor of 4.5–7), and with significant alcohol use. This last interaction is based on the results of alcohol-challenge study showing an increase in sedation, syncope, and hypotension in the treatment group, although alcohol was not restricted in the three major pivotal trials, and increases in these adverse effects were not found. As a result, the FDA required a boxed warning and an alcohol contraindication, and a postapproval risk evaluation management strategy that requires health-care prescribers and pharmacies to become certified to prescribe or dispense the medication. The first of three FDA-required postmarketing alcohol studies included 96 healthy premenopausal women who were randomized to 1 of 12 sequence groups for seven treatments: flibanserin 100 mg or placebo with ethanol 0.6 g/kg, 0.4 g/kg, or 0.2 g/kg or flibanserin 100 mg only. Dizziness with flibanserin plus alcohol was 39.8%, 34.1%, and 27.4% respectively, and 31.3% with flibanserin alone. There was no effect of ethanol concentration on orthostatic blood pressure, vertigo, hypotension, or somnolence, and no syncope was observed [237].

Other central nervous system active agents, approved for indications other than hypoactive sexual desire disorder, are used off-label for the treatment of hypoactive sexual desire disorder. Bupropion, approved as an antidepressant, has demonstrated improvement in sexual desire in premenopausal women with hypoactive sexual desire disorder at doses of 300–400 mg/d [238].

Finally, in case reports and one small open label trial, trazodone, a heterocyclic antidepressant with $5\text{-}HT_{1A}$ agonist, $5\text{-}HT_{2A}$ and $\alpha_1$-adrenergic receptor antagonist properties, has been reported to increase sexual desire in postmenopausal, nondepressed women with sleep and sexual complaints [239–241].

### Hormonal Management of Hypoactive Sexual Desire Disorder (Off-Label in United States)

As previously discussed, although low levels of androgens, including total and free testosterone, androstenedione, and dehydroepiandrosterone sulfate, have been associated with low sexual desire [107, 242, 243] (no cutoff level of these serum hormones has been established to identify women with hypoactive sexual desire disorder). Moreover, evidence does not support the routine use of systemic testosterone or other androgens (for example dehydroepiandrosterone) in women suffering from conditions associated with low androgen levels (Box 6.1) [216, 244]. Accordingly, a recent meta-analysis showed that systemic dehydroepiandrosterone treatment was not effective in improving libido and sexual function in postmenopausal women with normal adrenal function [244].

In contrast, compelling evidence consistently demonstrates that high physiologic doses of testosterone therapy improve desire, arousal, vaginal blood flow, orgasm frequency, and sexual satisfaction in surgically and naturally menopausal women either alone or in combination with menopausal estrogen therapy [110, 245–247]. In 24-week phase 3 clinical trials in naturally and surgically postmenopausal women with hypoactive sexual desire disorder, the 300 µg/d testosterone patch was found to significantly improve sexual desire as measured by the Profile of Female Sexual Function and frequency of satisfying sexual events versus placebo. Level of sexually-related distress using the Personal Distress Scale also decreased but did not differ significantly from placebo. The most common adverse events in descending order were application site reactions, acne, breast pain, headache, and hirsutism. Other than blood testosterone levels, laboratory findings (liver function tests, hematology, lipid profiles, clotting measures, and carbohydrate metabolism) remained essentially unchanged from baseline and did not differ among treatment groups. The Food and Drug Administration withheld approval of the 300 µg/d testosterone patch based on concerns about long-term negative effects that were not demonstrated in clinical use in the European Union. In fact, in a 12-month randomized controlled trial of a transdermal testosterone product (150 or 300 mg/d) or placebo in 814 naturally and surgically menopausal women not taking estrogen supplementation, 300 µg/d transdermal testosterone increased and sustained the number of satisfactory sexual events and was safely administered [248]. Data regarding the safety of testosterone in long-term studies (up to four years' duration) raised no concerns [249].

When serum levels of testosterone are maintained within the normal range for premenopausal women with a variety of sexual complaints, short-term safety data are reassuring [217, 248–251]. Presence of hirsutism, androgenic alopecia, and/or acne are contradictions to testosterone therapy. No increased breast cancer risk has been observed for current or past users [252–254] of parenteral testosterone therapy.

According to the recent Endocrine Society Guideline, a 3–6-month trial of testosterone treatment is suggested in postmenopausal women suffering from hypoactive sexual desire disorder [217]. However, testosterone formulations for women are not globally available, so the use of testosterone preparations formulated for men or those formulated by pharmacies can easily lead to supraphysiological concentrations and virilization (acne, hirsutism, voice deepening, clitoromegaly, and androgenic alopecia) [217]. Therefore, if testosterone therapy is prescribed, measurement of testosterone levels is recommended at baseline and every six months thereafter to identify supraphysiologic levels.

*Tibolone*, a selective estrogen receptor modulator, appears to exert weak estrogen, progestogen and/or androgen activities [255]. One of the major metabolites of tibolone is weakly androgenic and tibolone lowers sex hormone binding globulin, resulting in an increase in endogenous free testosterone, so it has been proposed as a potential off-label treatment for hypoactive sexual desire disorder. A recent meta-analysis showed that, in symptomatic or early postmenopausal women, tibolone appeared to have no effect to a small benefit on overall sexual function versus the control. Other subpopulation analyses have suggested a moderate benefit, but when pain was considered tibolone showed no effect to a small benefit [144], not unexpected with improvements in vaginal atrophy with a selective estrogen receptor modulator. Therefore, tibolone does not appear to have an independent effect on sexual desire.

## Conclusions

Neuroendocrine function associated with excitation and inhibition of sexual desire should be fully evaluated and modifiable factors addressed. Specific treatments may improve sexual desire in women with hypoactive sexual desire disorder.

## References

1 Gangestad S, Thornhill R, Garver-Apgar CE. Women's sexual interests across the ovulatory cycle depend on primary partner developmental instability. *Proc Biol Sci.* 2005;272(1576):2023–2027.

2 Penton-Voak I, Perrett DI, Castles DL, *et al.* Menstrual cycle alters face preference. *Nature.* 1999;399(6738):741–742.

3 Gangestad S, Simpson JA, Cousins AJ, *et al.* Women's preferences for male behavioral displays change across the menstrual cycle. *Psychol Sci.* 2004;15(3):203–207.

4 Gangestad S, Thornhill R, Garver CE. Changes in women's sexual interests and their partners' mate-retention tactics across the menstrual cycle: evidence for shifting conflicts of interest. *Proc Biol Sci.* 2002;269(1494):975–982.

5 Pillsworth E, Haselton MG, Buss DM. Ovulatory shifts in female sexual desire. *J Sex Res.* 2004;41(1):55–65.

6 Michl G, Török J, Griffith SC, Sheldon BC. Experimental analysis of sperm competition mechanisms in a wild bird population. *Proc Natl Acad Sci USA.* 2002;99(8):5466–5470.

7 Limoncin E, Ciocca G, Gravina GL, *et al.* Pregnant women's preferences for men's faces differ significantly from nonpregnant women. *J Sex Med.* 2015;12(5):1142–1151.

8 Fiers T, Kaufman J. Free and Bioavailable Testosterone Calculator. 2017. http://www.issam.ch/freetesto.htm (last accessed 18 December 2017).

9 Pohl C, deRidder CM, Plant TM. Gonadal and nongonadal mechanisms contribute to the prepubertal hiatus in gonadotropin secretion in the female rhesus monkey (Macaca mulatta). *J Clin Endocrinol Metab.* 1995;80(7):2094–2101.

10 Clarke S, Dhillo WS. Kisspeptin across the human lifespan: evidence from animal studies and beyond. *J Endocrinol Invest.* 2016;229(3):R83–98.

11 Herbison A. Control of puberty onset and fertility by gonadotropin-releasing hormone neurons. *Nat Rev Endocrinol.* 2016;12(8):451–466.

12 de Roux N. GnRH receptor and GPR54 inactivation in isolated gonadotropic deficiency. *Best Pract Res Clin Endocrinol Metab.* 2006;20(4):515–528.

13 George J, Seminara SB. Kisspeptin and the hypothalamic control of reproduction: lessons from the human. *Endocrinology.* 2012;153(11):5130–5136.

14 Li X, Kinsey-Jones JS, Cheng Y, *et al.* Kisspeptin signalling in the hypothalamic arcuate nucleus regulates GnRH pulse generator frequency in the rat. *PLoS One.* 2009; 4(12):e8334.

15 Han S, McLennan T, Czieselsky K, Herbison AE. Selective optogenetic activation of arcuate kisspeptin neurons generates pulsatile luteinizing hormone secretion. *Proc Natl Acad Sci USA.* 2015;112(42):13109–13114.

16 True C, Verma S, Grove KL, Smith MS. Cocaine- and amphetamine-regulated transcript is a potent stimulator of GnRH and kisspeptin cells and may contribute to negative energy balance-induced reproductive inhibition in females. *Endocrinology.* 2013;154(8):2821–2832.

17 Frazao R, Dungan Lemko HM, *et al.* Estradiol modulates Kiss1 neuronal response to ghrelin. *Am J Physiol Endocrinol Metab.* 2014;306(6):E606–614.

18 Nestor C, Kelly MJ, Rønnekleiv OK. Cross-talk between reproduction and energy homeostasis: central impact of estrogens, leptin and kisspeptin signaling. *Horm Mol Biol Clin Investig.* 2014;17(3):109–128.

19 Saenger P, Dimartino-Nardi J. Premature adrenarche. *J Endocrinol Invest.* 2001;24(9):724–733.

20 Smith M, Jennes L. Neural signals that regulate GnRH neurones directly during the oestrous cycle. *Reproduction.* 2001;122(1):1–10.

21 Li Q, Millar RP, Clarke IJ, Smith JT. Evidence that neurokinin B controls basal gonadotropin-releasing hormone secretion but is not critical for estrogen-positive feedback in sheep. *NeuroEndocrinology.* 2015;101(2):161–174.

22 Vuong C, Van Uum SH, O'Dell LE, *et al.* The effects of opioids and opioid analogs on animal and human endocrine systems. *Endocr Rev.* 2010;31(1):98–132.

23 Krsmanovic L, Hu L, Leung PK, *et al.* Pulsatile GnRH secretion: roles of G protein-coupled receptors, second messengers and ion channels. *Mol Cell Endocrinol.* 2010;314(2):158–163.

24 Araujo-Lopes R, Crampton JR, Aquino NS, *et al.* Prolactin regulates kisspeptin neurons in the arcuate nucleus to suppress LH secretion in female rats. *Endocrinology.* 2014;155(3):1010–1020.

25 Zuloaga D, Morris JA, Jordan CL, Breedlove SM. Mice with the testicular feminization mutation demonstrate a role for androgen receptors in the regulation of anxiety-related behaviors and the hypothalamic-pituitary-adrenal axis. *Horm Behav.* 2008;54(5):758–766.

26 Bakker J, De Mees C, Douhard Q, *et al.* Alpha-fetoprotein protects the developing female mouse brain from masculinization and defeminization by estrogens. *Nat Neurosci.* 2006;9(2):220–226.

27 Puts D, Jordan CL, Breedlove SM. Defending the brain from estrogen. *Nat Neurosci.* 2006;9(2):155–156.

28 Swartz S, Soloff MS. The lack of estrogen binding by human alpha-fetoprotein. *J Clin Endocrinol Metab.* 1974;39(3):589–591.

29 Imperato-McGinley J, Peterson RE, Gautier T, *et al.* Hormonal evaluation of a large kindred with complete androgen insensitivity: evidence for secondary 5 alpha-reductase deficiency. *J Clin Endocrinol Metab.* 1982;54(5):931–941.

30 Mazur T. Gender dysphoria and gender change in androgen insensitivity or micropenis. *Arch Sex Behav.* 2005;34(4):411–421.

31 Hines M. Sex steroids and human behavior: prenatal androgen exposure and sex-typical play behavior in children. *Ann NY Acad Sci.* 2003;1007:272–282.

32 Savic I, Frisen L, Manzouri A, *et al.* Role of testosterone and Y chromosome genes for the masculinization of the human brain. *Hum Brain Mapp.* 2017;38(4):1801–1814.

33 Grumbach M, Auchus RJ. Estrogen: consequences and implications of human mutations in synthesis and action. *J Clin Endocrinol Metab.* 1999;84(12):4677–4693.

34 Reinisch J, Mortensen EL, Saunders SA. Prenatal exposure to progesterone affects

sexual orientation in humans. *Arch Sex Behav.* 2017; 46(5):1239–1249.

35  Schulz K, Sisk CL. The organizing actions of adolescent gonadal steroid hormones on brain and behavioral development. *Neurosci Biobehav Rev.* 2016;70:148–158.

36  Maas M, Lefkowitz ES Sexual Esteem in emerging adulthood: associations with sexual behavior, contraception use, and romantic relationships. *J Sex Res.* 2015;52(7):795–806.

37  Vigil P, Orellana RF, Cortés ME, *et al.* Endocrine modulation of the adolescent brain: a review. *J Pediatr Adolesc Gynecol.* 2011;24(6):330–337.

38  Paus T. Sex differences in the human brain: a developmental perspective. *Prog Brain Res.* 2010;186:13–28.

39  Goddings A, Mills KL, Clasen LS, *et al.* The influence of puberty on subcortical brain development. *Neuroimage.* 2014;88:242–251.

40  Ahmed E, Zehr JL, Schulz KM, *et al.* Pubertal hormones modulate the addition of new cells to sexually dimorphic brain regions. *Nat Neurosci.* 2008;11(9): 995–997.

41  Juraska J, Markham JA. The cellular basis for volume changes in the rat cortex during puberty: white and gray matter. *Ann NY Acad Sci.* 2004;1021:431–435.

42  Herting M, Gautam P, Spielberg JM, *et al.* The role of testosterone and estradiol in brain volume changes across adolescence: a longitudinal structural MRI study. *Hum Brain Mapp.* 2014;35(11):5633–5645.

43  Ohman A. The role of the amygdala in human fear: automatic detection of threat. Psychoneuro *Endocrinology.* 2005;30(10): 953–958.

44  Garavan H, Pendergrass JC, Ross TJ, *et al.* Amygdala response to both positively and negatively valenced stimuli. 12. 2001;12(2779–2783).

45  Everitt B, Cardinal RN, Parkinson JA, Robbins TW. Appetitive behavior: impact of amygdala-dependent mechanisms of emotional learning. *Acad Sci.* 2003;985:233–250.

46  Rupp H, James TW, Ketterson ED, *et al.* Lower sexual interest in postpartum women: relationship to amygdala activation and intranasal oxytocin. *Horm Behav.* 2013;63(1):114–121.

47  Childress A, Ehrman RN, Wang Z, *et al.* Prelude to passion: limbic activation by "unseen" drug and sexual cues. *PLoS One.* 2008;3(1):e1506.

48  Song H, Zou Z, Kou J, *et al.* Love-related changes in the brain: a resting-state functional magnetic resonance imaging study. *Front Hum Neurosci.* 2015;9:71.

49  Barth C, Steele CJ, Mueller K, *et al.* In-vivo dynamics of the human hippocampus across the menstrual cycle. *Sci Rep.* 2016;6:32833. doi: 10.1038/srep32833.

50  Protopopescu X, Butler T, Pan H, *et al.* Hippocampal structural changes across the menstrual cycle. *Hippocampus.* 2008;18:985–958.

51  Franke K, Hagemann G, Schleussner E, Gaser C. Changes of individual Brain AGE during the course of the menstrual cycle. *Neuroimage.* 2008;115.

52  Hagemann G, Ugur T, Schleussner E, *et al.* Changes in brain size during the menstrual cycle. *PLoS One.* 2011;6(2):e14655.

53  Pletzer B, Kronbichler M, Aichhorn M, *et al.* Menstrual cycle and hormonal contraceptive use modulate human brain structure. *Brain Res.* 2010;1348:55–62.

54  Balu D, Lucki I. Adult hippocampal neurogenesis: regulation, functional implications, and contribution to disease pathology. *Neurosci Biobehav Rev.* 2009;33(3):232–252.

55  Stratmann M, Konrad C, Kugel H, *et al.* Insular and hippocampal gray matter volume reductions in patients with major depressive disorder. *PLoS One.* 2014;9(7):e102692.

56  Melcangi R, Panzica GC. Neuroactive steroids: old players in a new game. *Neuroscience.* 2006;183(3):733–739.

57  Mahmoud R, Wainwright SR, Galea LA. Sex hormones and adult hippocampal neurogenesis: Regulation, implications, and

potential mechanisms. *Front Neuroendocrinol.* 2016;41:129–152.

58 Eberling J, Wu C, Tong-Turnbeaugh R, Jagust WJ. Estrogen- and tamoxifen-associated effects on brain structure and function. *Neuroimage.* 2004;21(1):364–371.

59 Elbejjani M, Fuhrer R, Abrahamowicz M, *et al.* Hippocampal atrophy and subsequent depressive symptoms in older men and women: results from a 10-year prospective cohort. *Am J Epidemiol.* 2014;180(4): 385–393.

60 Vargas K, Milic J, Zaciragic A, *et al.* The functions of estrogen receptor beta in the female brain: A systematic review. *Maturitas.* 2016;93:41–57.

61 Kim G, Jeong GW. Menopause-related brain activation patterns during visual sexual arousal in menopausal women: An fMRI pilot study using time-course analysis. *Neuroscience.* 2017;343:449–458.

62 MacLusky N, Clark AS, Naftolin F, Goldman-Rakic PS. Estrogen formation in the mammalian brain: possible role of aromatase in sexual differentiation of the hippocampus and neocortex. *Steroids.* 1987;50(4–6):459–474.

63 Goldstein J, Seidman LJ, Horton NJ, *et al.* Normal sexual dimorphism of the adult human brain assessed by in vivo magnetic resonance imaging. *Cereb Cortex.* 2001;11(6):490–497.

64 Arnow B, Desmond JE, Banner LL, *et al.* Brain activation and sexual arousal in healthy, heterosexual males. *Brain.* 2002;125:1014–1023.

65 Abler B, Kumpfmüller D, Grön G, *et al.* Neural correlates of erotic stimulation under different levels of female sexual hormones. *PLoS One.* 2013;8(2):e54447.

66 Gingnell M, Engman J, Frick A, *et al.* Oral contraceptive use changes brain activity and mood in women with previous negative affect on the pill – a double-blinded, placebo-controlled randomized trial of a levonorgestrel-containing combined oral contraceptive. *PsychoneuroEndocrinology.* 2013;38(7):1133–1144.

67 Rossetti M, Cambiasso MJ, Holschbach MA, Cabrera R. Oestrogens and progestagens: synthesis and action in the brain. *J Neuroendocrinol.* 2016;28(7). doi: 10.1111.

68 Borrow AP, Cameron NM. Estrogenic mediation of serotonergic and neurotrophic systems: implications for female mood disorders. *Prog Neuropsychopharmacol Biol Psychiatry.* 2014;54:13–25.

69 Chavez C, Hollaus M, Scarr E, *et al.* The effect of estrogen on dopamine and serotonin receptor and transporter levels in the brain: an autoradiography study. *Brain Res.* 2010;1321:51–59.

70 Alexander A, Irving AJ, Harvey J. Emerging roles for the novel estrogen-sensing receptor GPER1 in the CNS. *Neuropharmacology.* 2017;113: 652–660.

71 Melmed S, Polonsky K, Reed Larsen P, Kronenberg H. Williams Textbook of Endocrinology. Elsevier; 2016.

72 Barth C, Villringer A, Sacher J. Sex hormones affect neurotransmitters and shape the adult female brain during hormonal transition periods. *Front Neurosci.* 2015;9:37.

73 Bäckström T, Bixo M, Johansson M, *et al.* Allopregnanolone and mood disorders. *Prog Neurobiol.* 2014;113:88–94.

74 Ekholm U, Turkmen S, Hammarbäck S, Bäckström T. Sexuality and androgens in women with cyclical mood changes and pre-menstrual syndrome. *Acta Obstet Gynecol Scand.* 2014;93(3):248–255.

75 Sánchez M, Bourque M, Morissette M, Di Paolo T. Steroids-dopamine interactions in the pathophysiology and treatment of CNS disorders. *CNS Neurosci Ther.* 2010; 16(3):e43–71.

76 Jacobs E, D'Esposito M. Estrogen shapes dopamine-dependent cognitive processes: implications for women's health. *J Neurosci.* 2011;31(14):5286–5293.

77 Uban K, Rummel J, Floresco SB, Galea LA. Estradiol modulates effort-based decision making in female rats.

*Neuropsychopharmacology.* 2012;37(2):390–401.

78 Rey C, Lipps J, Shansky RM. Dopamine D1 receptor activation rescues extinction impairments in low-estrogen female rats and induces cortical layer-specific activation changes in prefrontal-amygdala circuits. *Neuropsychopharmacology.* 2014;39(5):1282–1289.

79 Young E, Becker JB. Perspective: sex matters: gonadal steroids and the brain. *Neuropsychopharmacology.* 2009;34(3):537–538.

80 Quinlan M, Almey A, Caissie M, *et al.* Estradiol and striatal dopamine receptor antagonism influence memory system bias in the female rat. *Neurobiol Learn Mem.* 2013;106:221–229.

81 Bethea C, Reddy AP, Tokuyama Y, *et al.* Protective actions of ovarian hormones in the serotonin system of macaques. *Front Neuroendocrinol.* 2009;30(2):212–238.

82 Lanzenberger R, Mitterhauser M, Kranz GS, *et al.* Progesterone level predicts serotonin-1a receptor binding in the male human brain. *Neuro Endocrinology.* 2011;94(1):84–88.

83 Frye C, Rhodes ME, Petralia SM, *et al.* 3alpha-hydroxy-5alpha-pregnan-20-one in the midbrain ventral tegmental area mediates social, sexual, and affective behaviors. *Neuroscience.* 2006;138(3):1007–1014.

84 Benmansour S, Weaver RS, Barton AK, *et al.* Comparison of the effects of estradiol and progesterone on serotonergic function. *Biol Psychiatry.* 2012;71(7):633–641.

85 Gressier F, Verstuyft C, Hardy P, *et al.* Menopausal status could modulate the association between 5-HTTLPR and antidepressant efficacy in depressed women: a pilot study. *Arch Womens Ment Health.* 2014;17(6):569–573.

86 Pinto-Meza A, Usall J, Serrano-Blanco A, *et al.* Gender differences in response to antidepressant treatment prescribed in primary care. Does menopause make a difference? *J Affect Disord.* 2006;93(1–3):53–60.

87 Sramek J, Murphy MF, Cutler NR. Sex differences in the psychopharmacological treatment of depression. *Dialogues Clin Neurosci.* 2016;18(4):447–457.

88 Asberg M, Thoren P, Traskman L, *et al.* "Serotonin depression" a biochemical subgroup within the affective disorders? *Science.* 1976;191:478–480.

89 Gordon N, Goelman G. Understanding alterations in serotonin connectivity in a rat model of depression within the monoamine-deficiency and the hippocampal-neurogenesis frameworks. *Behav Brain Res.* 2016;296:141–148.

90 Clayton A, El Haddad, S, Iluonakhamhe, J, *et al.* Sexual dysfunction associated with major depressive disorder and antidepressant treatment. *Expert Opin Drug Saf.* 2014;13(10):1361–1374.

91 Schreiner-Engel P, Schiavi RC, Smith H, White D. Sexual arousability and the menstrual cycle. *Psychosom Med.* 1981;43(3):199–214.

92 Bancroft J, Sanders D, Davidson D, Warner P. Mood, sexuality, hormones, and the menstrual cycle. III. Sexuality and the role of androgens. *Psychosom Med.* 1983;45(6): 509–516.

93 Mhillaj E, Morgese MG, Tucci P, *et al.* Effects of anabolic-androgens on brain reward function. *Front Neurosci.* 2015;9:295.

94 Braams B, Peper JS, van der Heide D, *et al.* Nucleus accumbens response to rewards and testosterone levels are related to alcohol use in adolescents and young adults. *Dev Cogn Neurosci.* 2016;17:83–93.

95 Arnedo M, Salvador A, Martínez-Sanchís S, Pellicer O. Similar rewarding effects of testosterone in mice rated as short and long attack latency individuals. *Addict Biol.* 2002;7(4):373–379.

96 Huang E, Chen YH, Huang TY, *et al.* Chronic administration of nandrolone increases susceptibility to morphine dependence without correlation with LVV-hemorphin 7 in rats. *Neuropeptides.* 2016;59:63–69.

97 Frye C. The role of neurosteroids and non-genomic effects of progestins and androgens in mediating sexual receptivity of rodents. *Brain Res Brain Res Rev.* 2001;37(1–3):201–222.

98 Clark A, Lindenfeld RC, Gibbons CH. Anabolic-androgenic steroids and brain reward. *Pharmacol Biochem Behav.* 1996;53(3):741–745.

99 Schroeder J, Packard MG. Role of dopamine receptor subtypes in the acquisition of a testosterone conditioned place preference in rats. *Neurosci Lett.* 2000;282(1–2):17–20.

100 Suschinsky K, Bossio JA, Chivers ML. Women's genital sexual arousal to oral versus penetrative heterosexual sex varies with menstrual cycle phase at first exposure. *Horm Behav.* 2014;65(3): 319–327.

101 Gueguen N. The receptivity of women to courtship solicitation across the menstrual cycle: a field experiment. *Biol Psychol.* 2009;80(3):321–324.

102 Guillermo C, Manlove HA, Gray PB, *et al.* Female social and sexual interest across the menstrual cycle: the roles of pain, sleep and hormones. *BMC Womens Health.* 2010;10:19.

103 Alder E, Cook A, Davidson D, *et al.* Hormones, mood and sexuality in lactating women. *Br J Psychiatry.* 1986;148:74.

104 Appelt H, Strauss B. The psychoen-docrinology of female sexuality. *A research project. German J Psychol.* 1986;10:143.

105 Davis SR, Davison SL, Donath S, Bell RJ. Circulating androgen levels and self-reported sexual function in women. *JAMA.* 2005;294(1):91–96.

106 Wahlin-Jacobsen S, Pedersen AT, Kristensen E, *et al.* Is there a correlation between androgens and sexual desire in women? *J Sex Med.* 2015;12:358–373.

107 Randolph J, Jr., Zheng H, Avis NE, *et al.* Masturbation frequency and sexual function domains are associated with serum reproductive hormone levels across the menopausal transition. *J Clin Endocrinol Metab.* 2015;100:258–266.

108 Sherwin B, Gelfand MM, Brender W. Androgen enhances sexual motivation in females: a prospective, crossover study of sex steroid administration in the surgical menopause. *Psychosom Med.* 1985;47(4):339–351.

109 Sherwin B, Gelfand MM. The role of androgen in the maintenance of sexual functioning in oophorectomized women. *Psychosom Med.* 1987;49(4):397–409.

110 Buster J, Kingsberg SA, Aguirre O, *et al.* Testosterone patch for low sexual desire in surgically menopausal women: a randomized trial. *Obstet Gynecol.* 2005;105(5):944–952.

111 Archer J, Love-Geffen TE, Herbst-Damm KL, *et al.* Effect of estradiol versus estradiol and testosterone on brain-activation patterns in postmenopausal women. *Menopause.* 2006;13:528–537.

112 Davis S, Goldstat R, Papalia MA, *et al.* Effects of aromatase inhibition on sexual function and wellbeing in postmenopausal women treated with testosterone: a randomized placebo controlled trial. *Menopause.* 2006;13:37–45.

113 Davison S, Bell R, Donath S, *et al.* Androgen levels in adult females: changes with age, menopause, and oophorectomy. *J Clin Endocrinol Metab.* 2005;90(7):3847–3853.

114 Haring R, Hannemann A, John U, *et al.* Age-specific reference ranges for serum testosterone and androstenedione concentrations in women measured by liquid chromatography tandem mass spectrometry. *J Clin Endocrinol Metab.* 2012;97(2):408–415.

115 Pinilla L, Aguilar E, Dieguez C, *et al.* Kisspeptins and reproduction: physiological roles and regulatory mechanisms. *Physiol Rev.* 2012;92(3):1235–1316.

116 Comninos A, Wall MB, Demetriou L, *et al.* Kisspeptin modulates sexual and emotional brain processing in humans. *J Clin Invest.* 2017;127(2):709–719.

117 Feldman R. The neurobiology of human attachments. *Trends Cogn Sci.* 2017;21(2):80–99.

118 Kavaliers M, Matta R, Choleris E. Mate-choice copying, social information processing, and the roles of oxytocin. *Neurosci Biobehav Rev.* 2017;72:232–242.

119 Acevedo-Rodriguez. A MS, Handa RJ. Oxytocin and estrogen receptor β in the brain: an overview. *Front Endocrinol (Lausanne).* 2015;6:160.

120 Muin D, Wolzt M, Marculescu R, *et al.* Effect of long-term intranasal oxytocin on sexual dysfunction in premenopausal and postmenopausal women: a randomized trial. *Fertil Steril.* 2015;104(3):715–723.

121 Bancroft J. The Endocrinology of sexual arousal. *J Endocrinol Invest.* 2005;186(3):411–427.

122 Maggi M, Buvat J, Corona G, *et al.* Hormonal causes of male sexual dysfunctions and their management. *J Sex Med.* 2013;10(3):661–677.

123 Bauer M, Heinz A, Whybrow PC. Thyroid hormones, serotonin and mood: of synergy and significance in the adult brain. *Mol Psychiatry.* 2002;7(2):140–156.

124 Campos-Barros A, Hoell T, Musa A, *et al.* Phenolic and tyrosyl ring iodothyronine deiodination and thyroid hormone concentrations in the human central nervous system. *J Clin Endocrinol Metab.* 1996;81:2179–2185.

125 Gressier F, Trabado S, Verstuyft C, *et al.* Thyroid-stimulating hormone, 5-HTTLPR genotype, and antidepressant response in depressed women. *Psychiatr Genet.* 2011;21(5):253–256.

126 Cleare A, McGregor A, Chambers SM, *et al.* Thyroxine replacement increases central 5-hydroxytryptamine activity and reduces depressive symptoms in hypothyroidism. *NeuroEndocrinology.* 1996;64:65–69.

127 Cleare A, McGregor A, O'Keane V. Neuroendocrine evidence for an association between hypothyroidism, reduced central 5-HT activity and depression. *Clin Endocrinol (Oxf).* 1995;43:713–719.

128 Lifschytz T, Segman R, Shalom G, *et al.* Basic mechanisms of augmentation of antidepressant effects with thyroid hormone. *Curr Drug Targets.* 2006;7(2):203–210.

129 Rosner W, Aden DP, Khan MS. Hormonal influences on the secretion of steroid-binding proteins by a human hepatoma-derived cell line. *J Clin Endocrinol Metab.* 1984;59:806–808.

130 Jänne M, Deol HK, Power SGA, *et al.* Human sex hormone-binding globulin gene expression in transgenic mice. *Molecular Endocrinology.* 1998;12:123–136.

131 Selva D, Hammond GL. Thyroid hormones act indirectly to increase sex hormone-binding globulin production by liver via hepatocyte nuclear factor-4alpha. *J Mol Endocrinol.* 2009;43(1):19–27.

132 Maseroli E, Fanni E, Cipriani S, *et al.* Cardiometabolic risk and female sexuality: focus on clitoral vascular resistance. *J Sex Med.* 2016;13(11):1651–1661.

133 Both S, Ter Kuile M, Enzlin P, *et al.* Sexual response in women with type 1 diabetes mellitus: a controlled laboratory study measuring vaginal blood flow and subjective sexual arousal. *Arch Sex Behav.* 2015;44(6):1573–1587.

134 Chalas E. Ovaries, estrogen, and longevity. *Obstet Gynecol.* 2013;121:701–702.

135 Graziottin A, Koochaki PE, Rodenberg CA, Dennerstein L. The prevalence of hypoactive sexual desire disorder in surgically menopausal women: an epidemiological study of women in four European countries. *J Sex Med.* 2009;6(8):2143–2153.

136 Kokcu A, Kurtoglu E, Bildircin D, et al. Does surgical menopause affect sexual performance differently from natural menopause? *J Sex Med* 2015;12: 1407–1414.

137 Dennerstein L, Koochaki P, Barton I, *et al.* Hypoactive sexual desire disorder in menopausal women: a survey of Western European women. *J Sex Med.* 2006;3(2):212–222.

138 Laughlin G, Barrett-Connor E, Kritz-Silverstein D, von Mühlen D. Hysterectomy, oophorectomy, and endogenous sex hormone levels in older women: the Rancho Bernardo Study. *J Clin Endocrinol Metab.* 2000;85: 645–651.

139 Couzinet B, Meduri G, Lecce MG, *et al.* The postmenopausal ovary is not a major androgen-producing gland. *JCEM.* 2001;86:5080–5086.

140 Fogle R, Stanczyk FZ, Zhang X, Paulson RJ. Ovarian androgen production in postmenopausal women. *JCEM.* 2007;92:3040–3043.

141 Labrie F, Martel C, Balser J. Wide distribution of the serum dehydroepiandrosterone and sex steroid levels in postmenopausal women: role of the ovary? *Menopause.* 2011;18(1): 30–43.

142 Rodriguez M, Shoupe D. Surgical menopause. *Endocrinol Metab Clin North Am.* 2015;44:531–542.

143 Tucker P, Bulsara MK, Salfinger SG, *et al.* The effects of pre-operative menopausal status and hormone replacement therapy (HRT) on sexuality and quality of life after risk-reducing salpingo-oophorectomy. *Maturitas.* 2016;85:42–48.

144 Nastri C, Lara LA, Ferriani RA, *et al.* Hormone therapy for sexual function in perimenopausal and postmenopausal women. *Cochrane Database Syst Rev.* 2013;Jun 5(6):CD009672.

145 Nathorst-Böös J, von Schoultz B, Carlström K. Elective ovarian removal and estrogen replacement therapy- effects on sexual life, psychological well-being and androgen status. *J Psychosom Obstet Gynaecol.* 1993;14:283–293.

146 Fang C, Cherry C, Devarajan K, *et al.* A prospective study of quality of life among women undergoing risk-reducing salpingo-oophorectomy versus gynecologic screening for ovarian cancer. *Gynecol Oncol.* 2009;112:594–600.

147 Davis S, Worsley R, Miller KK, *et al.* Androgens and female sexual function and dysfunction findings from the Fourth International Consultation of Sexual Medicine. *J Sex Med.* 2016;13(2): 168–178.

148 Janse F, Tanahatoe SJ, Eijkemans MJ, Fauser BC. Testosterone concentrations, using different assays, in different types of ovarian insufficiency: a systematic review and meta-analysis. *Hum Reprod Update.* 2012;18:405–419.

149 van der Stege J, Groen H, van Zadelhoff SJ, *et al.* Decreased androgen concentrations and diminished general and sexual well-being in women with premature ovarian failure. *Menopause.* 2008;15:23–31.

150 Gravholt C, Svenstrup B, Bennett P, Sandahl Christiansen J. Reduced androgen levels in adult turner syndrome: influence of female sex steroids and growth hormone status. *Clin Endocrinol (Oxf).* 1999;50:791–800.

151 Gravholt C, Hjerrild BE, Mosekilde L, *et al.* Body composition is distinctly altered in Turner syndrome: relations to glucose metabolism, circulating adipokines, and endothelial adhesion molecules. *Eur J Endocrinol.* 2006;155:583–592.

152 Bou Khalil R, Souaiby L, Farès N. The importance of the hypothalamo-pituitary-adrenal axis as a therapeutic target in anorexia nervosa. *Physiol Behav.* 2017;15(171):13–20.

153 Castellini G, Lelli L, Ricca V, Maggi M. Sexuality in eating disorders patients: etiological factors, sexual dysfunction and identity issues. A systematic review. *Horm Mol Biol Clin Investig.* 2016;25(2):71–90.

154 Miller K, Sesmilo G, Schiller A, *et al.* Androgen deficiency in women with hypopituitarism. *J Clin Endocrinol Metab.* 2001;86:561–567.

155 Lundberg P, Hulter B. Sexual dysfunction in patients with hypothalamo-pituitary

disorders. *Exp Clin Endocrinol.* 1991;98(2):81–88.

156 Kadioglu P, Yalin AS, Tiryakioglu O, *et al.* Sexual dysfunction in women with hyperprolactinemia: a pilot study report. *J Urol.* 2005;174(5):1921–1925.

157 Krysiak R, Drosdzol-Cop A, Skrzypulec-Plinta V, Okopien B. Sexual function and depressive symptoms in young women with elevated macroprolactin content: a pilot study. *Endocrine.* 2016;53(1): 291–298.

158 Atis G, Dalkilinc A, Altuntas Y, *et al.* Sexual dysfunction in women with clinical hypothyroidism and subclinical hypothyroidism. *J Sex Med.* 2010;7:2583–2590.

159 Veronelli A, Mauri C, Zecchini B, *et al.* Sexual dysfunction is frequent in premenopausal women with diabetes, obesity, and hypothyroidism, and correlates with markers of increased cardiovascular risk. A preliminary report. *J Sex Med.* 2009;6(6):1561–1568.

160 Pasquali D, Maiorino MI, Renzullo A, *et al.* Female sexual dysfunction in women with thyroid disorders. *J Endocrinol Invest* 2013;36(6):729–733.

161 Krysiak R, Drosdzol-Cop A, Skrzypulec-Plinta V, Okopien B. Sexual function and depressive symptoms in young women with thyroid autoimmunity and subclinical hypothyroidism. *Clin Endocrinol* 2016;84(6):925–931.

162 Atis G, Dalkilinc A, Altuntas Y, *et al.* Hyperthyroidism: a risk factor for female sexual dysfunction. *J Sex Med.* 2011;8:2327–2333.

163 Jacobson A, Braffett BH, Cleary PA, *et al.* Relationship of urologic complications with health-related quality of life and perceived value of health in men and women with type 1 diabetes: the Diabetes Control and Complications/Epidemiology of Diabetes Interventions and Complications cohort. *Diabetes Care.* 2015;38:1904–12.

164 Pontiroli A, Cortelazzi D, Morabito A. Female sexual dysfunction and diabetes: a systematic review and meta-analysis. *J Sex Med.* 2013;10(4):1044–1051.

165 Enzlin P, Mathieu C, Van Den Bruel A, *et al.* Prevalence and predictors of sexual dysfunction in patients with type 1 diabetes. *Diabetes Care.* 2003;26(2):409–414.

166 Wincze J, Albert A, Bansal S. Sexual arousal in diabetic females: physiological and self-report measures. *Arch Sex Behav.* 1993;22:587–601.

167 Erol B, Tefekli A, Sanli O, *et al.* Does sexual dysfunction correlate with deterioration of somatic sensory system in diabetic women? *Int J Impot Res.* 2003;15:198–202.

168 Baldassarre M, Alvisi S, Berra M, *et al.* Changes in vaginal physiology of menopausal women with type 2 diabetes. *J Sex Med.* 2015;12(6):1346–1355.

169 Trompeter S, Bettencourt R, Barrett-Connor E. Metabolic syndrome and sexual function in postmenopausal women. *Am J Med.* 2016;129(12):1270–1277.

170 Esposito K, Ciotola M, Marfella R, *et al.* The metabolic syndrome: a cause of sexual dysfunction in women. *Int J Impot Res.* 2005;17(3):224–226.

171 Martelli V, Valisella S, Moscatiello S, *et al.* Prevalence of sexual dysfunction among postmenopausal women with and without metabolic syndrome. *J Sex Med.* 2012;9:434–441.

172 Politano CA, Valadares AL, Pinto-Neto A, Costa-Paiva L. The metabolic syndrome and sexual function in climacteric women: a cross-sectional study. *J Sex Med.* 2015;12(2):455–462.

173 Bajos N, Wellings K, Laborde C, *et al.* Sexuality and obesity, a gender perspective: results from French national random probability survey of sexual behaviour. *BMJ.* 2010;340:c2573.

174 Nackers L, Appelhans BM, Segawa E, *et al.* Associations between body mass index and sexual functioning in midlife women: the Study of Women's Health Across the Nation. *Menopause.* 2015;22(11):1175–1181.

175 Kolotkin R, Binks M, Crosby RD, *et al.* Obesity and sexual quality of life. *Obesity.* 2006;14(3):472–479.

176 Esposito K, Ciotola M, Giugliano F, *et al.* Association of body weight with sexual function in women. *Int J Impot Res.* 2007;19(4):353–357.

177 Castellini G, Mannucci E, Mazzei C, *et al.* Sexual function in obese women with and without binge eating disorder. *J Sex Med.* 2010;7(12):3969–3978.

178 Kinzl J, Trefalt E, Fiala M, *et al.* Partnership, sexuality and sexual disorders in morbidly obese women: consequences of weight loss after gastric banding. *Obes Surg.* 2001;11:455–458.

179 Sysko R, Devlin MJ, Walsh BT, *et al.* Satiety and test meal intake among women with binge eating disorder. *Int J Eat Disord.* 2007;40:554–561.

180 Borges R, Temido P, Sousa L, *et al.* Metabolic syndrome and sexual (dys) function. *J Sex Med.* 2009;6:2958–2975.

181 Bond D, Wing RR, Vithiananthan S, *et al.* Significant resolution of female sexual dysfunction after bariatric surgery. *Surg Obes Rel Dis.* 2011;7(1):1–7.

182 Kolotkin R, Binks M, Crosby RD, *et al.* Improvements in sexual quality of life after moderate weight loss. *Int J Impot Res.* 2008;20:487–492.

183 Wing R, Bond DS, Gendrano IN, *et al.* Effect of intensive lifestyle intervention on sexual dysfunction in women with type 2 diabetes: results from an ancillary Look AHEAD study. *Diabetes Care.* 2013;36:2937–2944.

184 Clayton A, Maserejian NN, Connor MK, *et al.* Depression in premenopausal women with HSDD: baseline findings from the HSDD Registry for Women. *Psychosom Med.* 2012;74(3):305–311.

185 Lorenz T, Rullo J, Faubion S. Antidepressant-Induced female sexual dysfunction. *Mayo Clin Proc.* 2016;91(9):1280–1286.

186 Clayton A, Alkis AR, Parikh NB, Votta JG. Sexual dysfunction due to psychotropic medications. *Psychiatr Clin North Am.* 2016;39(3):427–463.

187 Atlantis E, Sullivan T. Bidirectional association between depression and sexual dysfunction: a systematic review and meta-analysis. *J Sex Med.* 2012;9(6):1497–1507.

188 Markland A, Richter HE, Fwu CW, *et al.* Prevalence and trends of urinary incontinence in adults in the United States, 2001 to 2008. *J Urol.* 2011;186(2):589–593.

189 Zhu L, Cheng X, Sun J, *et al.* Association between Menopausal symptoms and overactive bladder: a cross-sectional questionnaire survey in China. *PLoS One.* 2015;10(10):e0139599.

190 Salonia A, Zanni G, Nappi RE, *et al.* Sexual dysfunction is common in women with lower urinary tract symptoms and urinary incontinence: results of a cross-sectional study. *Eur Urol.* 2004;45(5):642–648.

191 Patel V, Weiss HA, Kirkwood BR, *et al.* Common genital complaints in women: the contribution of psychosocial and infectious factors in a population-based cohort study in Goa, *India. Int J Epidemiol.* 2006;35(6):1478–1485.

192 Smith A. Female urinary incontinence and wellbeing: results from a multi-national survey. *BMC Urol.* 2016;16(1):22–28.

193 Nishizawa O. How serotonin is related with lower urinary dysfunction. *Adv Ther.* 2015;32(Suppl 1):1–2.

194 Matsumoto-Miyai K, Yoshizumi M, Kawatani M. Regulatory effects of 5-hydroxytryptamine receptors on voiding function. *Adv Ther.* 2015;32(Suppl 1):3–15.

195 Mitsui T, Kanno Y, Kitta T, *et al.* Supraspinal projection of serotonergic and noradrenergic pathways modulates nociceptive transmission in the lower urinary tract of rats. *Low Urin Tract Symptoms.* 2016;8(3):186–190.

196 Wood L, Anger JT. Urinary incontinence in women. *Br Med J.* 2014;349: g4531–4537.

197 Mohammadi K, Rahnama P, Mohseni SM, *et al*. Determinants of sexual dysfunction in women with multiple sclerosis. *BMC Neurol*. 2013;13(13):83–89.

198 Hajiaghababaei M, Javidan AN, Saberi H, *et al*. Female sexual dysfunction in patients with spinal cord injury: a study from Iran. *Spinal Cord*. 2014;52:646–649.

199 Melmed S, Casanueva FF, Hoffman AR, *et al*. Diagnosis and treatment of hyperprolactinemia: an Endocrine Society clinical practice guideline. *J Clin Endocrinol Metab*. 2011;96(2):273–288.

200 Pastor Z, Holla, K, Chmel, R. The influence of combined oral contraceptives on female sexual desire: a systematic review. *Eur J Contracept Reprod Health Care*. 2013;18(1):27–43.

201 Lopez L, Grey TW, Chen M, *et al*. Theory-based interventions for contraception. *Cochrane Database Syst Rev*. 2016;23(11):CD007249.

202 Zimmerman Y, Eijkemans MJ, Coelingh Bennink HJ, *et al*. The effect of combined oral contraception on testosterone levels in healthy women: a systematic review and meta-analysis. *Hum Reprod Update*. 2014;20(1):76–105.

203 Zethraeus N, Dreber A, Ranehill E, *et al*. Combined oral contraceptives and sexual function in women – a double-blind, randomized, placebo-controlled trial. *J Clin Endocrinol Metab*. 2016;101(11):4046–4053.

204 van Zuuren E, Fedorowicz Z. Interventions for hirsutism excluding laser and photoepilation therapy alone: abridged Cochrane systematic review including GRADE assessments. *Br J Dermatol*. 2016;175(1):45–61.

205 Grover S, Mattoo SK, Pendharkar S, Kandappan V. Sexual dysfunction in patients with alcohol and opioid dependence. *Indian J Psychol Med*. 2014;36(4):355–365.

206 Association American Psychiatric Association. Psychiatric Association agnostic and Statistical Manual of Mental Disorders IV, Text Revision (DSM-IV-TR). Washington, DC: American Psychiatric Association; 2003.

207 Clayton A, Goldfischer ER, Goldstein I, *et al*. Validation of the decreased sexual desire screener (DSDS): A brief diagnostic instrument for generalized acquired female hypoactive sexual desire disorder (HSDD). *J Sex Med*. 2009;6:730–738.

208 Wiegel M, Meston C, Rosen R. The female sexual function index (FSFI): cross-validation and development of clinical cutoff scores. *J Sex Marit Ther*. 2005;31:1–20.

209 Derogatis L, Clayton A, Lewis-D'Agostino D, *et al*. Validation of the female sexual distress scale-revised for assessing distress in women with hypoactive sexual desire disorder. *J Sex Med*. 2008;5(2):357–364.

210 Siu AL, US Preventive Services Task Force (USPSTF), Bibbins-Domingo K, *et al*. Screening for depression in adults: US Preventive Services Task Force recommendation statement. *JAMA*. 2016;315(4):380–387.

211 Roberts C, Ladenson PW. *Hypothyroidism. Lancet*. 2004;363(9411):793–803.

212 Cooper D. *Hyperthyroidism. Lancet*. 2003; 362(9382):459–468.

213 Clayton AH, Goldstein I, Kim NN, *et al*. The International Society for the Study of Women's Sexual Health Process of Care for Management of Hypoactive Sexual Desire Disorder in Women. Mayo Clinic Proceedings. doi: https://doi.org/10.1016/j.mayocp.2017.11.002.

214 De Leo S, Lee SY, Braverman LE. *Hyperthyroidis. Lancet*. 2016; 388(19947):906–918.

215 Arlt W, Callies F, van Vlijmen JC, *et al*. Dehydroepiandrosterone replacement in women with adrenal insufficiency. *N Engl J Med*. 1999;341:1013–1020.

216 Alkatib A, Cosma, M, Elamin, MB, *et al*. A systematic review and meta-analysis of randomized placebo-controlled trials of DHEA treatment effects on quality of life in women with adrenal insufficiency.

*J Clin Endocrinol Metab.* 2009;94(10): 3676–3681.

217 Wierman M, Arlt, W, Basson, R, *et al.* Androgen therapy in women: a reappraisal: an endocrine society clinical practice guideline. *J Clin Endocrinol Metab.* 2014;99:2489–3510.

218 Abler B, Seeringer A, Hartmann A, *et al.* Neural correlates of antidepressant-related sexual dysfunction: a placebo-controlled fMRI study on healthy males under subchronic paroxetine and bupropion. *Neuropsychopharmacology.* 2011;36:1837–1847.

219 Patel K, Allen S, Haque MN, *et al.* Bupropion: a systematic review and meta-analysis of effectiveness as an antidepressant. *Ther Adv Psychopharmacol.* 2016;6(2):99–144.

220 Taylor D, Sparshatt A, Varma S, Olofinjana O. Antidepressant efficacy of agomelatine: meta-analysis of published and unpublished studies. *Br Med J.* 2014;348:g1888–1907.

221 Montejo A, Majadas S, Rizvi SJ, Kennedy SH. The effects of agomelatine on sexual function in depressed patients and healthy volunteers. *Hum Psychopharmacol.* 2011;26(8):537–542.

222 Clayton A, Reddy S, Focht K, *et al.* An evaluation of sexual functioning in employed outpatients with major depressive disorder treated with desvenlafaxine 50 mg or placebo. *J Sex Med.* 2013;10:768–776.

223 Clayton A, Hwang E, Kornstein SG, *et al.* Effects of 50 and 100 mg desvenlafaxine versus placebo on sexual function in patients with major depressive disorder: a meta-analysis. *Int Clin Psychopharmacol.* 2015;30(6):307–315.

224 Sanchez C, Asin KE, Artigas F. Vortioxetine, a novel antidepressant with multimodal activity: Review of preclinical and clinical data. *Pharmacol Ther.* 2015;145:43–57.

225 Alvarez E, Perez V, Artigas F. Pharmacology and clinical potential of vortioxetine in the treatment of major depressive disorder. *Neuropsychiatr Dis Treat.* 2014;10:1297–1307.

226 Mahableshwarkar A, Jacobsen PL, Serenko M, *et al.* A randomized, double-blind, placebo-controlled study of the efficacy and safety of 2 doses of vortioxetine in adults with major depressive disorder. *J Clin Psychiatry.* 2015;76:583–591.

227 Jacobsen P, Mahableshwarkar AR, Chen Y, *et al.* Effect of vortioxetine vs. escitalopram on sexual functioning in adults with well-treated major depressive disorder experiencing SSRI-induced sexual dysfunction. *J Sex Med.* 2015;12(10):2036–2048.

228 Clayton A, Kennedy SH, Edwards JB, *et al.* The effect of vilazodone on sexual function during the treatment of major depressive disorder. *J Sex Med.* 2013;10(10):2465–2476.

229 Clayton A, Gommoll C, Chen D, *et al.* Sexual dysfunction during treatment of major depressive disorder with vilazodone, citalopram, or placebo: results from a phase IV clinical trial. *Int Clin Psychopharmacol.* 2015;30(4):216–223.

230 Keks N, Hope J, Culhane C. Management of antidepressant-induced sexual dysfunction. *Australas Psychiatry.* 2014;22:525–528.

231 Zisook S, Rush AJ, Haight BR, *et al.* Use of bupropion in combination with serotonin reuptake inhibitors. *Biol Psychiatry.* 2006;59:203–210.

232 González-Blanco L, Greenhalgh AM, Garcia-Rizo C, *et al.* Prolactin concentrations in antipsychotic-naïve patients with schizophrenia and related disorders: A meta-analysis. *Schizophr Res.* 2016;174(1–3):156–160.

233 Serretti A, Chiesa A. A meta-analysis of sexual dysfunction in psychiatric patients taking antipsychotics. *Int Clin Psychopharmacol.* 2011;26(3): 130–140.

234 Derogatis L, Komer L, Katz M, *et al.* Treatment of hypoactive sexual desire disorder in premenopausal women: efficacy of flibanserin in the VIOLET Study. *J Sex Med.* 2012;9(4):1074–1085.

235 Thorp J, Simon J, Dattani D, *et al.* Treatment of hypoactive sexual desire disorder in premenopausal women: efficacy of flibanserin in the DAISY study. *J Sex Med.* 2012;9(3):793–804.

236 Katz M, DeRogatis, LR, Ackerman, R, *et al.* Efficacy of flibanserin in women with hypoactive sexual desire disorder: results from the BEGONIA trial. *J Sex Med.* 2013;10:1807–1815.

237 Sicard E, Raimondo D, Vittitow J, *et al.* Effect of alcohol administered with flibanserin on dizziness, syncope, and hypotension in healthy premenopausal women. 23rd Congress of the World Association for Sexual Health; Prague, 2017.

238 Segraves R, Clayton, A, Croft, H, *et al.* Bupropion sustained release for the treatment of hypoactive sexual desire disorder in premenopausal women. *J Clin Psychopharmacol.* 2004;24:339–342.

239 Eraslan D, Ertekin E, Ertekin BA, Oztürk O. Treatment of insomnia with hypnotics resulting in improved sexual functioning in post-menopausal women. *Psychiatr Danub.* 2014;26(4):353–357.

240 Medina C. Clitoral priapism: a rare condition presenting as a cause of vulvar pain. *Obstet Gynecol.* 2002;100:1089–1091.

241 Michael A, O'Donnell EA. Fluoxetine-induced sexual dysfunction reversed by trazodone. *Can J Psychiatry.* 2000;45:847–848.

242 Davis S, Davison SL, Donath S, Bell RJ. Circulating androgen levels and self-reported sexual function in women. *JAMA.* 2005;294:91–96.

243 Wahlin-Jacobsen S, Pedersen AT, Kristensen E, *et al.* Is there a correlation between androgens and sexual desire in women? *J Sex Med.* 2014. Epub

2014/12/06. doi: 10.1111/jsm.12774. PubMed PMID: 25475395.

244 Elraiyah T, Sonbol, MB, Wang, Z, *et al.* Clinical review: The benefits and harms of systemic dehydroepiandrosterone (DHEA) in postmenopausal women with normal adrenal function: a systematic review and meta-analysis. *J Clin Endocrinol Metab.* 2014; 99(10):3536–3542.

245 Simon J, Braunstein G, Nachtigall L, *et al.* Testosterone patch increases sexual activity and desire in surgically menopausal women with hypoactive sexual desire disorder. *J Clin Endocrinol Metab.* 2005;90(9):5226–5233.

246 Braunstein G, Sundwall DA, Katz M, *et al.* Safety and efficacy of a testosterone patch for the treatment of hypoactive sexual desire disorder in surgically menopausal women. *Arch Intern Med.* 2005;165:1582–1589.

247 Shifren J, Davis S, Moreau M, *et al.* Testosterone patch for the treatment of hypoactive sexual desire disorder in naturally menopausal women: Results from the INTIMATE NM1 Study. *Menopause.* 2006;13(5):770–779.

248 Davis S, Moreau, M, Kroll, R, *et al.* Testosterone for low libido in menopausal women not taking estrogen therapy. *N Eng J Med.* 2008;359:2005–2017.

249 Nachtigall L, Casson P, Lucas J, *et al.* Safety and tolerabililty of testosterone patch therapy for up to 4 years in surgically menopausal women receiving oral or transdermal oestrogen. *Gynecol Endocrinol.* 2011;27(1):39–48.

250 Davis S, Hirschberg, AL, Wagner, LK, *et al.* The effect of transdermal testosterone on mammographic density in postmenopausal women not receiving systemic estrogen therapy. *J Clin Endocrinol Metab.* 2009;94:4907–4913.

251 Davis S. Cardiovascular and cancer safety of testosterone in women. *Curr Opin Endocrinol Diabetes Obe.* 2011;18:198–203.

252 Dimitrakakis C, Jones, R, Liu, A, *et al.* Breast cancer incidence in postmenopausal women using testosterone in addition to usual hormone therapy. *Menopause.* 2004;11(5):531–535.

253 Davis S, Wolfe R, Farrugia H, *et al.* The incidence of invasive breast cancer among women prescribed testosterone for low libido. *J Sex Med.* 2009;6:1850–1856.

254 Glaser RL, Dimitrakakis C. Reduced breast cancer incidence in women treated with subcutaneous testosterone, or testosterone with anastrozole: A prospective, observational study. *Maturitas.* 2013;76:342–349.

255 Modelska K, Cummings S. Tibolone for postmenopausal women: systematic review of randomized trials. *J Clin Endocrinol Metab.* 2002;87(1):16–23.

**Part II**

**Arousal Disorders**

# 7

# Nosology and Epidemiology of Arousal Disorders in Women

*Leonard R. Derogatis*

### Abstract

This chapter reviews the history and development of the diagnosis female sexual arousal disorder (FSAD) and discusses its close ties to the evolution of the diagnostic system of the American Psychiatric Association (i.e. DSM-I to DSM-5). It reviews the principal criteria underlying the diagnosis and their underlying significance. The chapter also discusses the widespread dissatisfaction with the current DSM-5 system, and the development, in response, of the new ISSWSH diagnostic system for female sexual dysfunctions. Diagnostic standards for the FSAD diagnosis in the ISSWSH system are described and elucidated as an alternative to the DSM-5 system. In addition, the chapter provides a brief review of the current status of epidemiological research focused on the prevalence of FSAD as defined in contemporary nosological systems.

**Keywords:**  *diagnosis; prevalence; nosology; nomenclature; FSD; FSAD*

## Nosology

As with other categories of female sexual dysfunction, the formal nosologic definition of arousal disorders in women has evolved over time with the progression of the Diagnostic and Statistical Manual of Mental Disorders (DSM) diagnostic system. Female sexual arousal disorder (FSAD) began in a relatively undifferentiated state as one of a number of categories of "psychophysiological autonomic and visceral disorders" termed "psychophysiological genitourinary reactions" [1]. The second iteration of the DSM as it relates to female sexual arousal disorder maintained this undifferentiated delineation, "psychophysiological genitourinary reactions" [1].

It was not until the DSM-III [2] in 1980 that significant nosological changes appeared in female sexual arousal disorder. In the DSM-III [2], a superordinate category of "psychosexual disorders" was introduced, of which "Inhibited sexual excitement" was one constituent category. Inhibited sexual excitement was defined as: "Recurrent and persistent inhibition of sexual excitement during sexual activity". The principal manifestation was, "...complete failure to attain or maintain the lubrication-swelling response of sexual excitement until the completion of the sexual act" (p. 156). This characterization focused exclusively on genital response and characterizes the first clear representation of arousal dysfunction in the woman.

With the DSM-III-R [3], published seven years later, the label of the superordinate category was modified to simply "sexual dysfunctions", and the label of "female sexual arousal disorder" was first introduced. In this edition, the woman could manifest the

*Textbook of Female Sexual Function and Dysfunction: Diagnosis and Treatment*, First Edition. Edited by Irwin Goldstein, Anita H. Clayton, Andrew T. Goldstein, Noel N. Kim, and Sheryl A. Kingsberg.
© 2018 John Wiley & Sons Ltd. Published 2018 by John Wiley & Sons Ltd.

condition in one of two ways: either, "persistent or recurrent complete or partial failure to attain or maintain the lubrication-swelling response of sexual excitement until completion of the sexual activity", or "persistent or recurrent lack of a subjective sense of sexual excitement and pleasure during sexual activity" (p. 165). Thus, a cognitive-subjective component was introduced for women that was also present in the male definition of arousal disorder. In addition, the generic specifiers of "lifelong versus acquired" and "generalized versus situational" were introduced in the DSM-III-R.

In the DSM-IV [4], the definition of female sexual arousal disorder again returned to an exclusively physical genital portrayal. It was described as: "a persistent or recurrent inability to attain or maintain until completion of the sexual activity, an adequate lubrication-swelling response of sexual excitement" (p. 500). In addition, a second criterion, the required presence of "manifest personal distress" was added at this time. The specifiers, *lifelong/acquired* and *generalized/situational* were characterized as specifying *subtypes* in this edition.

The DSM-5 [5] does not represent arousal disorder as a distinct diagnostic entity, but rather merges it with hypoactive sexual desire disorder, to create the combined diagnostic entity female sexual interest/arousal disorder (FSIAD). The diagnosis requires that the patient manifest at least three of six possible diagnostic characteristics for a minimum period of at least six months, and that these symptoms be accompanied by manifest personal distress. In addition, the level of severity of the condition must be specified by characterizing it as "mild", "moderate" or "severe".

The introduction of the diagnosis of female sexual interest/arousal disorder in the DSM-5 has been met with a substantial measure of concern by experts in the area of sexual medicine [6, 7]. Difficulties with the merged diagnostic indication have been reviewed in other sections of this book (Chapter 3). However, to focus on a more positive perspective,

dissatisfaction with the DSM-5 nomenclature for female sexual dysfunction has ultimately served as a strong influence in bringing about the development of the new more rigorous and scientific ISSWSH nosology [8] for female sexual dysfunction.

As has been outlined in detail [8], there have been numerous previous attempts to define female sexual arousal disorder, some focused solely on genital physiology, others concentrating on the subjective emotional response, and still others featuring a combined genital and subjective/emotional response. Each definition carries with it both strengths and weaknesses, which are too numerous to examine here.

The new ISSWSH nosology defines female genital arousal disorder (FGAD) as follows: "Female genital arousal disorder is defined as the inability to develop or maintain an adequate genital response, including vulvovaginal lubrication, engorgement of the genitalia, and sensitivity of the genitals associated with the sexual activity for a minimum of six months" (p. 8) [8]. Subcategories are identified as (i) related to vascular injury or dysfunction and/or (ii) neurological injury or dysfunction. Clinically significant personal distress remains a required feature of the presentation, and previous traditional specifiers from the DSM-IV and DSM-5 remain as aspects of the new definition as well.

An exclusionary caution is appended to the diagnosis of female genital arousal disorder involving the conditions of vulvovaginal atrophy, vulvovaginal infection, inflammatory disorders of the vulva or vagina, vestibulodynia and clitorodynia. Any of these conditions would preclude a specific diagnosis of female genital arousal disorder.

A strength of the diagnostic category of female genital arousal disorder is that measurement of the vascular and neural status of the patient may be achieved by much more precise objective instruments that provide highly reliable ratio scale measurement as compared to questionnaire-based assessments. Evaluations of the complex subjective-emotional status of the patient are avoided in this definition, thereby avoiding a controversial component of prior female sexual arousal disorder definitions. Although there should be no problem in implementing these assessments in clinical trials and research protocols, it is true that the instruments required for these measurements are not typically found in the practitioner's office. However, a careful history and clinical examination will enable a diagnosis to be made in most instances.

## Epidemiology

The epidemiology of female sexual arousal disorder suffers from the same limitations as other diagnostic categories of female sexual dysfunction: imprecise nomenclature, equivocal diagnostic criteria, and nonstandardized study designs or outcomes measurement. In addition, as with other categories of female sexual dysfunction, there is the introduction of the disjunctive personal distress criterion that separates prevalence rates into those estimated with a distress criterion as part of the diagnostic definition and those where the distress criterion is omitted. The distress criterion has become a pivotal element of contemporary approaches to female sexual dysfunction nomenclature, distinguishing between true cases of persistent dysfunction versus transient sexual difficulty. Thus, only epidemiological studies that include the distress criterion are discussed here.

As was the case with hypoactive sexual desire disorder, the most comprehensive recent study of the prevalence of female sex-ual arousal disorder was the PRESIDE study conducted by Shifren [9] and her colleagues, who surveyed over 31,000 respondents from over 50,000 US households. In PRESIDE, the unadjusted prevalence of the problem of low sexual arousal, regardless of the presence of distress, was 26.1%. The overall prevalence of low arousal *with* distress was 5.4%, with the intermediate age subgroup (45–64 years) having the highest prevalence of 7.5%, and the youngest age group having the lowest prevalence of 3.3%. The oldest age group (≥65) had a prevalence of 6.0%.

Hayes [10] and colleagues published a review in 2006 of female sexual difficulties in which they attempted to integrate information on duration of the difficulty into their analysis. Only 11 out of 1248 studies met their inclusion criteria and only two of them included a distress criterion. Based on this data, 31% of the women experienced sexual arousal difficulties with distress and 28% experienced difficulties with a duration of ≥6 months. The authors indicated that while rates of the specific types of sexual difficulties varied widely, a consistent pattern emerged across the studies with prevalence rates decreasing from desire > orgasm > arousal > pain.

Obviously, it is too soon to have any data available on the prevalence rates of the new diagnostic categories in the ISSWSH nosology; however, because of the articulation of much more rigorous criterion and use of explicit specifiers, it is anticipated that prevalence data will be more precise and reliable than historical estimates have been in the past.

## References

1 American Psychiatric Association. *The Diagnostic and Statistical Manual of Mental Disorders*. Washington, DC: American Psychiatric Association; 1952.

2 American Psychiatric Association. *DSM-III: Diagnostic and Statistical Manual of Mental Disorders*. 3rd edn. Washington, DC: American Psychiatric Association; 1980.

3 American Psychiatric Association. *DSM-III-R: Diagnostic and Statistical Manual of Mental Disorders*. 3rd edn Revised. Washington, DC: American Psychiatric Association; 1987.

4 American Psychiatric Association. *DSM-IV: Diagnostic and Statistical Manual of Mental Disorders*. 4th Ed. Washington, DC: American Psychiatric Association; 1994.

5 American Psychiatric Association. *DSM-5: Diagnostic and Statistical Manual of Mental Disorders*. 5th edn. Washington, DC: American Psychiatric Association; 2013.

6 Clayton AH, Derogatis LR, Rosen R, *et al*. Does clinical research data support sexual desire and arousal disorders as distinct diagnoses? *J Sex Med*. 2010;7(S3):143–144.

7 Derogatis LR, Clayton AH, Rosen R, *et al*. Do multiple convergent measures of female sexual dysfunction support sexual desire and arousal disorders as distinct diagnoses? *J Sex Med*. 2010;7(S3):142–143.

8 Parish SJ, Goldstein AT, Goldstein SW, *et al*. Toward a more evidence-based nosology and nomenclature for female sexual dysfunctions – Part II. *J. Sex. Med*. 2016;13:1888–1906.

9 Shifren JL, Monz BU, Russo PA, *et al*. Sexual problems and distress in United States women: prevalence and correlates. *Obstet Gynecol*. 2008;112(5):970–978.

10 Hayes RD, Bennett CM, Fairly CK, *et al*. What can prevalence studies tell us about female sexual difficulty and dysfunction. *J. Sex. Med*. 2006;3:589–595.

# 8

# Anatomy and Physiology of Arousal

*Kwangsung Park and Noel N. Kim*

### Abstract

Sexual arousal is a physiological response to internal and external stimuli and is mediated by both central and peripheral nervous systems. This chapter focuses specifically on genital arousal, which is characterized by changes in sensation, tissue contractility, vasocongestion, and lubrication. The physiological events of the sexual arousal response in women are related to the structural integrity of genital tissues and the function of vascular, neural, and hormonal systems. The strongest evidence, thus far, indicates that the adrenergic and nitric oxide signaling systems play important roles in acutely regulating genital blood flow but sex steroid hormones are also critical for maintaining genital tissue health. The additive, synergistic or antagonistic interactions of cellular processes will ultimately determine the overall physiological responses manifested as blood flow, lubrication or tissue contractility.

**Keywords:** *sexual arousal; genital engorgement; parasympathetic; nonadrenergic noncholinergic; nitric oxide; vasoactive intestinal polypeptide; vaginal lubrication; aquaporin; androgen; estrogen*

---

Sexual arousal is a physiological response to internal and external stimuli and is mediated by both central and peripheral nervous systems.

Genital arousal is characterized by changes in sensation, tissue contractility, vasocongestion, and lubrication.

Neural, endocrine, and vascular factors affect specific and distinct cellular components within genital tissues to maintain their function.

---

## Introduction

Sexual arousal comprises both genital and extragenital responses that anticipate sexual activity and continue up to the point of orgasm [1–4]. These responses result from the processing of internal stimuli (e.g., dreams, fantasies, memories, love, intimacy needs, libido) and external stimuli (e.g., auditory, visual, olfactory, tactile), leading to increased activity in the central and peripheral nervous systems (Figure 8.1) [5, 6]. Characteristic physiological changes in the genitals include vulvovaginal lubrication (vaginal fluids and secretions of paraurethral and Bartholin's glands), genital engorgement, and increased sensitivity of the genitalia. Extragenital changes include erection of the nipples, flushing of the skin, and increases in heart rate, blood pressure, and respiration rate.

While subjective arousal has been assessed in clinical studies apart from the physical responses of genital arousal, recent expert opinion has raised the possibility that subjective

*Textbook of Female Sexual Function and Dysfunction: Diagnosis and Treatment*, First Edition. Edited by Irwin Goldstein, Anita H. Clayton, Andrew T. Goldstein, Noel N. Kim, and Sheryl A. Kingsberg.
© 2018 John Wiley & Sons Ltd. Published 2018 by John Wiley & Sons Ltd.

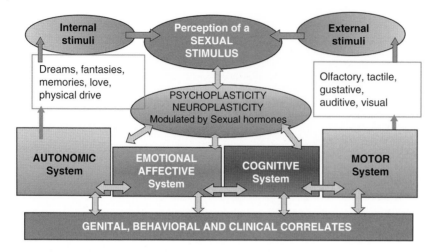

**Figure 8.1** Physiology of sexual desire/interest and central arousal. (Adapted from [6].) (*See plate section for color representation of the figure*)

arousal can be more consistently understood as a manifestation of sexual desire [7; *also see Chapter 4, Desire: CNS Anatomy and Neurochemistry of Sexual Desire*]. This perspective arises from several lines of evidence that suggest that women often conflate their experience of sexual arousal and desire [8] and, generally, have less cognitive awareness of their own genital arousal that is an autonomic response and can occur in the absence of subjective arousal [9–11]. In part, this discordance may be a function of decreased proprioception of internal genital organs in women, as evidenced by the observation that subjective sexual arousal is more strongly correlated with vulvar blood flow than vaginal vasocongestion [12]. Further, men (who have full visual and sensory feedback from their genitals) have a higher degree of concordance between subjective sexual arousal and genital arousal when compared to women [13–15]. However, other mechanistic explanations cannot be ruled out and the nature of subjective sexual arousal remains under active investigation.

This chapter focuses exclusively on the mechanisms regulating genital sexual arousal. The physiologic events of the sexual arousal response in women are related to the structural integrity of genital tissues and the function of vascular, neural, and hormonal systems [16, 17]. Thus, relevant anatomy will be integrated into discussions of mechanism.

## Hemodynamic Considerations for Genital Sexual Arousal

The genital arousal response is manifested by increased blood flow to the genital tissues, which results in clitoral engorgement and accompanying vulvar swelling [18–20]. With sexual stimulation, increased blood flow to the clitoral cavernosal and labial arteries results in increased clitoral intracavernosal pressure, protrusion of the glans clitoris, and engorgement of the labia minora [21, 22]. The clitoris is an important organ for female sexual arousal and the contemporary understanding of clitoral anatomy is the functional entity of the clitoral complex, composed of the distal vagina, urethra, and clitoris [18]. This functional grouping of tissues has also been termed the "clitoral urethral complex" [23] or "clitourethrovaginal complex" [24]. These associated structures have common

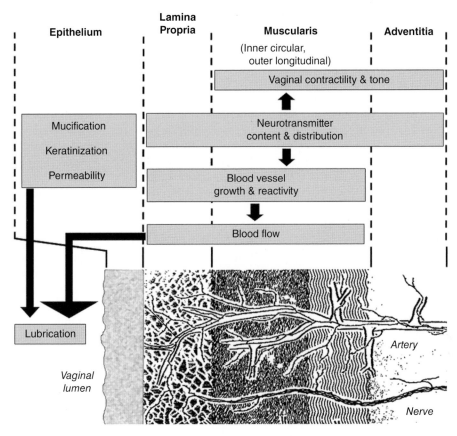

**Figure 8.2** Interaction between cellular constituents of the vagina and the physiological processes mediated by them. (Adapted from [17].)

vasculature and innervation and move in unity during sexual activity [19, 24].

Magnetic resonance imaging technology has enabled better access to understanding the female sexual response. Dynamic magnetic resonance imaging scans of pelvis and genitals showed a change in engorgement that occurred within three minutes of audiovisual sexual stimulation and reached a peak level at about nine minutes [25, 26]. The clitoral volume can be increased by 50–300% when engorged [25]. Engorgement of the clitoris is achieved with minimal corporal veno-occlusion. This is consistent with the function of the clitoris, which is primarily a sensory organ that engorges during sexual activity. Only in the pathologic state of clitoral priapism is there significant corporal veno-occlusion.

The vagina consists of distinct layers of tissue defined by the epithelium, lamina propria, muscularis, and the adventitia (Figure 8.2). The vagina also has an extensive vascular network, primarily within the lamina propria (submucosal) layer and vaginal engorgement is critical for the production of lubricating fluids during sexual arousal (Figure 8.2) [27]. Vascular corrosion cast studies in rats have demonstrated that the subepithelial region of the vagina contains a dense and rich network of capillaries that perfuse the epithelium and larger venous sinuses that can functionally imbue the vagina with erectile tissue-like qualities [28]. Noninvasive anatomical study of the vaginal microvessel architecture showed that the vaginal microcirculation consisted of homogenously distributed hairpin-shaped capillary loops [29]. In the nonaroused state, this microcirculation of the vagina exhibits a phenomenon called vasomotion (detected as pseudorandomly distributed low and high amplitude signals by photoplethysmography) that decreases when vaginal blood flow increases during sexual stimulation [30]. While this serves as a sensitive measure of sexual arousal in research studies, the clinical significance of this phenomenon remains to be determined.

## Neural Regulation of Sexual Arousal

Increased activation of the autonomic nervous system stimulates parasympathetic outflow from the sacral nerves (S2, S3, S4) to allow genital engorgement and vaginal lubrication. Stimulation of sympathetic activity causes increases in heart rate and blood pressure, as well as activation of striated muscle that participates in sexual activity. Within female genital tissues, multiple studies have demonstrated the presence of adrenergic, cholinergic and nonadrenergic noncholinergic (NANC) neurotransmitters (neuropeptide Y, vasoactive intestinal polypeptide, peptide histidine methionine, nitric oxide, calcitonin gene-related peptide, substance P) [31–47]. While the roles of each of these neurotransmitters remains incompletely characterized, the strongest evidence, thus far, indicates that the adrenergic and nitric oxide signaling systems play important roles in regulating genital blood flow.

### Adrenergic Regulation of Genital Arousal

In the basal, nonstimulated state, norepinephrine from sympathetic nerve terminals constricts vascular and nonvascular smooth muscle to maintain low genital blood flow and a high degree of tone to the vaginal wall. *In vitro* and *in vivo* animal studies have demonstrated the presence of functional $\alpha_1$- and $\alpha_2$-adrenergic receptors in vaginal and clitoral

tissue and intravaginal injection of $\alpha$-adrenergic receptor antagonists causes a marked increase in the amplitude and duration of the engorgement response with and without pelvic nerve stimulation [39, 48–50]. In clinical studies, the $\alpha_1$-adrenergic receptor antagonist phentolamine has been reported to improve vaginal lubrication in postmenopausal women with female sexual arousal disorder [51] while the $\alpha_2$-adrenergic receptor agonist clonidine impaired both vaginal engorgement and subjective sexual response when administered to healthy volunteers [52].

Interestingly, mild systemic activation of the sympathetic system (15–30 minutes postexercise) can also facilitate the genital arousal response in women [53]. While exercise-induced sympathetic activation by itself does not cause increased vaginal engorgement, moderate sympathetic activation followed by visual sexual stimulation enhances vaginal blood volume and vasocongestion to a greater extent than visual sexual stimulation alone [54]. In healthy women, it is likely that erotic stimulation specifically results in relaxation of smooth muscle within the genital organs, even in the face of increased systemic sympathetic output. Elevated systemic blood pressure and positive chronotropic/inotropic effects on the heart, secondary to moderate sympathetic activation, would facilitate genital engorgement by increasing the pressure gradient between the larger resistance arteries and the local genital circulation.

### Nitrergic Regulation of Genital Arousal

Studies have demonstrated the presence of neuronal and endothelial nitric oxide synthase (NOS) in clitoral and vaginal tissues, as well as functional changes to blood flow after administration of drugs that interfere with nitric oxide synthesis/signaling or nitric oxide-liberating compounds [33, 40, 48, 55–61]. In human vaginal tissue, immunoreactivity for phosphodiesterase type 5 was localized in the endothelium and smooth muscle of blood vessels [57].

In addition, vaginal and clitoral smooth muscle cells in culture have been shown to express phosphodiesterase type 5 [62, 63]. Clinical studies have shown that in healthy women, the phosphodiesterase type 5 inhibitor sildenafil significantly improved arousal, orgasm, and enjoyment when compared with placebo [64–67]. However, other clinical studies have shown no improvement in women's sexual function [68, 69]. Thus, while the physiological significance of the nitric oxide-cyclic GMP system is well established, the clinical efficacy of phosphodiesterase type 5 inhibitors in treating female sexual dysfunction may depend upon appropriate screening and identification of patients most likely to benefit from such therapy.

## Regulation of Genital Arousal by other Nonadrenergic Noncholinergic (NANC) Neurotransmitters

With regard to other nonadrenergic noncholinergic neurotransmitters, several reports have suggested that exogenous vasoactive intestinal polypeptide can relax clitoral and vaginal smooth muscle and increase blood flow [44, 46, 50, 70–72]. However, there has been no conclusive experimental evidence for the functional involvement of endogenous vasoactive intestinal polypeptide due to the lack of specific and selective antagonists for vasoactive intestinal polypeptide receptors. Peptide histidine methionine is a vasoactive intestinal polypeptide precursor and is colocalized in nerve fibers with vasoactive intestinal polypeptide in the female reproductive tract. In the vagina, peptide histidine methionine is present in higher concentrations than vasoactive intestinal polypeptide and can cause relaxation of the nonvascular smooth muscle by acting through the same receptors as vasoactive intestinal polypeptide [44, 73]. Peptide histidine methionine has also been reported to increase vaginal blood flow in women [45].

Neuropeptide Y has been detected at relatively high concentrations in human, rabbit, and rat vagina [34, 38, 74–76]. Due to its primary localization within nerve fibers near blood vessels, it has been postulated that neuropeptide Y regulates blood flow in the vagina. In isolated tissue studies, neuropeptide Y was shown to constrict small arteries from human cervix and have an additive effect to norepinephrine [74], suggesting that neuropeptide Y has vasoconstrictor activity and may have a similar function in the vagina. While substance P and calcitonin gene-related peptide are known to be involved primarily in sensory pathways, these peptide neurotransmitters have been shown to mediate vasodilation in specific vascular beds of the brain and ovaries [77, 78]. Their roles in modulating the sexual arousal response remain to be elucidated.

## Afferent Pathways Influencing Genital Arousal

Sensory input from the genitals can initiate and/or propagate the arousal response. Different genital tissues and organs have different sensitivities to varying stimuli. These include mechanosensitivity (pressure stimulus), chemosensitivity (irritant stimulus), and thermosensitivity (cool or warm stimulus). Mechanical and chemical stimulation of the cervix is associated with intense and "touch" sensations mediated by the vagus, hypogastric (T11-L3), and pelvic (L6-S1) nerves [79, 80]. Mechanical and chemical stimulation of the vagina elicits gentle to intense sensations of distension, which are mediated by the pelvic nerve [79, 80]. Touch and thermal stimulation of the clitoris (skin sensitivity) are mediated by the pudendal nerve (L6) [79, 80]. The pudendal nerve also carries sensory information to the spinal cord from the vulva and striated pelvic and perineal muscles [79, 80].

Nerve transection and tracer studies in animal models have provided valuable information regarding both the neuroanatomy and neurophysiology of the genital organs and the sexual response. Afferent fibers from the clitoris travel in the pudendal nerve. The conduction velocity of myelinated clitoral afferent fibers is slightly slower than skin afferent pathways (about 10–15 m/s) [81]. In comparison, conduction velocities of nerves from the vagina and uterus are significantly slower (2 m/s), corresponding to the conduction velocity of C-fibers [81]. The receptive fields of vaginal afferent fibers are smallest at the orifice and progressively increase in size up the vaginal canal to the vagino-cervical junction [82]. This translates to poorer localization of sensation internally. In relative terms, the anterior vaginal wall has denser innervation than the posterior wall and the distal vagina has denser innervation than the proximal vagina (relative to the cervix) [82]. The vagus nerve is important for analgesia and pupil dilation and may be activated by vagino-cervical stimulation. Women with spinal cord injury can experience orgasm with vagino-cervical stimulation through the vagal pathways but it remains unclear whether the vagus serves as a supplemental sensory pathway or whether it may only be activated after spinal cord injury [83–86].

## Regulation of Vaginal Lubrication

The vagina has a potential space covered by a film of fluid, which is usually insufficient to allow painless penile penetration and thrusting [87]. Comfortable or pleasurable sexual intercourse requires vaginal lubrication, which is part of the sexual arousal response and reflects a women's sexual health [88, 89]. Vaginal fluid is derived from several sources, including vaginal transudate and fluids from the upper reproductive tract, such as cervical mucus and endometrial and tubal fluids [90]. The chemical composition of vaginal fluid is represented by a mixture of ions ($Na^+$, $K^+$, $Cl^-$ and $Ca^{2+}$), glycerol, lactic acid, acetic acid, and glycogen [90–92].

## Possible Mechanisms of Vaginal Transudation

As discussed previously, vaginal vasocongestion enhances the production of lubricating fluid. This fluid primarily consists of plasma transudate that is produced as follows: (i) the capillaries of microcirculation become dilated, resulting in increased hydrostatic pressure; (ii) plasma transudate (ultrafiltrate) is forced into the interstitial space around the blood vessels; and (iii) the transudate passes through the vaginal epithelium onto the mucosa of the vagina [93].

As summarized in Figure 8.3, three separate mechanisms have been proposed to explain transvaginal epithelial permeability. Firstly, the ionic transcellular transport mechanism accounts for plasma transudate being filtered from the submucosal capillaries by actively transferring $Na^+$ from the capillary lumen to the interstitial fluid with water absorption following osmotic drag [94].

Secondly, transcellular fluid transport may also occur through aquaporin (AQP) water channels. Aquaporins are water channel proteins that are expressed in many fluid-containing tissues such as kidney tubules and glandular epithelia, including the human vaginal epithelium and subepithelial capillaries [95–97]. A subset of aquaporins called aquaglyceroporins have also been identified in the human vaginal epithelium and can transport glycerol and some solutes, as well as water [95, 96, 98]. In animal studies, specific aquaporin proteins translocate from the cytoplasm to the plasma membrane after pelvic nerve stimulation [99], suggesting that aquaporins are dynamically regulated to increase membrane permeability to water upon sexual stimulation.

Thirdly, plasma transudate may move through the epithelial paracellular (intercellular) space and is controlled by the resistance of the epithelial tight junction ($R_{TJ}$) and the epithelial lateral intercellular space ($R_{LIS}$) [100–102]. This paracellular permeability is regulated by estrogen through the expression of intracellular structural proteins and

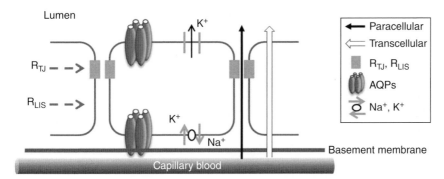

**Figure 8.3** Mechanisms of transvaginal epithelial permeability. (*See plate section for color representation of the figure*)

extracellular tight junction proteins [100, 103]. This estrogen response occurs more rapidly in vaginal epithelial cells from premenopausal women compared to those from postmenopausal women [100].

### Purinergic Receptors and Vaginal Moisture

Purinergic receptor ligands have been studied for their effects on the physiology of various systems throughout the body [104]. Gorodeski *et al.* first reported P2Y receptor responses in human endocervical cells *in vitro* and have presented evidence of P2Y$_2$ receptor gene expression in these cells [105, 106]. In animal studies, P2Y$_2$ receptor mRNA was localized to endocervical and cervical gland, epithelium, and stratified squamous epithelium of the vagina and topical application of P2Y$_2$ receptor agonists increased vaginal moisture in ovariectomized animals to levels that were comparable to or significantly higher than control animals [107]. Studies of cervical mucus quantity and composition in response to fluctuating hormone levels in women has shown that certain mucin subtypes are upregulated during ovulation [108]. Stimulation of the P2Y$_2$ receptor activates phospholipase C, which results in increased inositol trisphosphate levels and release of calcium from the endoplasmic reticulum. This stimulates cellular functions such as increased mucin secretion and chloride efflux, resulting in increased surface liquid and hydration of secretions.

## Modulation of Female Genital Arousal by Sex Steroid Hormones

Sex steroid hormones may regulate distinct cellular components of the vagina (Figure 8.4). Each of these cellular interactions influences specific physiological events such as growth and function of neurons, blood vessels, smooth muscle, and epithelial cells. Preclinical and clinical studies suggest that estrogens modulate genital hemodynamics and are critical for maintaining structural and functional integrity of vaginal tissues [109–112]. Estrogen deprivation may lead to decreased pelvic blood flow, resulting in diminished vaginal lubrication, clitoral fibrosis, thinning of the vaginal wall, and decreased vaginal submucosal vasculature [113, 114]. In addition, estrogen deficiency leads to involution and atrophy of the genital organs, adversely affecting cervical, endocervical, and glandular mucin production. In contrast, estrogen replacement in postmenopausal women increases pelvic blood flow, re-establishing vaginal structural integrity and lubrication.

Androgens are not only essential for the development of reproductive function in women and hormonal homeostasis but also

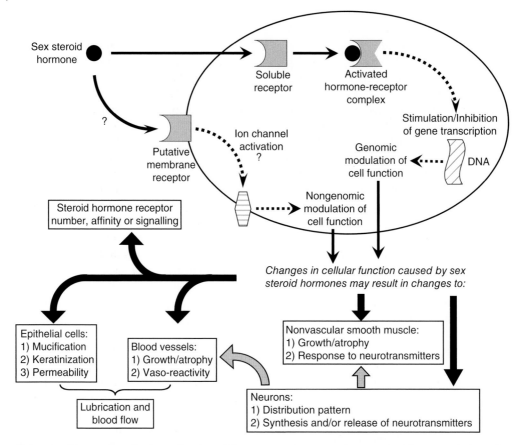

**Figure 8.4** Proposed mechanisms of sex steroid hormone action in regulating vaginal function. Binding of steroid hormones to specific receptors (intracellular or membrane bound) leads to genomic and nongenomic activation of cellular processes. These include regulation of steroid receptor synthesis, activation of ion channels, increased DNA synthesis, regulation of growth factors, and neurotransmitter synthesis. The cascade of events triggered by sex steroid hormone binding brings about changes in vaginal tissue structure and function that modulate the vaginal arousal response to sexual stimulation. (Reprinted from [17].)

represent the immediate precursors for the biosynthesis of estrogens [115]. Although clinical studies have indicated that androgens modulate sexual arousal responses [116–126], the precise mechanisms by which androgens facilitate such responses is not fully characterized. In addition, progesterone is an important signaling molecule in peripheral nerves, where it promotes myelin sheath formation by activating expression of specific hormone sensitive genes [127]. However, the role of progesterone on peripheral vaginal arousal remains poorly understood.

The role of steroid hormones in modulating tissue structure, blood flow, lubrication

and mucification, neurotransmitter biosynthesis and function, smooth muscle contractility, and expression of sex steroid receptors in genital tissue is discussed in greater detail in the following subsections.

### Effect of Sex Steroid Hormones on Genital Tissue Structure

In addition to the long established effects of estrogen on vaginal epithelium [128], ovariectomy can also reduce the volume of the vaginal muscularis layer with a considerable increase in connective tissue between muscle bundles [129]. Other studies in rats and rabbits have also consistently noted decreased smooth muscle content and increased connective tissue in both the vagina and clitoris after ovariectomy [130, 131]. Estradiol supplementation in ovariectomized animals can restore smooth muscle content in the vaginal wall and decrease interstitial fibrosis but under histological examination, the tissue can be qualitatively different in appearance from control animals [129]. Testosterone treatment may also restore muscularis fiber bundles but to a lesser extent than estradiol [129]. A combination of estradiol and testosterone or a combination of estradiol and progesterone was necessary to restore vaginal muscularis fiber bundles in ovariectomized animals to an appearance that was similar to control intact animals [129]. Thus, while the vaginal epithelium is primarily responsive to estrogen, these findings suggest that estrogens, androgens, and progestins have additive effects in submucosal structures of the vaginal wall that cannot be replicated by any individual hormone.

## Effect of Sex Steroid Hormones on Genital Blood Flow and Vaginal Lubrication

In animal studies, hormone depletion by ovariectomy resulted in a significant reduction in vaginal blood flow in response to pelvic nerve stimulation when compared to controls [58, 110, 132]. Estradiol or estradiol plus testosterone treatment of ovariectomized animals restored genital blood flow responses to pelvic nerve-stimulation. Treatment of ovariectomized animals with testosterone alone did not result in increased genital blood flow in the rabbit [58] but was effective in increasing blood flow in the rat [133]. These observations suggest that estrogens and androgens regulate the vascular components of genital tissues, but these effects may be species specific.

In the vasculature, estrogen is known to generally be beneficial in maintaining endothelial function and has been demonstrated to upregulate nitric oxide synthase (NOS) in endothelial cells, oocytes, heart, kidney, skeletal muscle, esophagus, and cerebellum [134–137]. In a similar fashion, sex steroid hormones may modulate genital blood flow through the regulation of nitric oxide synthase (NOS). Yet, ovariectomy increases enzymatic activity and protein levels of NOS in the vagina and clitoris [130, 131, 138] while estrogen supplementation given for various periods of time (3–14 days), beginning two weeks after ovariectomy, reversed these changes [130, 131, 138, 139]. It has been postulated that the upregulation of NOS may be a compensatory mechanism to mitigate the adverse changes occurring throughout the vaginal wall, but it is unknown if these changes are transient or stable and it remains unclear if this occurs in women after surgical or natural menopause. Further, specific changes in the endothelium of the vaginal submucosal vasculature have not been examined with regard to NOS activity and expression.

NOS expression in the proximal (upper) vagina may be more sensitive to estrogen than the distal (lower) vagina, potentially reflecting the different embryonic origins of upper vagina that arises from the Müllerian duct, whereas the lower vagina is derived from the urogenital sinus [140]. Interestingly, estrogen downregulated NOS activity in the rabbit lower urinary tract (bladder and urethra) but not in upper urinary tract (kidney) [141]. Thus, estrogen may exert similar regulation over NOS in genital and lower urinary tissues. Similar to estrogen, progesterone also increases NOS activity in rat and rabbit vagina [142, 143] but androgens (testosterone, dihydrotestosterone, delta-5-androstenediol) do not reverse the upregulation of NOS in the vagina after ovariectomy [138].

In addition to modulating NOS, sex steroid hormones may also modulate blood flow by regulating the activity of vasoactive intestinal polypeptide in the vagina [131, 138, 139, 141–145]. For example, the binding affinity of vasoactive intestinal polypeptide to tissues of the genital tract was greatest in ovariectomized rabbits treated with estrogen and progesterone [144]. Furthermore, administration of vasoactive intestinal polypeptide to postmenopausal women receiving no hormone replacement failed to increase vaginal blood flow, whereas those receiving hormone replacement exhibited increases in blood flow that were comparable to premenopausal women [145].

Genital atrophy and diminished genital blood flow, secondary to declining estrogen (as occurs during peri- and postmenopause), negatively affects vaginal lubrication in women [146, 147]. These clinical observations are further supported by laboratory studies. In estrogen-deprived animals, production of vaginal transudate was markedly decreased compared to controls and was restored by estrogen treatment [148]. Vaginal mucin production has been reported to be stimulated by low doses of estrogen but reduced by high doses of estrogen [149–151]. Androgens have also been shown to increase vaginal mucification in the rat [152, 153]. Treatment of ovariectomized rats with topical dehydroepiandrosterone, which can be converted within tissues to more active androgens and estrogens, resulted in complete reversal of vaginal atrophy and stimulated proliferation and mucification of the vaginal epithelium [154].

## Effects of Androgens and Estrogens on Vaginal Innervation and Smooth Muscle Contractility

Genital sexual arousal induces changes in the tissue properties of the vaginal canal that are in part regulated by the tone of the smooth muscle within the muscularis layer. Ovariectomy reduces relaxation of vaginal smooth muscle to electric field stimulation (neurogenic response) and to exogenous vasoactive intestinal polypeptide in organ bath studies [50]. While estrogen supplementation was ineffective, androgen treatment enhanced relaxation to electrical stimulation and restored vasoactive intestinal polypeptide-induced relaxation, suggesting that androgens may modulate

neurotransmitter function. In addition, vaginal tissue from testosterone-treated animals developed significantly greater contractile force to exogenous noradrenaline. These observations suggest that testosterone may be an important regulator of vaginal nonvascular smooth muscle contractility. Contrasted with the positive effects of estrogen and progesterone on vasoactive intestinal polypeptide-induced blood flow in the vagina (previous section), different hormones clearly have very specific and localized effects (e.g., the vasculature within the lamina propria versus the smooth muscle in the muscularis layer).

Adrenergic nerves of the female genital tract are also sensitive to changes in the hormonal milieu. In animal studies, treatment with estrogen alone or a mixture of estradiol and progesterone increased the norepinephrine content of adrenergic nerves in the vagina [155–157]. In contrast to the effects of estrogen on adrenergic neurotransmitter content, the density of overall innervation has been observed to increase in the rat vagina subsequent to ovariectomy and decrease after estrogen administration [158]. These changes consisted of adrenergic, cholinergic, and calcitonin gene-related peptide-containing nerves, which can mediate vasoconstriction and nociception. It was suggested that similar changes may explain the sensitivity and hyperalgesia of the vagina in postmenopausal women. In other studies using rats, testosterone significantly increased the density of adrenergic nerve fibers and this effect was attenuated when estradiol was co-administered with testosterone [129]. These observations suggest differential regulation of both motor and sensory nerves in the vagina by sex steroid hormones.

## Effects of Androgens and Estrogens on Androgen and Estrogen Receptors

While the effects of steroid hormones on the regulation of estrogen and progesterone receptors in reproductive organs have been extensively investigated [159, 160], there are limited studies on the regulation of expression of sex steroid hormone receptors in the vagina [161]. In ovariectomized rats, estrogen receptor (ER) protein and specific binding of estradiol to estrogen receptor was increased in the vagina after four weeks, whereas estradiol replacement (at physiological concentrations) decreased estrogen receptor [132]. Given the critical role of the estrogen receptor in maintaining vaginal tissue structure and function, this may represent a compensatory upregulation of receptor in response to low systemic estrogen. Importantly, a subphysiological dose of estradiol did not prevent the upregulation of estrogen receptor in ovariectomized rats and this low dose of estradiol restored vaginal blood flow responses to levels that were similar to control animals [132]. This suggests that a critical level of estrogen is required in the vagina to impact estrogen receptor levels and that low dose estradiol may exert beneficial effects on vaginal tissue structure and function in the postmenopausal state. These findings are consistent with the efficacy of intravaginal low dose estrogen for vaginal atrophy in postmenopausal women [162, 163]. In contrast, androgen receptors in the vagina are downregulated after ovariectomy and testosterone treatment of ovariectomized rats prevented this downregulation [133]. Estrogen receptor in the vagina remained elevated in ovariectomized rats irrespective of testosterone treatment.

Thus, the estrogen receptor undergoes reciprocal regulation by estrogen in the vagina, whereas the androgen receptor is positively regulated by testosterone. Similar phenomena have also been observed in clinical studies. Messenger RNA for the estrogen receptor-α isoform increases in the vagina of postmenopausal women and decreases after systemic hormone replacement therapy, but not with local intravaginal administration of low dose estradiol [164]. Also, when compared to pre- or postmenopausal women, androgen receptor protein levels increased in the vagina of women treated with long-term, high dose testosterone prior to undergoing transgender surgery [165].

## Summary and Conclusions

Genital arousal is dependent upon the proper function of neural, endocrine, and vascular systems. The content and distribution of nerve fibers, blood vessels, nonvascular smooth muscle, extracellular matrix, and the health of the epithelium can impact upon normal vaginal responses (engorgement and lubrication) during sexual arousal. The additive, synergistic or antagonistic interactions of cellular processes will ultimately determine the overall physiological responses manifested as blood flow, lubrication or tissue contractility. Thus, pathological changes in any of the processes discussed in this chapter may lead to alterations in neurotransmitter function, tissue composition/structure, and smooth muscle contractility, with concomitant decreases in vaginal blood flow, lubrication, and sensation, resulting in diminished vaginal arousal. A detailed discussion of arousal disorder is provided in a separate chapter.

## References

1 Giraldi A, Rellini AH, Pfaus J, Laan E. 2013. Female sexual arousal disorders. *J Sex Med.* 10:58–73.

2 Kinsey AC, Pomeroy WB, Martin CE, Gebhard PH. 1953. *Sexual Behavior in the Human Female*. Philadelphia, PA: W.B. Saunders.

3 Masters WH, Johnson V. 1966. *Human Sexual Response*. Boston, MA: Little, Brown.

4 Miner M, Esposito K, Guay A, *et al.* 2012. Cardiometabolic risk and female sexual health. *J Sex Med.* 9:641–651.

5 Graziottin A, Giraldi A. 2006. Anatomy and physiology of women's sexual function. In:

Porst H, Buvat J. (eds), *ISSM (International Society of Sexual Medicine) Standard Committee Book, Standard Practice in Sexual Medicine*. Oxford: Blackwell. pp. 289–304.

6 Graziottin A, Gambini D. 2015. Anatomy and physiology of genital organs – women. *Handb Clin Neurol.* 130:39–60.

7 Parish SJ, Goldstein AT, Goldstein SW, *et al.* 2016. Toward a more evidence-based nosology and nomenclature for female sexual dysfunctions – Part II. *J Sex Med.* 13:1888–1906.

8 Brotto LA. 2010. The DSM diagnostic criteria for hypoactive sexual desire disorder in women. *Arch Sex Behav.* 39:221–239.

9 Both S, Everaerd W, Laan E. 2003. Modulation of spinal reflexes by aversive and sexually appetitive stimuli. *Psychophysiology.* 40:174–183.

10 Chivers ML, Rieger G, Latty E, *et al.* 2004. A sex difference in the specificity of sexual arousal. *Psychol Sci.* 15:736–744.

11 Laan E, Everaerd W, Evers A. 1995. Assessment of female sexual arousal: Response specificity and construct validity. *Psychophysiology.* 32:476–485.

12 Bouchard KN, Chivers ML, Pukall CF. 2017. Effects of genital response measurement device and stimulus characteristics on sexual concordance in women. *J Sex Res.* 54(9):1197–1208. doi: 10.1080/00224499.2016.1265641.

13 Kukkonen TM, Binik YM, Amsel R, Carrier S. 2007. Thermography as a physiological measure of sexual arousal in both men and women. *J Sex Med.* 4:93–105.

14 Suschinsky KD, Lalumière ML, Chivers ML. 2009. Sex differences in patterns of genital sexual arousal: measurement artifacts or true phenomena? *Arch Sex Behav.* 38:559–573.

15 Wincze JP, Venditti E, Barlow D, Mavissakalian M. 1980. The effects of a subjective monitoring task in the physiological measure of genital response to erotic stimulation. *Arch Sex Behav.* 9:533–545.

16 Imbimbo C, Gentile V, Palmieri A, *et al.* 2003. Female sexual dysfunction: An update on physiopathology. *J Endocrinol Invest.* 26(Suppl 3):102–104.

17 Traish AM, Kim NN, Munarriz R, Goldstein I. 2004. Female genital sexual arousal: biochemical mediators and potential mechanisms of dysfunction. *Drug Discov Today Dis Mech.* 1:91–97.

18 O'Connell HE, Eizenberg N, Rahman M, Cleeve J. 2008. The anatomy of the distal vagina: Towards unity. *J Sex Med.* 5:1883–1891.

19 Pauls RN. 2015. Anatomy of the clitoris and the female sexual response. *Clin Anat.* 28:376–384.

20 Puppo V. 2013. Anatomy and physiology of the clitoris, vestibular bulbs, and labia minora with a review of the female orgasm and the prevention of female sexual dysfunction. *Clin Anat.* 26:134–152.

21 Berman JR. 2005. Physiology of female sexual function and dysfunction. *Int J Impot Res.* 17 (Suppl 1):S44–S51.

22 Park K, Goldstein I, Andry C, *et al.* 1997. Vasculogenic female sexual dysfunction: The hemodynamic basis for vaginal engorgement insufficiency and clitoral erectile insufficiency. *Int J Impot Res.* 9:27–37.

23 Oakley SH, Mutema GK, Crisp CC, *et al.* 2013. Innervation and histology of the clitoral-urethral complex: A cross-sectional cadaver study. *J Sex Med.* 10:2211–2218.

24 Jannini EA, Buisson O, Rubio-Casillas A. 2014. Beyond the G-spot: Clitourethrovaginal complex anatomy in female orgasm. *Nat Rev Urol.* 11:531–538.

25 Maravilla KR, Yang CC. 2008. Magnetic resonance imaging and the female sexual response: overview of techniques, results, and future directions. *J Sex Med.* 5:1559–1571.

26 Vaccaro CM. 2015. The use of magnetic resonance imaging for studying female sexual function: A review. *Clin Anat.* 28:324–330.

27 Traish AM, Botchevar E, Kim NN. 2010. Biochemical factors modulating female genital sexual arousal physiology. *J Sex Med.* 7:2925–2946.

28 Shabsigh A, Buttyan R, Burchardt T, *et al.* 1999. The microvascular architecture of the rat vagina revealed by image analysis of vascular corrosion casts. *Int J Impot Res.* 11(Suppl 1):S23–S30.

29 Weber MA, Milstein DM, Ince C, *et al.* 2015. Vaginal microcirculation: Non-invasive anatomical examination of the micro-vessel architecture, tortuosity and capillary density. *Neurourol Urodyn.* 34:723–729.

30 Levin RJ, Wylie K. 2008. Vaginal vasomotion – its appearance, measurement, and usefulness in assessing the mechanisms of vasodilatation. *J Sex Med.* 5:377–386.

31 Amenta F, Porcelli F, Ferrante F, Cavallotti C. 1979. Cholinergic nerves in blood vessels of the female reproductive system. *Acta Histochemica.* 65:133–137.

32 Blank MA, Gu J, Allen JM, *et al.* 1986. The regional distribution of NPY-, PHM-, and VIP-containing nerves in the human female genital tract. *Int J Fertil.* 31:218–222.

33 Burnett AL, Calvin DC, Silver RI, *et al.* 1997. Immunohistochemical description of nitric oxide synthase isoforms in human clitoris, *J Urol.* 158:75–78.

34 Giraldi A, Alm P, Werkstrom V, *et al.* 2002. Morphological and functional characterization of a rat vaginal smooth muscle sphincter. *Int J Impot Res.* 14:271–282.

35 Giuliano F, Allard J, Compagnie S, *et al.* 2001. Vaginal physiological changes in a model of sexual arousal in anesthetized rats. *Am J Physiol.* 281:R140–R149.

36 Giuliano F, Rampin O, Allard J. 2002. Neurophysiology and pharmacology of female genital sexual response. *J Sex Marital Ther..* 28(Suppl 1):101–121.

37 Hauser-Kronberger C, Cheung A, Hacker GW, *et al.* 1999. Peptidergic innervation of the human clitoris. *Peptides.* 20:539–543.

38 Hoyle CH, Stones RW, Robson T, *et al.* 1996. Innervation of vasculature and microvasculature of the human vagina by NOS and neuropeptide-containing nerves. *J Anat.* 188:633–644.

39 Kim NN, Min K, Huang YH, *et al.* 2002. Biochemical and functional characterization of alpha-adrenergic receptors in the rabbit vagina. *Life Sci.* 71:2909–2920.

40 Kim SW, Jeong SJ, Munarriz R, *et al.* 2003. Role of the nitric oxide-cyclic GMP pathway in regulation of vaginal blood flow. *Int J Impot Res.* 15:355–361.

41 Lakomy M, Szatkowska C, Chmielewski S. 1987. The adrenergic and AChE-positive nerves in pig vagina. *Anatomischer Anzeiger.* 164:39–46.

42 Lakomy M, Happola O, Majewski M, Kaleczyc J. 1994. Immunohistochemical localization of neuropeptides in nerve fibers of the porcine vagina and uterine cervix. *Folia Histochem Cytobiol.* 32:167–175.

43 Owman C, Rosenbren E, Sjöberg NO. 1967. Adrenergic innervation of the human female reproductive organs: a histochemical and chemical investigation. *Obstet Gynecol.* 30:763–773.

44 Palle C, Ottesen B, Jorgensen J, Fahrenkrug J. 1989. Peptide histidine methionine and vasoactive intestinal peptide: Occurrence and relaxant effect in the human female reproductive tract. *Biol Reprod.* 41:1103–1111.

45 Palle C, Bredkjaer HE, Ottesen B, Fahrenkrug J. 1990. Peptide histidine methionine (PHM) increases vaginal blood flow in normal women. *Peptides.* 11:401–404.

46 Palle C, Bredkjaer HE, Ottesen B, Fahrenkrug J. 1990. Vasoactive intestinal polypeptide and human vaginal blood flow: comparison between transvaginal and intravenous administration. *Clin Exp Pharmacol Physiol.* 17:61–68.

47 Papka RE, Cotton JP, Traurig HH. 1985. Comparative distribution of neuropeptide tyrosine, vasoactive intestinal peptide, substance P-immunoreactive, acetylcholinesterase-positive and noradrenergic nerves in the reproductive tract of the female rat. *Cell Tissue Res.* 242:475–490.

48 Cellek S, Moncada S. 1998. Nitrergic neurotransmission mediates the non-adrenergic non-cholinergic responses in the clitoral corpus cavernosum of the rabbit. *Br J Pharmacol.* 125:1627–1629.

49 Giraldi A, Persson K, Werkström V, *et al.* 2001. Effects of diabetes on neurotransmission in rat vaginal smooth muscle, *Int J Impot Res.* 13:58–66.

50 Kim NN, Min K, Pessina MA, *et al.* 2004. Effects of ovariectomy and steroid hormones on vaginal smooth muscle contractility. *Int J Impot Res.* 16:43–50.

51 Rosen RC, Phillips NA, Gendrano NC 3rd, Ferguson DM. 1999. Oral phentolamine and female sexual arousal disorder: A pilot study. *J Sex Marital Ther.* 25:137–144.

52 Meston CM, Gorzalka BB, Wright JM. 1997. Inhibition of subjective and physiological sexual arousal in women by clonidine. *Psychosom Med.* 59:399–407.

53 Meston CM. 2000. Sympathetic nervous system activity and female sexual arousal. *Am J Cardiol.* 86(Suppl):30F–34F.

54 Meston CM, Gorzalka BB. 1995. The effects of sympathetic activation following acute exercise on physiological and subjective sexual arousal in women. i. 33:651–664.

55 Angulo J, Cuevas P, Cuevas B, *et al.* 2003. Vardenafil enhances clitoral and vaginal blood flow responses to pelvic nerve stimulation in female dogs. *Int J Impot Res.* 15:137–141.

56 Cama E, Colleluori DM, Emig FA, *et al.* 2003. Human arginase II: Crystal structure and physiological role in male and female sexual arousal. *Biochemistry.* 42:8445–8451.

57 D'Amati G, di Gioia CR, Bologna M, *et al.* 2002. Type 5 phosphodiesterase expression in the human vagina. *Urology.* 60:191–195.

58 Min K, Munarriz R, Kim NN, *et al.* 2002. Effects of ovariectomy and estrogen and androgen treatment on sildenafil-mediated changes in female genital blood flow and vaginal lubrication in the animal model. *Am J Obstet Gynecol.* 187:1370–1376.

59 Pacher P, Mabley JG, Liaudet L, *et al.* 2003. Topical administration of a novel nitric oxide donor, linear poly-ethylenimine-nitric oxide/nucleophile adduct (DS1), selectively increases vaginal blood flow in anesthetized rats. *Int J Impot Res.* 15:461–464.

60 Park JK, Kim JU, Lee SO, *et al.* 2002. Nitric oxide-cyclic GMP signaling pathway in the regulation of rabbit clitoral cavernosum tone. *Exp Biol Med (Maywood).* 227:1022–1030.

61 Vemulapalli S, Kurowski S. 2000. Sildenafil relaxes rabbit clitoral corpus cavernosum. *Life Sci.* 67:23–29.

62 Park K, Moreland RB, Goldstein I, *et al.* 1998. Sildenafil inhibits phosphodiesterase type 5 in human clitoral corpus cavernosum smooth muscle. *Biochem Biophys Res Commun.* 249:612–617.

63 Traish A, Moreland RB, Huang YH, *et al.* 1999. Development of human and rabbit vaginal smooth muscle cell cultures: effects of vasoactive agents on intracellular levels of cyclic nucleotides. *Mol Cell Biol Res Commun.* 2:131–137.

64 Berman JR, Berman LA, Toler SM, *et al.* 2003. Safety and efficacy of sildenafil citrate for the treatment of female sexual arousal disorder: A double-blind, placebo controlled study. *J Urol.* 170:2333–2338.

65 Caruso S, Intelisano G, Lupo L, Agnello C. 2001. Premenopausal women affected by sexual arousal disorder treated with sildenafil: A double-blind, cross-over, placebo-controlled study. *BJOG.* 108:623–628.

66 Caruso S, Intelisano G, Farina M, *et al.* 2003. The function of sildenafil on female sexual pathways: A double-blind, cross-over, placebo-controlled study. *Eur J Obstet Gynecol Reprod Biol.* 110:201–206.

67 Laan E, van Lunsen RH, Everaerd W, *et al.* 2002. The enhancement of vaginal vasocongestion by sildenafil in healthy premenopausal women. *J Womens Health Gend Based Med.* 11:357–365.

68 Basson R, McInnes R, Smith MD, *et al.* 2002. Efficacy and safety of sildenafil citrate

in women with sexual dysfunction associated with female sexual arousal disorder. *J Womens Health Gend Based Med.* 11:367–377.

69 Kaplan SA, Reis RB, Kohn IJ, *et al.* 1999. Safety and efficacy of sildenafil in postmenopausal women with sexual dysfunction, *Urology.* 53:481–486.

70 Levin RJ. 1991. VIP, vagina, clitoral and periurethral glans – an update on human female genital arousal. *Exp Clin Endocrinol.* 98:61–69.

71 Ottesen B. 1983. Vasoactive intestinal polypeptide as a neurotransmitter in the female genital tract. *Am J Obstet Gynecol.* 147:208–224.

72 Ottesen B, Pedersen B, Nielsen J, *et al.* 1987. Vasoactive intestinal polypeptide (VIP) provokes vaginal lubrication in normal women. *Peptides.* 8:797–800.

73 Ziessen T, Moncada S, Cellek S. 2002. Characterization of the non-nitrergic NANC relaxation responses in the rabbit vaginal wall. *Br J Pharmacol.* 135:546–554.

74 Jorgensen JC, Sheikh SP, Forman A, *et al.* 1989. Neuropeptide Y in the human female genital tract: Localization and biological action. *Am J Physiol.* 257:E220–E227.

75 Jorgensen JC. 1994. Neuropeptide Y in mammalian genital tract: Localization and biological action. *Dan Med Bull.* 41:294–305.

76 Tenmoku S, Ottesen B, O'Hare MM, *et al.* 1988. Interaction of NPY and VIP in regulation of myometrial blood flow and mechanical activity. *Peptides.* 9:269–275.

77 Busse R, Trogisch G, Bassenge E. 1985. The role of endothelium in the control of vascular tone. *Basic Res Cardiol.* 80:475–490.

78 Brain SD, Grant AD. 2004. Vascular actions of calcitonin gene-related peptide and adrenomedullin. *Physiol Rev.* 84:903–934.

79 Berkley KJ, Hotta H, Robbins A, Sato Y. 1990. Functional properties of afferent fibers supplying reproductive and other pelvic organs in pelvic nerve of female rat. *J Neurophysiol.* 63:256–272.

80 Berkley KJ, Robbins A, Sato Y. 1993. Functional differences between afferent fibers in the hypogastric and pelvic nerves innervating female reproductive organs in the rat. *J Neurophysiol.* 36:533–544.

81 Kawatani M, Tanowitz M, de Groat WC. 1994. Morphological and electrophysiological analysis of the peripheral and central afferent pathways from the clitoris of the cat. *Brain Res.* 646:26–36.

82 Hilliges M, Falconer C, Ekman-Ordeberg G, *et al.* 1995. Innervation of the human vaginal mucosa as revealed by PGP 9.5 immunohistochemistry. *Acta Anat (Basel).* 153:119–126.

83 Sipski ML, Alexander CJ. 1993. Sexual activities, response and satisfaction in women pre- and post-spinal cord injury. *Arch Phys Med Rehabil.* 74:1025–1029.

84 Sipski ML, Alexander CJ, Rosen R. 2001. Sexual arousal and orgasm in women: effects of spinal cord injury. *Ann Neurol.* 49:35–44.

85 Whipple B, Komisaruk BR. 2002. Brain (PET) responses to vaginal-cervical self-stimulation in women with complete spinal cord injury: preliminary findings. *J Sex Marital Ther.* 28:79–86.

86 Whipple B, Gerdes CA, Komisaruk BR. 2004. Sexual response to self-stimulation in women with complete spinal cord injury. *J Sex Res.* 33:231–240.

87 Levin RJ, Both S, Georgiadis J, *et al.* 2016. The physiology of female sexual function and the pathophysiology of female sexual dysfunction (Committee 13A). *J Sex Med.* 13:733–759.

88 Jozkowski KN, Herbenick D, Schick V, *et al.* 2013. Women's perceptions about lubricant use and vaginal wetness during sexual activities. *J Sex Med.* 10:484–492.

89 Rosen R, Brown C, Heiman J, *et al.* 2000. The Female Sexual Function Index (FSFI): A multidimensional self-report instrument for the assessment of female sexual function. *J Sex Marital Ther.* 26:191–208.

90 Owen DH, Katz DF. 1999. A vaginal fluid simulant. *Contraception.* 59:91–95.

91 Levin RJ. 2003. A journey through two lumens! *Int J Impot Res.* 15:2–9.

92 Wagner G, Levin RJ. 1980. Electrolytes in vaginal fluid during the menstrual cycle of coitally active and inactive women. *J Reprod Fertil.* 60:17–27.

93 Salonia A, Giraldi A, Chivers ML, *et al.* 2010. Physiology of women's sexual function: Basic knowledge and new findings. *J Sex Med.* 7:2637–2660.

94 Levin RJ. 1997. Actions of spermicidal and virucidal agents on electrogenic ion transfer across human vaginal epithelium in vitro. *Pharmacol Toxicol.* 81:219–225.

95 Kim SO, Oh KJ, Lee HS, *et al.* 2011. Expression of aquaporin water channels in the vagina in premenopausal women. *J Sex Med.* 8:1925–1930.

96 Verkman AS. 2005. More than just water channels: unexpected cellular roles of aquaporins. *J Cell Sci.* 118:3225–3232.

97 Wang F, Feng XC, Li YM, *et al.* 2006. Aquaporins as potential drug targets. *Acta Pharmacol Sin.* 27:395–401.

98 Lee HS, Kim SO, Ahn K, Park K. 2016. All-trans retinoic acid increases aquaporin 3 expression in human vaginal epithelial cells. *Sex Med.* 4:e249–e254

99 Park K, Han HJ, Kim SW, *et al.* 2008. Expression of aquaporin water channels in rat vagina: Potential role in vaginal lubrication. *J Sex Med.* 5:77–82.

100 Gorodeski GI. 2007. Estrogen modulation of epithelial permeability in cervical-vaginal cells of premenopausal and postmenopausal women. *Menopause.* 14:1012–1019.

101 Spring KR, Hope A. 1978. Size and shape of the lateral intercellular spaces in a living epithelium. *Science.* 200:54–58.

102 Ussing HH, Zerahn K. 1951. Active transport of sodium as the source of electric current in the short-circuited isolated frog skin. *Acta Physiol Scand.* 23:110–127.

103 Oh KJ, Lee HS, Ahn K, Park K. 2016. Estrogen modulates expression of tight junction proteins in rat vagina. *Biomed Res Int.* doi: 10.1155/2016/4394702.

104 Ralevic V, Burnstock G. 1998. Receptors for purines and pyrimidines. *Pharmacol Rev.* 50:413–492.

105 Gorodeski GI, Hopfer U, De Santis BJ, *et al.* 1995. Biphasic regulation of paracellular permeability in human cervical cells by two distinct nucleotide receptors, *Am J Physiol.* 268:C1215–C1226.

106 Gorodeski GI. 2002. Regulation of transcervical permeability by two distinct P2 purinergic receptor mechanisms, *Am J Physiol.* 282:C75–C83.

107 Min K, Munarriz R, Yerxa BR, *et al.* 2003. Selective P2Y$_2$ receptor agonists stimulate vaginal moisture in ovariectomized rabbits. *Fertil Steril.* 79:393–398.

108 Gipson IK, Moccia R, Spurr-Michaud S, *et al.* 2001. The amount of MUC5B mucin in cervical mucus peaks at midcycle, *J Clin Endocrinol Metab.* 86:594–600.

109 Bachmann GA, Ebert GA, Burd ID. 1999. Vulvovaginal complaints. In: Lobo RA (ed) *Treatment of the Postmenopausal Woman: Basic and Clinical Aspects.* Philadelphia, PA: Lippincott Williams & Wilkins, pp. 195–201.

110 Park K, Ahn K, Lee S, *et al.* 2001. Decreased circulating levels of estrogen alter vaginal and clitoral blood flow and structure in the rabbit. *Int J Impot Res.* 13:116–124.

111 Park K, Ryu SB, Park YI, *et al.* 2001. Diabetes mellitus induces vaginal tissue fibrosis by TGF-β$_1$ expression in the rat model. *J Sex Marital Ther.* 27:577–587.

112 Sarrel PM, Wiita B. 1997. Vasodilator effects of estrogen are not diminished by androgen in postmenopausal women. *Fertil Steril.* 68:1125–1127.

113 Bachmann GA. The impact of vaginal health on sexual function. 1990. *J Clin Pract.* Sexual Special Issue:18–21.

114 Sarrel PM. 1998. Ovarian hormones and vaginal blood flow: using laser Doppler velocimetry to measure effects in a clinical trial of post-menopausal women, *Int J Impot Res.* 10(Suppl 2):S91–S93.

115 Dorfman RI, Shipley RA. 1956. *Androgens: Biochemistry, Physiology and Clinical Significance.* New York: Wiley.

116 Arlt W, Callies F, van Vlijmen JC, *et al.* 1999. Dehydroepiandrosterone replacement in women with adrenal insufficiency. *New Engl J Med.* 341:1013–1020.

117 Arlt W, Callies F, Allolio B. 2000. DHEA replacement in women with adrenal insufficiency: Pharmacokinetics, bioconversion and clinical effects on well-being, sexuality and cognition. *Endocr Res.* 26:505–511.

118 Davis SR, McCloud P, Strauss BJ, Burger H. 1995. Testosterone enhances estradiol's effects on postmenopausal bone density and sexuality. *Maturitas.* 21:227–236.

119 Davis SR, Burger HG. 1998. The rationale for physiological testosterone replacement in women. *Baillieres Clin Endocrinol Metab.* 12:391–405.

120 Greenblatt RB, Mortara F, Torpin R. 1942. Sexual libido in the female. *Am J Obstet Gynecol.* 44:658–663.

121 Munarriz R, Talakoub L, Flaherty E, *et al.* 2002. Androgen replacement therapy with dehydroepiandrosterone for androgen insufficiency and female sexual dysfunction: Androgen and questionnaire results. *J Sex Marital Ther.* 28(Suppl 1):165–173.

122 Sherwin BB, Gelfand MM, Brender W. 1985. Androgen enhances sexual motivation in females: a prospective, crossover study of sex steroid administration in the surgical menopause. *Psychosom Med.* 47:339–351.

123 Sherwin BB, Gelfand MM. 1987. The role of androgen in the maintenance of sexual functioning in oophorectomized women. *Psychosom Med.* 49:397–409.

124 Sherwin BB. 1991. The impact of different doses of estrogen and progestin on mood and sexual behavior in postmenopausal women. *J Clin Endocrinol Metab.* 72:336–343.

125 Shifren JL, Braunstein GD, Simon JA, *et al.* 2000. Transdermal testosterone treatment in women with impaired sexual function after oophorectomy. *N Engl J Med.* 343:682–688.

126 Shifren JL. 2004. The role of androgens in female sexual dysfunction. *Mayo Clin Proc.* 79(Suppl):S19–S24.

127 Schumacher M, Guennoun R, Mercier G, *et al.* 2001. Progesterone synthesis and myelin formation in peripheral nerves. *Brain Res Brain Res Rev.* 37:343–359.

128 Utian WH. 1989. Biosynthesis and physiologic effects of estrogen and pathophysiologic effects of estrogen deficiency: a review. *Am J Obstet Gynecol.*;161:1828–1831.

129 Pessina MA, Hoyt RF Jr, Goldstein I, Traish AM. 2006. Differential effects of estradiol, progesterone, and testosterone on vaginal structural integrity. *Endocrinology.* 147:61–69.

130 Berman JR, McCarthy MM, Kyprianou N. 1998. Effect of estrogen withdrawal on nitric oxide synthase expression and apoptosis in the rat vagina. *Urology.* 51:650–656.

131 Yoon HN, Chung WS, Park YY, *et al.* 2001. Effects of estrogen on nitric oxide synthase and histological composition in the rabbit clitoris and vagina. *Int J Impot Res.* 13:205–211.

132 Kim SW, Kim NN, Jeong SJ, *et al.* 2004. Modulation of rat vaginal blood flow and estrogen receptor by estradiol. *J Urol.* 172:1538–1543.

133 Traish AM, Kim SW, Stankovic M, *et al.* 2007. Testosterone increases blood flow and expression of androgen and estrogen receptors in the rat vagina. *J Sex Med.* 4:609–619.

134 Goetz RM, Morano I, Calovini T, *et al.* 1994. Increased expression of endothelial constitutive nitric oxide synthase in rat aorta during pregnancy. *Biochem Biophys Res Commun.* 205:905–910.

135 Hattori MA, Arai M, Saruwatari K, Kato Y. 2004. Estrogen regulation of nitric oxide synthesis in the porcine oocyte. *Mol Cell Biochem.* 260:13–19.

136 Hishikawa K, Nakaki T, Marumo T, *et al.* 1995. Upregulation of nitric oxide synthase by estradiol in human aortic endothelial cells. *FEBS Lett.* 360:291–293.

137 Weiner CP, Lizasoain I, Baylis SA, *et al.* 1994. Induction of calcium-dependent nitric oxide synthases by sex hormones. *Proc Natl Acad Sci USA.* 91:5212–5216.

138 Traish AM, Kim NN, Huang YH, *et al.* 2003. Sex steroid hormones differentially regulate nitric oxide synthase and arginase activities in the proximal and distal rabbit vagina. *Int J Impot Res.* 15:397–404.

139 Batra S, Al-Hijji J. 1998. Characterization of nitric oxide synthase activity in rabbit uterus and vagina: downregulation by estrogen. *Life Sci.* 62:2093–2100.

140 Healey A. 2012. Embryology of the female reproductive tract. In: Mann GS, Blair JC, Garden AS (eds) *Imaging of Gynecological Disorders in Infants and Children.* Berlin/ Heidelberg: Springer-Verlag. pp. 21–30.

141 Al-Hijji J, Batra S. 1999. Down regulation by estrogen of nitric oxide synthase activity in the female rabbit lower urinary tract. *Urology.* 53:637–641.

142 Al-Hijji J, Larsson B, Batra S. 2000. Nitric oxide synthase in the rabbit uterus and vagina: hormonal regulation and functional significance. *Biol Reprod.* 62:1387–1392.

143 Al-Hijji J, Larsson I, Batra S. 2001. Effect of ovarian steroids on nitric oxide synthase in the rat uterus, cervix and vagina. *Life Sci.* 69:1133–1142.

144 Ottesen B, Larsen JJ, Staun-Olsen P, *et al.* 1985. Influence of pregnancy and sex steroids on concentration, motor effect and receptor binding of VIP in the rabbit female genital tract. *Regul Pept.* 11:83–92.

145 Palle C, Bredkjaer HE, Fahrenkrug J, Ottesen B. 1991. Vasoactive intestinal polypeptide loses its ability to increase vaginal blood flow after menopause. *Am J Obstet Gynecol.* 164:556–558.

146 Goldstein I, Alexander JL. 2005. Practical aspects in the management of vaginal atrophy and sexual dysfunction in perimenopausal and postmenopausal women. *J Sex Med.* 2(Suppl 3):154–165.

147 Graziottin A, Leiblum SR. 2005. Biological and psychosocial pathophysiology of female sexual dysfunction during the menopausal transition. *J Sex Med.* 2(Suppl 3):133–145.

148 Min K, Munarriz R, Kim NN, *et al.* 2003. Effects of ovariectomy and estrogen replacement on basal and pelvic nerve stimulated vaginal lubrication in an animal model. *J Sex Marital Ther.* 29(Suppl 1):77–84.

149 Carlborg L. 1969. Comparative action of various oestrogenic compounds on mouse vaginal sialic acids II. *Acta Endocrinol (Copenh).* 62:663–670.

150 Galletti F, Gardi R. 1973. Effect of ovarian hormones and synthetic progestins on vaginal sialic acid in the rat. *J Endocrinol.* 57:193–198.

151 Nishino Y, Neumann F. 1974. The sialic acid content in mouse female reproductive organs as a quantitative parameter for testing the estrogenic and antiestrogenic effect, antiestrogenic depot effect, and dissociated effect of estrogens on the uterus and vagina. *Acta Endocrinol Suppl (Copenh).* 187:3–62.

152 Kennedy TG. 1974. Vaginal mucification in the ovariectomized rat in response to 5alpha-pregnane-3,20-dione, testosterone and 5alpha-androstan-17beta-ol-3-one: Test for progestogenic activity. *J Endocrinol.* 61:293–300.

153 Kennedy TG, Armstrong DT. 1976. Induction of vaginal mucification in rats with testosterone and 17beta-hydroxy-5alpha-androstan-3-one. *Steroids.* 27:423–430.

154 Sourla A, Flamand M, Belanger A, Labrie F. 1998. Effect of dehydroepiandrosterone on vaginal and uterine histomorphology in the rat. *J Steroid Biochem Mol Biol.* 66:137–149.

155 Kaleczyc J. 1994. Effect of estradiol and progesterone on noradrenaline content in nerves of the oviduct, uterus and vagina

in ovariectomized pigs. *Folia Histochem Cytobiol.* 32:119–126.

156 Rosengren E, Sjoberg NO. 1968. Changes in the amount of adrenergic transmitter in the female genital tract of rabbit during pregnancy. *Acta Physiol Scand.* 72:412–424.

157 Sjoberg NO. 1968. Increase in transmitter content of adrenergic nerves in the reproductive tract of female rabbits after oestrogen treatment. *Acta Endocrinol (Copenh).* 57:405–413.

158 Ting AY, Blacklock AD, Smith PG. 2004. Estrogen regulates vaginal sensory and autonomic nerve density in the rat. *Biol Reprod.* 71:1397–1404.

159 Clark JH, Peck EJ Jr. 1979. Female sex steroids: Receptors and function. *Monogr Endocrinol.* 14:I–XII, 1–245.

160 Mowa CN, Iwanaga T. 2000. Differential distribution of oestrogen receptor-alpha and -beta mRNAs in the female reproductive organ of rats as revealed by in situ hybridization. *J Endocrinol.* 165:59–66.

161 Chen GD, Oliver RH, Leung BS, *et al.* 1999. Estrogen receptor alpha and beta expression in the vaginal walls and uterosacral ligaments of premenopausal and postmenopausal women. *Fertil Steril.* 71:1099–1102.

162 Simon JA, Maamari RV. 2013. Ultra-low-dose vaginal estrogen tablets for the treatment of postmenopausal vaginal atrophy. *Climacteric.* 16(Suppl 1):37–43.

163 North American Menopause Society. 2007. The role of local vaginal estrogen for treatment of vaginal atrophy in postmenopausal women: 2007 position statement of The North American Menopause Society. *Menopause.* 14:355–369.

164 Skala CE, Petry IB, Albrich SB, *et al.* 2010. The effect of hormonal status on the expression of estrogen and progesterone receptor in vaginal wall and periurethral tissue in urogynecological patients. *Eur J Obstet Gynecol Reprod Biol.* 153:99–103.

165 Baldassarre M, Perrone AM, Giannone FA, *et al.* 2013. Androgen receptor expression in the human vagina under different physiological and treatment conditions. *Int J Impot Res.* 25:7–11.

# 9

# Psychological Management of Arousal Disorders

*Isbelia Segnini and Tuuli M. Kukkonen*

### Abstract

There are a number of psychosocial, relational, and contextual factors that impact female sexual arousal. Although there are no studies that establish causality, numerous significant correlational relationships exist and it follows that addressing these variables in evaluation and psychological treatment can help improve sexual functioning in women. For example, treatment of a female patient whose dysfunction stems from changes related to aging should have a different focus than that of a survivor of abuse. This chapter offers an exploration of the factors that affect sexual desire and arousal disorders in women, as well as tools available for diagnosis and treatment of sexual dysfunction.

**Keywords:**  *sexual desire; sexual arousal; arousal disorder; psychological treatment; psychological factors that impact sexual arousal; effects of partner dysfunction in women; relationship effects of erectile dysfunction; cognitive behavioral sexual therapy; treatment of sexual dysfunction; female sexual arousal*

---

Psychosocial, emotional, and partner factors that impact female sexual arousal.

Tools for assessment and diagnosis of dysfunction.

Comparison of common treatments of dysfunction.

---

## Introduction

During a woman's lifetime, the female sexual response is greatly influenced by both biological issues including hormonal, neurologic, and vascular factors, and by sociocultural factors. It follows then, that female sexuality depends on multiple elements, including those that govern couple relationships. As many of these variables as possible should be taken into account when evaluating a patient with a sexual health disorder.

Female sexual arousal was first measured by gynecologist William Masters and sexologist Virginia Johnson who conducted laboratory observations of sexual behaviors, including masturbation and intercourse [1]. They identified psychological and physiological aspects of sexual behavior, describing four main phases of the sexual response: excitement, plateau, orgasm, and resolution. One relevant finding was that, in women, an emotional component is of paramount importance. In other words, according to Masters and Johnson, women must be

*Textbook of Female Sexual Function and Dysfunction: Diagnosis and Treatment*, First Edition. Edited by Irwin Goldstein, Anita H. Clayton, Andrew T. Goldstein, Noel N. Kim, and Sheryl A. Kingsberg.
© 2018 John Wiley & Sons Ltd. Published 2018 by John Wiley & Sons Ltd.

emotionally involved in order to enter the first phase (excitement) [1].

In the 1970s, sex therapist Helen Singer Kaplan developed a three-phase model of the human sexual response: desire, excitement, and orgasm [2]. The innovation of this cognitive-physiological model was the inclusion of desire as the first stage. The incorporation of desire as a part of the sexual response provided the foundation for research in sexual function and dysfunction over almost 40 years. In 2013, the DSM-5 united the desire and excitement stages for the purposes of diagnosis of dysfunction, which gave rise to the present controversy on the topic [3].

Both Masters and Johnson's and Kaplan's models considered that arousal can begin with emotional and/or physical stimulation [1, 2]. This phase can last any length of time, from a few minutes to several hours. On the other hand, Basson described a new model of the human sexual response cycle [4]. She affirmed that, in women, there are reasons beyond plain sexual hunger to engage in sexual actions with a partner, such as to increase emotional closeness, attachment, and commitment. The cycle can be described as follows: (i) a woman begins in a neutral stage; (ii) she could wish an intimate contact or she could be responsive to a partner's proposition; (iii) this self-initiation or responsiveness enables an immediate biological and/or psychological response, which functions as a stimulus for sexual arousal [4].

The mental aspect of sexual arousal may be as important as the attention to genital vasocongestion and other physical sexual responses [4]. The awareness of desire and physical arousal induces a feedback loop that potentially increases the level of excitement. This leads to emotional and/or physical satisfaction, which could, in turn, augment the couple's level of emotional intimacy. Thus, the Basson model incorporates positive or negative experiences within the cycle to have an emotional impact on future encounters [4]. Nevertheless, it is important to emphasize that the Masters and Johnson model and

the Kaplan model remain valuable in understanding sexual responses in women. In two separate studies, that included 133 nurses in the United States and 429 women in Denmark, about two-thirds of the women in either population did not endorse the Basson model, favoring the Masters and Johnson or the Kaplan models [5, 6]. Further, in these nonclinical study samples, women who endorsed the Basson model tended to have lower scores on the Female Sexual Function Index (FSFI) [5, 6].

To conclude, sexual arousal in women involves multiple variables and stimuli, which provoke a physical and/or emotional response, leading to (further) sexual interactions between a woman and her partner. Additionally, female sexual function and dysfunction can impact a woman's self-esteem, well-being, and relationships. It is important to stress the role of biological, psychological, developmental and contextual elements, personal history, couple interaction, and partners' possible sexual dysfunction both in evaluation and treatment of possible dysfunction [7, 8].

## Etiology: Psychological Factors that Impact Sexual Arousal

The relationship between various psychological factors and female sexual arousal has been well established, albeit through correlational and self-report studies. In particular, research examining negative moods, anxiety and stress has demonstrated significant links to sexual dysfunction [9]. Less frequently studied has been the association between positive mood and sexual arousal. Laboratory induced positive moods have significantly increased subsequent self-reported sexual arousal to sexual stimuli, and pre-existing positive affect has also been shown to predict increased sexual arousal in a laboratory setting [10–13].

Additionally, a daily diary study in a sample of women found a bidirectional relationship between mood and sexual activity, with positive mood predicting next day sexual activity and sexual activity predicting next day lower levels of stress and negative mood [14]. Although the studies looking at general positive affect were conducted on women without sexual arousal difficulties, it is conceivable that examining and encouraging positive affect in women with arousal difficulties might be worthwhile.

## Depression

Various studies have examined the link between self-reported sexual functioning and depression and have found a significant relationship across different life stages. Higher levels of depression are associated with poorer sexual functioning in college-aged adults, pregnant, and postpartum women, as well as women in middle age and later stages of life [15–21]. Moreover, a nationally representative sample of over 31 000 respondents in the United States found that approximately 40% of women with sexual arousal disorders had comorbid depression and the link between depression and sexual functioning is maintained even when controlling for antdepressant medication use [22–24].

## Anxiety

In addition to depression, women's self-reported sexual functioning is also related to anxiety disorders [25, 26]. Specifically, women with anxiety disorders report significantly worse sexual functioning than those without anxiety disorders [27]. It is important to note, however, that moderate levels of anxiety in nonclinical populations have been shown to facilitate sexual arousal and interest [10, 17, 28, 29]. The degree of anxiety, therefore, and not just its presence, is likely relevant in the assessment of sexual arousal difficulties.

## Body Image

A number of other variables have been linked to poorer sexual functioning in women. Internal perceptions such as negative self-schemas and poor body image have been linked to lower sexual satisfaction and higher levels of sexual dysfunction [12, 30–34]. In a recent study examining 88 women between the ages of 18 and 25 years, Quinn-Nilas and colleagues found that poorer ratings on various body image scales significantly predicted lower levels of sexual arousal as measured by the FSFI. Specifically, body dissatisfaction and negative feelings about one's appearance were predictive of decreased ratings of sexual arousal. Further, they found that body image concerns specific to sexual encounters were the strongest predictor of arousal difficulties.

## Environmental Stressors

Environmental or external stressors, such as financial worries and work-related deadlines, are also associated with higher levels of sexual dysfunction [35–40]. For example, in a recent factor analysis on daily stressors in a sample of 246 participants, researchers found that financial stressors and stresses related to low socioeconomic status were significantly related to lower scores of sexual functioning in women [36].

## Culture and Religion

Furthermore, culture and attitudes towards sexuality can interact to predict sexual dysfunction. For example, in a study of East Asian and Euro-Canadian women, sexual conservatism was a significant predictor of sexual dysfunction in the East Asian sample of women but not the Euro-Canadian sample [41]. Religiosity can also impact sexual dysfunction, with one study of 223 women demonstrating that higher religious adherence was a significant risk factor for female sexual dysfunction [42]. Additionally, higher levels of sexual guilt and religiosity were significantly associated with lower levels of sexual desire in both Euro-Canadian and East Asian women [43], and higher levels of sexual guilt in general have also been found to be significantly related to lower levels of sexual arousal [44–46].

Although the large majority of studies examining factors that affect sexual functioning are conducted on women who identify as heterosexual, a comprehensive review of the literature suggests that many of the same variables are also important to the sexual functioning of women who have sex with women [47]. Factors such as age, religion, cultural recognition, relationship duration, sexual satisfaction, psychological well-being, and relationship satisfaction are similar to those found in heterosexual women. Additionally, there are a number of factors that might be unique to lesbian couples, such as internalized homonegativity, degree of being "out", power, and social support, that could indirectly impact the experience of sexual dysfunction [48].

## Relational Factors that Impact Sexual Arousal

Sexual dysfunction in men and women may be diagnosed and treated in isolation but it is more effectively addressed within the context in which it was acquired. Relationally-motivated sexual dysfunction in women could be a function of relationship commitment and duration, sexual abuse as a child or of a sexual dysfunction suffered by her partner, which can affect her emotional state during sexual arousal and/or interactions. In general, negative expectations related to sexual life can have a direct effect on how women will respond to sexual stimuli [48].

## Relationship Commitment and Duration

Marital gratification has an important role in sexual satisfaction and vice versa, especially in women. For example, if her partner has been unfaithful, a woman could feel angry or depressed, which may reduce sexual desire and arousal. Another potential reaction is low self-esteem, body image, and self-confidence, resulting in similarly decreased levels of arousal.

In clinical practice, women sometimes talk about communication differences between the sexes. They express difficulty understand-ing "how men can have sex almost every day and/or want sex after having an argument." In general, women prioritize levels of affection and intimacy rather than the frequency of coitus in their sexual encounters.

At the beginning of a relationship, new stimuli, context, and the process of getting to know each other incentivize frequent sexual contact for a couple. Over time, a lack of behavioral variation reduces intensity of feelings and less time is spent promoting intimacy, thus patient complaints are related to the routine, shorter precoitus time and lower quality of sexual play [49]. Marital satisfaction and duration of the relationship can thus profoundly affect a woman's capacity to feel and express arousal.

## Childhood Sexual Abuse

Female sexual function and dysfunction are greatly affected in different ways by the experience of sexual abuse. Multiple factors have to be accounted for when dealing with this type of occurrence: age, frequency and intensity of contact, the sociocultural context, body image, body-related esteem, mood, physical damage, relationship with the abuser, the appearance of violence, and kind of treatment received, if any. There are immediate, intermediate, and long-term consequences to emotional and physical sexual health, which can be rooted in any of the previously listed factors. For example, guilt associated with childhood sexual abuse is an immediate psychological outcome; lowered body esteem may be considered an intermediate consequence, which leads to the ongoing result of depression and sexual aversion or rejection.

Clinical experience shows that depression is a common consequence of sexual abuse. In a 2016 study, it was found that significantly more symptoms of depression were reported in those women with a history of childhood sexual abuse [50]. Additionally, lower body esteem was associated with sexual inhibition and decreased sexual excitement. Both clinical practice and research have found that cognitive and affective factors, such as guilt related to childhood sexual abuse, may result in a fear of or aversion to sexuality [11].

## The Effects of Partner Dysfunction in Women

Any sexual impairment present in an individual can affect both members of the couple. In that sense, clinicians should work as a multidisciplinary team in order to have the breadth of experience to provide an accurate diagnosis, as well as efficacious treatment to the patient and her partner. In this section, selected male sexual impairments and their effects on female sexual and emotional health are discussed, including: erectile dysfunction, premature ejaculation, delayed or absent ejaculation, and Peyronie's Disease. Each of these has a physical and emotional effect on the male half of the pair, but also on the female by impacting her self-esteem, emotional perception of sexual intercourse, and, ultimately, her response to future sexual stimulation whether or not she remains with the same partner.

- *Erectile dysfunction*: the arousal phase in men is manifested principally by the erection of the penis. Any chronic impairment can result in stress to the man, reducing his self-confidence, and straining the couple's relationship [51].
  - Immediate psychological effects for the woman include worry that she is not attractive enough for her partner to become completely aroused, that he is no longer in love with her, that he has found another (more attractive or adventurous) partner, or that he has been/become homosexual. "…She may feel lonely, emotionally abandoned…" [52].
  - Long-term psychological effects for the woman may include a decrease in arousal, as she feels that coitus will be impossible or intercourse will only last for a short time. She may focus all of her attention during sexual activities on her partner's erection rather than her own sexual feelings or needs. Lastly, a woman whose partner experiences erectile dysfunction may come to reject sexual propositions entirely out of her belief that "nothing would happen and/or both of us will be frustrated," thus sexual contact becomes "an ordeal to be endured" [52].
  - Long-term relationship effects of erectile dysfunction are largely negative. The stress experienced by the female partner results in magnification of the impact of the condition on the male partner. The male partner, in this case, may also decrease the frequency of propositions in response to the woman's apathy or disgust. This outcome places the relationship under ongoing strain.
- *Premature ejaculation*: sexual function as well as satisfaction is affected by premature ejaculation. This condition places stress and a feeling of personal distress on the man, which contributes to a deterioration of intimacy.
  - Immediate psychological effects for the woman include sexual dissatisfaction, the feeling that something is missing from the relationship, frustration that her wishes and needs are not met [52].
  - In the long term, one or both partners may intentionally reduce the time and scope of pre-intercourse activities, provoking chronic difficulties in arousal and excitement of the woman, and affecting her ability to reach orgasm during coitus. This can result in a female sexual dysfunction, such as hypoactive sexual desire disorder or anorgasmia.
  - Long-term relationship effects of premature ejaculation are mostly negative. Psychological stress of the man and woman may decrease overall relationship satisfaction.
- *Delayed or absent ejaculation*: a delay or absent ejaculation is the least understood and least studied male dysfunction [53]. In clinical practice, women express that "something is happening with her partner's

feeling toward her, because he has delayed or no ejaculation". This kind of condition can cause interpersonal problems and in some cases presents a barrier to fertility.

There may also be physical side effects for the woman – patients complain that the "time it takes for their partner inside the vagina makes it dry and sometimes the skin gets irritated, provoking pain even when lubricant is used."

- For the woman, immediate negative psychological effects are related to the pain caused during intercourse. Women who orgasm multiple times during intercourse or who need a longer time to become aroused are less likely to complain or suffer when their male partner experiences delayed or absent ejaculation.

- Long term, the pain of intercourse may motivate the woman to refuse a sexual proposition until her vaginal tissue has recovered or longer.

- The relationship effects of delayed or absent ejaculation generally depend on whether pain is experienced and its severity. As stated earlier, some women have complementary sexual needs or desires that may reward this condition.

- *Peyronie's disease*: several research studies have focused on the effect of Peyronie's disease on the female partner in a relationship. However, studies have found that the physical interference on sexual activity imposed by Peyronie's disease affects not only the diagnosed male but also his female partner [54, 55]. Female partners of men who received treatment for their penile curvature demonstrated improvement on all domains of the female sexual function index, as well as reporting global improvement in their sex lives and their relationships [55]. There may be a feeling of helplessness related to partner frustration and/or sadness connected to intimacy [16]. It is important that both partners discuss the condition in an open manner, which can reduce feelings of fear

or confusion regarding future sexual interactions.

- Immediate psychological effects on the female partner of a man suffering from Peyronie's disease are typically concerned with penetration impairment. As a consequence, there can be less connection and intimacy, low satisfaction, and sexual relationship withdrawal.

- In the long term, the female partner of a man with Peyronie's disease may experience diminished sexual function, mood, and satisfaction.

- Surprisingly, overall relationship satisfaction of couples was not significantly affected by Peyronie's disease.

## Health and Lifespan Considerations

At any given stage in life, there may be challenges that impact sexual arousal as seen from the various factors discussed previously. Individual, relational, and sociocultural variables can all impact a woman's sexual response and must be considered regardless of life stage in the assessment of sexual dysfunction. Additionally, there are certain health issues and lifespan considerations that have a higher risk for sexual dysfunction that may impact the type of treatment that is undertaken.

### Pregnancy

Pregnancy has consistently been linked to poorer sexual functioning in women [56–58]. One prospective study of 63 women demonstrated decreased sexual functioning, as measured on the female sexual function index, as pregnancy progressed and functioning continued to be poorer than at baseline six months postpartum. Other self-report studies have demonstrated that women in their third trimester had poorer sexual functioning than those in their first and second trimesters [58, 59]. Additionally, research examining postpartum sexual functioning demonstrated that nearly two-thirds of study respondents experienced sexual dysfunction within the first year postpartum and, of those, approximately half complained of sexual arousal difficulties [60]. Moreover, voluntary and medically necessary termination of pregnancy resulted in significantly poorer sexual functioning for women, with women undergoing voluntary termination being worse off [61]. Although mode of delivery (vaginal versus cesarean section) has not been found to significantly impact female sexual functioning overall, vaginal delivery is associated with significantly decreased scores on the sexual arousal domain of the female sexual function index [62, 63].

## Infertility

In addition to pregnancy, women struggling with infertility are at higher risk for sexual dysfunction than those without infertility [64, 65]. One case control study of 119 women with infertility and 99 healthy controls found that 40% of women with infertility met the criteria for sexual dysfunction on the female sexual function index, as compared to 25% of the control group. Their scores on the sexual arousal and desire domains were significantly lower. Furthermore, the women with infertility retrospectively indicated that their level of sexual functioning prior to their diagnosis was similar to that of healthy controls [65]. More recent research suggests that a lack of sexual interest or desire is the most common complaint for women undergoing *in vitro* fertilization [66].

## Aging and Menopause

Aging and going through the menopausal transition are significantly related to increased incidence of sexual arousal difficulties. The National Social Life, Health and Aging Project, which examined a probability sample of over 3000 individuals from the ages of 57–85 years, found that the incidence of sexual dysfunction increases significantly with age [66]. Additionally, across all age groups, women were less likely than men to be engaging in sexual activity and, for those who were, approximately half indicated that they had a sexual dysfunction that they found bothersome. A review of population-based studies found significant declines in sexual functioning associated specifically with the menopausal transition, with rates of reported dysfunction doubling from early to late menopause [67]. More recently, another community-based study of 3302 women aged 42–52 years found modest associations between reported sexual arousal and follicle stimulating hormone in this age group, suggesting that hormonal changes specific to menopause, and not just age, can contribute to arousal difficulties [68].

## Diabetes

There are numerous studies that suggest poorer sexual functioning in women with diabetes (both types 1 and 2) as compared to healthy controls [69, 70]; however, a recent meta-analysis suggests that other factors, such as levels of depression, body mass index and age are important variables that could be partially accounting for this relationship [71]. Pontiroli and colleagues included 26 studies in their meta-analysis with over 3000 diabetic women and found that although there was an increased risk for female sexual dysfunction in women with diabetes as compared to controls, this risk was restricted to premenopausal women. Furthermore, body mass index was the only independent variable to be associated with female sexual function scores, suggesting that when assessing female sexual dysfunction in women with diabetes, these other variables play an important role.

## Metabolic Syndrome

There are studies that have found a link between poor sexual functioning and metabolic syndrome in women [72–75]. A study examining postmenopausal women found that those with metabolic syndrome had significantly higher rates of female sexual dysfunction with worse scores on all domains of the female sexual function index as compared to women without metabolic syndrome [76]. Other studies, however, have not found this association. For example, in women with polycystic ovarian syndrome, body weight was not related to sexual functioning; rather, polycystic ovarian syndrome itself was associated with significantly poorer sexual arousal on the female sexual function index as compared to women without polycystic ovarian syndrome [77]. Additionally, studies comparing sexually active obese premenopausal women with healthy controls found no significant differences in the various domains of the female sexual function index [78, 79].

### Cancer

Sexual arousal difficulties are common in women with various cancers, although most research has focused on breast and gynecological cancers [80]. In general, estimates of female sexual arousal disorder range from 25 to 50%, depending on the type of cancer [81–84]. These difficulties with sexual arousal have been shown to persist long after treatment is terminated [85–87]. A recent study of 2178 adult female survivors of childhood cancer and 408 siblings found that the cancer survivors had significantly lower sexual functioning, including poorer sexual arousal, as measured on the sexual functioning questionnaire, than their siblings, even after controlling for various demographic variables [88].

## Assessment of Sexual Response

As discussed previously, there are many factors to be considered in order to accurately assess human sexual health. They may be subjective (quality of sexual encounters) or objective (frequency of defined sexual experiences). Patient psychological interviews and sexual histories are the predominant methods used to collect subjective data concerning patients' sexual health, while a variety of assessment tools exist to collect more objective data.

### Sexual History

Although there are no standardized clinical interviews to assess sexual response, guidelines for structuring the assessment typically recommend a biopsychosocial approach, whereby the clinician will obtain diagnostically relevant information in various domains [89–91].

This assessment should include information on the nature of the problem, the extent and the context in which it occurs, as well as a history of the presenting issue. Getting a sense of perceived impairment across every activity in which the problem is present can be useful to highlight whether there are variations or exceptions to the problem (e.g. Are the difficulties with sexual arousal consistent in partnered versus unpartnered activities? Are there some activities that seem less affected by the problem?). Understanding the history of the difficulty allows for the determination of a timeline (e.g. Has this difficulty always been present or has it developed over time? Were there periods in the patient's life where this problem was not present?) The degree of impairment across various domains of the patient's life is key to determining how intrusive this difficulty has become (e.g. Is the patient experiencing interruptions to work, social, and other nonsexual areas of functioning as a result of the arousal difficulties?). Additionally, it is essential that clinicians get a sense of the degree of distress within the individual as it relates to the problem, as well as the motivation to seek treatment at this particular time.

A more general sexual history should include background and current information on the various relational and psychosocial variables mentioned throughout this chapter (Table 9.1). Understanding relationship history, current relationship strengths and

**Table 9.1** Sexual history.

| | |
|---|---|
| Current sexual arousal issues | Sexual activities in which the problem does and does not occur (e.g. various partnered activities, masturbation, etc) |
| | History of the current problem |
| | Degree of perceived impairment |
| | Level of distress |
| | Any situations or factors that have improved sexual functioning |
| | Any previous treatments and degree of success |
| | Motivation for treatment |
| Biological factors | Age |
| | Medical conditions, surgeries, medical treatments |
| | Lifestyle |
| Psychosocial factors | Depression |
| | Anxiety |
| | Environmental stressors |
| | Attitudes towards sexuality |
| | Body image |
| | Culture, religion |
| | Previous trauma |
| Relational Factors | Relationship commitment and duration |
| | Partner support |
| | Partner dysfunction |
| | Couple communication |

struggles, and partner dysfunction will help determine the course of treatment. Any concurrent health (physical or psychological) conditions need to be taken into consideration, as well as medications that might be interfering with arousal (see Chapter 10 for additional information). Finally, psychosocial variables, cultural and religious background, as well as more general information on social location, can help determine extraneous variables that might influence treatment.

While a wide variety of assessment instruments exist to evaluate female sexuality, sex response, desire, and other elements of sexual health, none are concerned primarily nor exclusively with female arousal. Table 9.2 shows more information about arousal-dedicated items found in five well-known assessments.

## Nonpharmacological Treatments

Although there are a number of different lubricants and creams that have been employed to treat female sexual arousal disor-der, none have published studies supporting their long-term use. Topical lubricants, vitamin E, mineral oils, and creams can serve to augment lubrication during sexual activity. While they do not enhance vasocongestion or address underlying causes of female sexual arousal disorder, these treatments are relatively low risk and tolerated by patients across the lifespan and across different medical conditions. One study examining a botanical massage oil (Zestra) found that its use did lead to increased self-reported sexual arousal in both women with and without female sexual arousal disorder, although no physical measures of arousal were obtained [92]. Assessing patients for any allergies, skin sensitivities or medical contraindications is important prior to suggesting such treatments.

Another alternative to topical agents are suction devices used to increase blood flow to the genital area. The use of an EROS therapy device (NuGyn, Saint Paul, MN) has demonstrated improvement in female sexual function index scores [93, 94] and, more recently, a proof of concept study on Fiera (Aytu Women's Health LLC, Englewood, CO)

**Table 9.2** Common female sexual health assessment instruments and arousal-related items.

| Assessment instrument | Items that relate to female arousal |
| --- | --- |
| Brief Index of Sexual functioning (BISF-W) [106] | 5,13,14 |
| Sexual Functions Questionnaire (SFQ) [107] | 7,8,9,10,11,12,13,14 |
| Female Arousal and Desire Inventory (SADI) [108] | N/A* |
| Sexual Interest and Desire Inventory (SIDI) [109] | 11,12 |
| Female Sexual Functions Index (FSFI) [110] | 3,4,5,6 |

*The items are not numbered and all may apply to measurement of female arousal function and dysfunction.

has produced positive results in premenopausal women [95]. Finally, lifestyle improvements, such as the addition of exercise routines, can also improve sexual functioning in patients with comorbid medical conditions [96, 97].

## Psychological Treatment

In clinical practice, a basic principle for any kind of psychological treatment is to establish a trusting, empathetic, and respectful relationship with the patient. In treatment of sexual dysfunctions, it should also be common practice to individualize each patient and his/her partner to identify etiology and reach a more accurate diagnosis from a multidimensional model.

Any sexual dysfunction produces psychological distress and relationship difficulties that can stimulate performance problems and anxiety [98]. In order to prevent these negative outcomes, patients and their partners may require a baseline sexual education primer and the safety to express their needs and expectations. On the other hand, it is important to be aware that intimacy and a loving connection are essential elements in order to allow men and women to reach a functional, satisfactory, and (sexually) active relationship. Thus, the interrelation between a dysfunctional or unsatisfactory relationship and sexual difficulties can be unclear – at times, the relationship status is the cause, and sometimes it is the consequence [21].

Patients presenting any sexual dysfunction are typically requested to temporarily discontinue sexual relations in order to redirect attention from the issue. Instead, it is suggested that patients spend time cultivating intimate, nonsexual encounters to increase harmony and affective physical contact. It is also recommended, in some cases, to watch and read erotic materials and use sexual toys to stimulate sexual consideration.

Female arousal disorder is often associated with emotional distress related to sexual anxiety, poor couple interaction, sexual aversion, and/or pain before and/or during sexual contact.

### Cognitive Behavioral Therapy

The foundation of cognitive behavioral therapy is rooted in the role of cognitive factors in the way people react, feel, and behave. Thoughts, beliefs, ideas, and cognitive schema are developed during the learning years and persist throughout our lives. When these elements are negative, they constitute automatic thoughts, images, and feelings that interfere with sexual pleasure in both men and women. The objective of cognitive behavioral therapy is to identify the cognitive schema or beliefs for better understanding of the psychological processes. This implies: approach and revision of thoughts, identification and elimination of undesirable behaviors, and their substitution for desirable ones and positive communication. Through this technique, patients change their attitudes in a positive manner toward sex, making their sexual lives more pleasurable and focusing on the quality of their sexual relationships instead of other factors such as intercourse frequency [99]. The main tool in cognitive behavioral sexual therapy is maieutics – use of the Socratic method to question the patient, challenging her ideas, schema, and beliefs, with the final goal of modifying the cognitions in order to cause changes in her behavior [100].

## Mindfulness Therapy

Associated with ancient practices such as meditation, mindfulness has been used to treat chronic pain, stress, depression, and other ailments. It can be combined with cognitive behavioral therapy (discussed in the previous section), cognitive coaching, and other methods to achieve promising results [101]. Recent research has examined the integration of mindfulness as part of the treatment of sexual dysfunction in women following gynecological cancer [102], sexual distress, and a history of sexual abuse. In the last decade, mindfulness has also been incorporated into psychological treatments for desire/arousal disorders in women.

The objective of mindfulness therapy is awareness and acceptance of sensations, emotions, and thoughts, focusing one's complete attention on the present. A 2011 study by Silverstein *et al.* [103] affirms that the practice and mastery of this technique should carry benefits for overall patient well-being, but also allows the patient to recognize and experience all physical interoceptive and sexual signals during sexual encounters. This study confirmed that mindfulness training allows women to develop their ability to focus, reduce depression and anxiety, and improve their self-image and general satisfaction. As a consequence, women can attain consonance between physical and emotional responses, thus ameliorating female sexual arousal disorders.

## Couples' and Individual Therapy

Treatment of sexual dysfunction can be approached with varying etiologies – organic, psychological, or a combination of the two. Sex therapy is an important tool in the psychological treatment of arousal-related problems. Through this technique, clinicians evaluate underlying factors and triggers to a patient's arousal-related sexual dysfunction. However, as noted previously, arousal and other sexual dysfunctions affect both members of a couple and, thus, treatment may be appropriate for a single patient and/or for a patient and her partner. While patients may elect to attend sessions alone or with a partner before even beginning therapy, clinicians may also recommend that a patient coming in alone bring her partner or vice versa.

When Kaplan wrote *The New Sex Therapy*, she designed a set of exercises for the treatment of sexual dysfunctions based on Masters and Johnson's indications for sex therapy [1, 104]. In couples' therapy, the first recommendation is to stop sexual contact between partners in order to redirect mutual attention away from the dysfunction. During this stage, the couple is also given mutual massage exercises with no genital touching, which are meant to encourage focus on their bodies' sensations, increase good communication of sexual needs, and to allow the patients to give and receive pleasure without the expectation that "something has to happen." Ultimately, the goal is to help the patient and her partner feel comfortable with one another.

When the first goals are reached, the next couples' exercise includes genital contact without any evaluation of the physical response. In successive sessions, the physical contact includes coitus with no expectation of experiencing an orgasm. The objective is to have the patients concentrate on sensations, then share them with their partner. The final step is for the couple to have a complete sexual encounter, starting with sexual play. This exercise may incorporate any of those previously completed. The main objective is that both members of the couple feel comfortable and fulfilled throughout the experience.

In contrast, individuals' sex therapy begins with exploration of the patient's sexual history, then sexual education (as needed) and a program of exercises to be completed at home, in private. The goal of individual therapy is for the patient to resolve her sexual conflicts through self-knowledge of her body, sexual needs, and personal growth. Progress will allow her to express and communicate her sexual excitement and needs to her partner. Individual sex therapy is carried out through a customized treatment plan, which is designed in the first few sessions, while her background, sexual history, and complaints are introduced and explored. Weekly therapy sessions are recommended for the first few months.

The home exercises center around familiarizing the patient with her anatomy and the way that she experiences sensations [105]. When she is comfortable with her genitals, it is recommended that she touch them, with and without lubricant (in order to redirect attention from the amount of natural wetting). Female patients are directed to finish their exploration with or without an orgasm.

While couples' therapy removes undesirable sexual experiences and then reacquaints the patient and her partner sexually through structured mutual experiences, individuals' therapy focuses on empowering self-knowledge with education and does not recommend abstinence. In general, patients presenting with sexual dysfunction are recommended to begin with individual sex therapy (which may or may not include psychotherapy). Following that, if the patient has a partner, it becomes important to incorporate them into the therapeutic plan, as described above.

There may be cases when a woman's partner refuses to attend therapy because the dysfunction is perceived as 'her'

problem only. In these cases, it is still recommended that the therapist engage the partner. Successful efforts may offer the partner the opportunity to describe the patient's symptoms, then leading them to discuss their own reactions and impressions.

Potential treatments for arousal dysfunction in women must incorporate a wide variety of contextual elements. For example, the effects of dysfunction and those of intense relationship dissatisfaction are so similar that they can easily be mistaken for each other. However, the treatment options available, including combinations of cognitive behavioral therapy, mindfulness therapy, and traditional sex therapy, allow clinicians to tailor therapeutic plans to their patients' needs. In general, it is important to recognize that dysfunction may be diagnosed in a woman or her partner but that the most likely case is that both members of the pair suffer emotional and/or physical effects of the diagnosis.

## Conclusions

In summary, there are a number of psychosocial, relational, and contextual factors that impact female sexual arousal. Although there are no studies that establish causality, numerous significant correlational relationships exist and it follows that addressing these variables in therapy can help improve sexual functioning in women. Therapists must consider the factors discussed in this chapter in conjunction with medical conditions and any physiological findings (Chapter 10). Ultimately, a comprehensive biopsychosocial assessment and treatment plan will provide women with the most holistic approach to ameliorating their sexual arousal difficulties. Thus, diagnosis and treatment by a multidisciplinary team could be the best way to deal with a woman's sexual dysfunction.

# References

1 Masters WH, Johnson VE. *Human Sexual Response*. Boston: Little Brown; 1966, pp. 3–8.

2 Kaplan HS. *Disorders of sexual desire and other new concepts and techniques in sex therapy*. New York: Brunner/Mazel Publication; 1979, pp. 3–18.

3 American Psychiatric Association. *Diagnostic and Statistical Manual of Mental Disorders*, Fifth Edition. Arlington, VA, American Psychiatric Association: 2013, pp. 433–437.

4 Basson, R. Human sex-response cycles. *J Sex Marital Ther.* 2001;27:33–43.

5 Giraldi A, Kristensen E, Sand M. Endorsement of models describing sexual response of men and women with a sexual partner: an online survey in a population sample of Danish adults ages 20-65 years. *J Sex Med.* 2015;12:116–128.

6 Sand M, Fisher WA. Women's endorsement of models of female sexual response: the nurses' sexuality study. *J Sex Med.* 2007;4:708–719.

7 Parish S. Role of the primary care and internal medicine clinician. In: Goldstein I, Meston CM, Davis S, Traish A (eds) *Women´s Sexual Function and Dysfunction: Study, Diagnosis and Treatment*. London: Taylor and Francis Group; 2006, pp. 689–695.

8 Kang D, Ducharme S. Integration of medical and psychologic diagnosis and treatment. In: Goldstein I, Meston CM, Davis S, Traish A (eds) *Women´s Sexual Function and Dysfunction: Study, Diagnosis and Treatment*. London: Taylor and Francis Group; 2006, pp. 721–728.

9 Brotto LA, Blitzer J, Laan E, *et al*. Women's sexual desire and arousal disorders. *J Sex Med.* 2010;7:586–614.

10 Hodgson B, Kukkonen TM, Binik YM, Carrier S. Using the dual control model to investigate the relationship between mood, physiological and self-reported sexual arousal in men and women. *J Sex Res.* 2016;53:979–993.

11 Peterson ZD, Janssen E. Ambivalent affect and sexual response: The impact of co-occurring positive and negative emotions on subjective and physiological sexual responses to erotic stimuli. *Arch Sex Behav.* 2007;36:793–807.

12 McCabe MP, Giles K. Differences between sexually functional and dysfunctional women in childhood experiences and individual and relationship domains. *Int J Sex Health.* 2012;24:181–194.

13 Ter Kuile MM, Both S, van Uden J. The effects of experimentally-induced sad and happy mood on sexual arousal in sexually healthy women. *J Sex Med.* 2010;7:1177–1184.

14 Burleson MH, Trevathan WR, Todd M. In the mood for love or vice versa? Exploring the relations among sexual activity, physical affection, affect, and stress in the daily lives of mid-aged women. *Arch Sex Behav.* 2007;36:357–368.

15 Kalmbach DA, Ciesla JA, Janata, JW, Kingsberg SA. Specificity of anhedonic depression and anxious arousal with sexual problems among sexually healthy young adults. *J Sex Med.* 2012;9:505–513.

16 Kalmbach DA, Pillai V, Kingsberg SA, Ciesla JA. The transaction between depression and anxiety symptoms and sexual functioning: A prospective study of premenopausal, healthy women. *Arch Sex Behav.* 2015;44:1635–1649.

17 Lykins AD, Janssen E, Graham C. The relationship between negative mood and sexuality in heterosexual college women and men. *J Sex Res.* 2006;43:136–143.

18 Chang S-R, Ho H-N, Chen K-H, *et al*. Depressive symptoms as a predictor of sexual function during pregnancy. *J Sex Med.* 2012;9:2582–2589.

19 Chivers ML, Pittini R, Grigoriadis S, *et al*. The relationship between sexual functioning and depressive symptomatology in postpartum women: A pilot study. *J Sex Med.* 2011;8:792–799.

20  Laumann EO, Nicolosi A, Glasser DB, *et al*. Sexual problems among women and men aged 40–80 y: Prevalence and correlates identified in the Global Study of Sexual Attitudes and Behaviors. *Int J Impot Res*. 2005;17:39–57.

21  Shifren JL, Monz BU, Russo PA, *et al*. Sexual problems and distress in United States women: Prevalence and correlates. *Obstet Gynecol*. 2008;112:970–978.

22  Clayton AH, Montejo AL. Major depressive disorder, antidepressants, and sexual dysfunction. *J Clin Psychiatry*. 2006;67(Suppl 6):33–37.

23  Johannes CB, Clayton AH, Odom DM, *et al*. Distressing sexual problems in United States women revisted: Prevalence after accounting for depression. *J Clin Psychiatry*. 2009;70:1698–1706.

24  Montgomery SA, Baldwin DS, Riley A. Antidepressant medications: A review of the evidence for drug-induced sexual dysfunction. *J Affective Disorders*. 2002;69:119–140.

25  Brotto L, Klein C. Psychological factors involved with women's sexual dysfunctions. *Expert Rev Obstet Gynecol*. 2010;5:93–104.

26  Laurent SM, Sims AD. Sexual dysfunction in depression and anxiety: Conceptualizing sexual dysfunction as part of an internalizing dimension. *Clin Psych Rev*. 2009;29:573–585.

27  Dettore D, Pucciarelli M, Santarnecchi E. Anxiety and female sexual functioning: An empirical study. *J Sex Marital Ther*. 2013;39:216–240.

28  Bradford A, Meston CM. The impact of anxiety on sexual arousal in women. *Behav Res Ther*. 2006;44:1067–1077.

29  Lorenz T, Harte CB, Hamilton LD, Meston CM. Evidence for a curvilinear relationship between sympathetic nervous system activation and women's physiological sexual arousal. *Psychophysiology*. 2012;49:111–117.

30  Pujols Y, Meston CM, Seal BN. The association between sexual satisfaction and body image in women. *J Sex Med*. 2010;7:905–916.

31  Woertman L, van den Brink F. Body image and female sexual functioning and behavior: A review. *J Sex Res*. 2012;49:184–211.

32  Satinsky S, Reece M, Dennis B, *et al*. An assessment of body appreciation and its relationship to sexual function in women. *Body Image*. 2012;9:137–144.

33  Middleton LS, Kuffel SW, Heiman JR. Effects of experimentally adopted sexual schemas on vaginal response and subjective sexual arousal: A comparison between women with sexual arousal disorder and healthy women. *Arch Sex Behav*. 2008;37:950–961.

34  Quinn-Nilas C, Benson L, Milhausen RR, *et al*. The relationship between body image and domains of sexual functioning among heterosexual, emerging adult women. *Sex Med*. 2016;4:e182–e189.

35  Hamilton LD, Julian AM. The relationship between daily hassles and sexual function in men and women. *J Sex Marital Ther*. 2014;40:375–395.

36  Hamilton LD, Meston CM. Chronic stress and sexual function in women. *J Sex Med*. 2013;10:2443–2454.

37  Bodenmann G, Ledermann T, Blattner D, Galluzzo C. Associations among everyday stress, critical life events, and sexual problems. *J Nerv Ment Dis*. 2006;194:494–501.

38  Bodenmann G, Ledermann T, Bradbury T. Stress, sex, and satisfaction in marriage. *Personal Relationships*. 2007;14:551–569.

39  Bodenmann G, Atkins D, Schär M, Poffet V. The association between daily stress and sexual activity. *J Fam Psychol*. 2010;24:271–279.

40  Ter Kuile M, Vigeveno, D, Laan E. Preliminary evidence that acute and chronic daily psychological stress affect sexual arousal in sexually functional women. *Behav Res Ther*. 2007;45:2078–2089.

41  Morton H, Gorzalka BB. Cognitive aspects of sexual functioning: Differences between East Asian-Canadian and Euro-Canadian

women. *Arch Sex Behav.* 2013;42:1615–1625.

42  Perez AV, Sigler G, Genoves S. Female sexual function and related factors. *Aten Primaria.* 2006;15 339–344.

43  Woo JST, Morshedian N, Brotto LA, Gorzalka BB. Sex guilt mediates the relationship between religiosity and sexual desire in East Asian and Euro-Canadian college-aged women. *Arch Sex Behav.* 2012;41:1485–1495.

44  Cado S, Leitenberg H. Guilt reactions to sexual fantasies during intercourse. *Arch Sex Behav.* 1990;19:49–63.

45  Darling CA, Davidson JK, Passarello LC. The mystique of first intercourse among college youth: The role of partners, contraceptive practices, and psychological reactions. *J Youth Adolescence.* 1992;1:97–117.

46  Morokoff PJ. Effects of sex guilt, repression, sexual "arousability" and sexual experience on female sexual arousal during erotica and fantasy. *J Personality Social Psych.* 1985;49:177–187.

47  Armstrong HL, Reissing ED. Women who have sex with women: A comprehensive review of the literature and conceptual model of sexual function. *Sex Relation Ther.* 2013;28:364–399.

48  Giraldi A, Rellini AH, Pfaus J, Laan E. Female sexual arousal disorders. *J Sex Med.* 2013;1:58–73.

49  Moore D, Heiman J. Women´s sexuality in context: relationship factors and female sexual function. In: Goldstein I, Meston CM, Davis S, Traish A (eds) *Women´s Sexual Function and Dysfunction: Study, Diagnosis and Treatment.* London: Taylor and Francis Group; 2006, pp. 64–84.

50  Kilimnik C, Meston C. Role of body esteem in the sexual excitation and inhibition responses of women with and without a history of childhood sexual abuse. *J Sex Med.* 2016;13:1718–1728.

51  Metz M, McCarthy B. *Coping with Erectile Dysfunctions: How to Regain Confidence and Enjoy Great Sex.* Oakland, CA: New Harbinger Publications; 2004.

52  Metz M, McCarthy B. *Coping with Premature Ejaculation: How to Overcome PE, Please Your Partner and Have Great Sex.* Oakland, CA: New Harbinger Publications; 2003, pp. 21–24.

53  Perelman M. Understanding and treating retarded ejaculation: A sex therapist's perspective. International Society for Sexual Medicine, 2009. http://www.issm.info/news/review-reports/understanding-and-treating-retarded-ejaculation; last accessed 20 December 2017.

54  Davis S, Ferrar S, Sadikaj G, *et al.* Female partners of men with Peyronie's disease have impaired sexual function, satisfaction, and mood while degree of sexual interference is associated with worse outcomes. *J Sex Med.* 2016;13:1095–1103.

55  Goldstein I, Knoll LD, Lipshultz LI, *et al.* Changes in the effects of Peyronie's disease after treatment with collagenase Clostridium histolyticum: Male patients and their female partners. *Sex Med.* 2017;5:e124–e130.

56  Pauls RN, Occhino JA, Dryfhout VL. Effects of pregnancy on female sexual function and body image: A prospective study. *J Sex Med.* 2008;5:1915–1922.

57  Erol B, Sanli O, Korkmaz D, *et al.* A cross-sectional study of female sexual function and dysfunction during pregnancy. *J Sex Med.* 2007;4:1381–1387.

58  Serati M, Salvatore S, Siesto G, *et al.* Female sexual function during pregnancy and after childbirth. *J Sex Med.* 2010;7:2782–2790.

59  Esmer AC, Akca A, Akbayir O, *et al.* Female sexual function and associated factors during pregnancy. *J Obstet Gynecol Res.* 2013;39:1165–1172.

60  Khajehei M, Doherty M, Tilley PJM, Sauer K. Prevalence and risk factors of sexual dysfunction in postpartum Australian women. *J Sex Med.* 2015;12:1415–1426.

61 Dundar B, Dilbaz B, Karadag B. Comparison of the effects of voluntary termination of pregnancy and uterine evacuation for medical reasons on female sexual function. *Eur J Obstet Gynecol Reprod Biol.* 2016;199:11–15.

62 Eid Ma, Sayed A, Abdel-Rehim R, Mostafa T. Impact of the mode of delivery on female sexual function after childbirth. *Int J Impot Res.* 2015;27:118–120.

63 Lurie S, Aizenberg M, Sulema V, *et al.* Sexual function after childbirth by the mode of delivery: A prospective study. *Arch Gynecol Obstet.* 2013;288:785–792.

64 Millheiser LS, Helmer AE, Quntero RB, *et al.* Is infertility a risk factor for female sexual dysfunction? A case-control study. *Fertil Steril.* 2010;94:2022–2025.

65 Iris A, Aydogan Kirmizi D, Taner CE. Effects of infertility and infertility duration on female sexual functions. *Arch Gynecol Obstet.* 2013;287:809–812.

66 Lindau ST, SChumm P, Laumann EO, *et al.* A study of sexuality and health among older adults in the United States. *New Engl J Med.* 2007;357:762–774.

67 Dennerstein L, Alexander JL, Kotz K. The menopause and sexual functioning: A review of the population-based studies. *Ann Rev Sex Res.* 2012;14:64–82.

68 Randolph JF Jr, Zheng H, Avis NE, *et al.* Masturbation frequency and sexual function domains are associated with serum reproductive hormone levels across the menopausal transition. *J Clin Endocrinol Metab.* 2015;100:258–266.

69 Enzlin P, Rosen R, Wiegel M, *et al.* Sexual dysfunction in women with type 1 diabetes: Long-term findings from the DCCT/EDIC study cohort. *Diabetes Care.* 2009;32:780–785.

70 Enzlin P, Mathieu C, Van Den Bruel A, *et al.* Prevalence and predictors of sexual dysfunction in patients with type 1 diabetes. *Diabetes Care.* 2003;26:409–414

71 Pontiroli AE, Cortelazzi D, Morabito A. Female sexual dysfunction and diabetes: A systematic review and meta–analysis. *J Sex Med.* 2013;10:1044–1051.

72 Esposito K., Ciotola M., Marfella R, *et al.* The metabolic syndrome: A cause of sexual dysfunction in women. *Int J Impot Res.* 2005;17:224–226.

73 Esposito K, Ciotola M, Giugliano F, *et al.* Association of body weight with sexual function in women. *Int J Impot Res.* 2007;19:353–357.

74 Kolotkin RL, Binks M, Crosby RD, *et al.* Obesity and sexual quality of life. *Obesity.* 2006;14:472–479.

75 Miner M, Esposito K, Guay A, *et al.* Cardiometabolic risk and female sexual health: The Princeton III summary. *J Sex Med.* 2012;9:641–651.

76 Martelli V, Valisella S, Moscatiello S, *et al.* Prevalence of sexual dysfunction among postmenopausal women with and without metabolic syndrome. *J Sex Med.* 2012;9:434–441.

77 Benetti–Pinto CL, Ferreira SR, Antunes A, Yela DA. The influence of body weight on sexual function and quality of life in women with polycystic ovary syndrome. *Arch Gynecol Obstet.* 2015; 291:451–455.

78 Kadioglu P, Yetkin DO, Sanli O, *et al.* Obesity might not be a risk factor for female sexual dysfunction. *BJU Int.* 2010;106:1357–1361.

79 Adolfsson B, Elofsson S, Rossner S, Unden AL. Are sexual dissatisfaction and sexual abuse associated with obesity? A population-based study. *Obes Res.* 2004;12:1702–1709.

80 Jeffrey DD, Tzeng JP, Keefe FJ, *et al.* Initial report of the cancer Patient-Reported Outcomes Measurement Information System (PROMIS) sexual function committee: Review of sexual function measures and domains used in oncology. *Cancer.* 2009;115:1142–1153.

81 Huyghe E, Sui D, Odensky E, Schover LR. Needs assessment survey to justify establishing a reproductive health clinic at a comprehensive cancer center. *J Sex Med.* 2009;6: 149–163.

82 Tierney KD, Facione N, Padilla G, *et al.* Altered sexual health and quality of life in women prior to hematopoietic cell transplantation. *Eur J Oncol Nurs.* 2007;11:298–308.

83 McKee AL Jr, Schover LR. Sexuality rehabilitation. *Cancer.* 2001;92(4 Suppl):1008–1012.

84 Fobair P, Stewart SL, Chang SL, *et al.* Body image and sexual problems in young women with breast cancer. *Psycho-Oncol.* 2006;15:579–594.

85 Hayden PJ, Keogh F, Ni Conghaile M, *et al.* A single-centre assessment of long-term quality-of-life status after sibling allogeneic stem cell transplantation for chronic myeloid leukemia in first chronic phase. *Bone Marrow Transplant.* 2004;34:545–556.

86 Andersen BL, Woods XA, Copeland LJ. Sexual self-schema and sexual morbidity among gynecologic cancer survivors. *J Consult Clin Psych.* 1997;65:221–229.

87 Speer JJ, Hillenberg B, Sugrue DP, *et al.* Study of sexual functioning determinants in breast cancer survivors. *Breast J.* 2005; 11:440–447.

88 Ford JS, Kawashima T, Whitton J, *et al.* Psychosexual functioning among adult female survivors of childhood cancer: A report from the childhood cancer survivor study. *J Clin Oncol.* 2014;28:3126–3138.

89 Wincze JP, Carey MP. *Sexual Dysfunction: A Guide for Assessment and Treatment.* New York: Guilford Press; 2001.

90 Basson R. ClinicaL practice. Sexual desire and arousal disorders in women. *New Engl J Med.* 2006;354:1497–1506.

91 Meana M, Binik YM, Thaler L. Sexual dysfunctions. In: Hunsley J, Mash EJ (eds) *A Guide to Assessments that Work.* New York: Oxford University Press; 2008, pp. 464–487.

92 Ferguson DM, Steidle CP, Singh GS, *et al.* Randomized placebo-controlled, double-blind, crossover design trial of the efficacy and safety of Zestra for women with and without female sexual arousal disorder. *J Sex Marital Ther.* 2003;29:33–44.

93 Munarriz R, Maitland S, Garcia SP, *et al.* A prospective duplex Doppler ultrasonographic study in women with sexual arousal disorder to objectively assess genital engorgement induced by EROS therapy. *J Sex Marital Ther.* 2003;29(Suppl 1):85–94.

94 Schroder M, Mell LK, Hurteau JA, *et al.* Clitoral therapy device for treatment of sexual dysfunction in irradiated cervical cancer patients. *Int J Radiat Oncol Biol Phys.* 2005;61:1078–1086.

95 Goldstein S., Goldstein I., Millheiser L. The impact of Fiera™, a women's sexual health consumer product, on premenopausal genital engorgement as measured by thermography: A proof of concept study. *J Sex Med.* 2016;13(Suppl 6):S249–S250.

96 Karvinen KH, Courneya KS, North S, Venner P. Associations between exercise and quality of life in bladder cancer survivors: A population-based study. *Cancer Epidemiol Biomarkers Prev.* 2007;16:984–990.

97 Lorenz TA, Meston CM. Exercise improves sexual function in women taking antidepressants: Results from a randomized crossover trial. *Depress Anxiety.* 2014;31:188–195.

98 Althof S, Rosen R, Rubio-Aurioles R, *et al.* Psychological and interpersonal aspects and their management. In: Porst H, Buvat J (eds) *Standard Practice in Sexual Medicine.* International Society for Sexual Medicine. Massachusetts: Blackwell Publishing; 2006, pp 18–24.

99 McCabe M. Evaluation of a cognitive behavior therapy program for people with sexual dysfunction. *J Sex Marital Ther.* 2001;27:259–271.

100 Partarrieu, A. Diálogo Socrático en psicoterapia cognitiva. III Congreso Internacional de Investigación y Práctica Profesional en Psicología en XVIII Jornadas de Investigación Séptimo Encuentro de Investigadores en Psicología del MERCOSUR. Buenos Aires. 2011; https://www.aacademica.org/000-052/236.pdf; last accessed 31 December 2017.

101  Collard P. *La biblia del mindfulness: Una guía completa para reducir el estrés en tu vida. Edición en Castellano.* Hong Kong: Gaia Ediciones; 2015, pp. 64–79.

102  Brotto LA, Heiman JR. Mindfulness in sex therapy: Applications for women with sexual difficulties following gynecologic cancer. *J Sex Relationship Ther.* 2007;22:3–11.

103  Silverstein RG, Brown AC, Roth HD, Britton WB. Effects of mindfulness on body awareness to sexual stimuli: Implications for female sexual dysfunction. *Psychosom Med.* 2011;73:817–825.

104  Kaplan H. *The New Sex Therapy: Active Treatment of Sexual Dysfunctions.* New York: Brunner/Mazel, Inc. 1974.

105  Berman J, Berman L. *For Women Only: A Revolutionary Guide to Overcoming Sexual Dysfunction and Reclaiming Your Sex Life.* New York: Henry Holt and Company; 2001.

106  Taylor J, Rosen R, Leiblum S. Self-report assessment of female sexual function: Psychometric evaluation of Brief Index of Sexual Functioning for women. *Arch Sex Behav.* 2004;23:627–643.

107  Quirk FH, Heiman JR, Rosen RC, *et al.* Development of a sexual function questionnaire for clinical trials of female sexual dysfunction. *J Womens Health Gender Based Med.* 2002;11: 277–289.

108  Toledano R, Pfaus J. The Sexual Arousal and Desire Inventory (SADI): A multidimensional scale to assess subjective sexual arousal and desire. *J Sex Med.* 2006;3:853–877.

109  Clayton A, Leiblum S, Evans K, *et al. Sexual Interest and Desire Inventory.* Ingelheim Pharmaceuticals, Inc.; 2004.

110  Rosen R, Brown C, Heiman J, *et al.* The Female Sexual Function Index (FSFI): A multidimensional self-report instrument for the assessment of female sexual function. *J Sex Marital Ther.* 2000;26:191–208.

# 10

# Pathophysiology and Medical Management of Female Genital Arousal Disorder

*Irwin Goldstein*

### Abstract

Female genital arousal disorder is considered to be the inability to develop or maintain adequate genital responses, including vulvovaginal lubrication, engorgement of the genitalia, and sensitivity of the genitalia, associated with sexual activity and causes distress for a minimum of six months. Sexual arousal of genital tissues occurs, in part, secondary to the central nervous system processing of both physical and emotional stimuli before and during sexual activity. This enhanced neurologic activity in the sympathetic and parasympathetic autonomic nervous systems results in multiple central and peripheral physiological changes. Female cognitive arousal disorder is defined as difficulty or inability to attain or maintain adequate mental excitement associated with sexual activity as manifested by problems with feeling turned on, engaged, and/or mentally sexually aroused for a minimum of six months. Treatments include psychologic strategies, vaginal lubricants, and/or vaginal moisturizers, devices, local and systemic vasodilation agents, local and systemic hormones, systemic agonists to central nervous system excitatory neurochemicals and central nervous system antagonists to inhibitory neurochemicals, and neurologic interventions.

**Keywords:** *genital arousal; cognitive arousal; sympathetic hypogastric nerve; parasympathetic pelvic nerve; vaginal lubrication; clitoral engorgement; cardiovascular health; genitourinary syndrome of menopause; testosterone; estradiol; local and systemic vasodilation agents*

---

Peripheral genital arousal responses are associated with tumescence of the labia minora, vaginal introitus, glans clitoris, corpora cavernosa of the clitoral shaft and crura, periurethral glans including the urethral meatus, anterior vaginal wall structures including the periurethral region and prostatic tissue, and Halban's fascia.

Risk factors include cardiovascular and neurologic disorders.

Biological-based treatment strategies include vaginal lubricants and/or moisturizers, devices, vasodilation agents, hormone agents, systemic agonists or antagonists to central nervous system excitatory or inhibitory neurochemicals, neurological interventions.

---

*Textbook of Female Sexual Function and Dysfunction: Diagnosis and Treatment*, First Edition. Edited by Irwin Goldstein, Anita H. Clayton, Andrew T. Goldstein, Noel N. Kim, and Sheryl A. Kingsberg.
© 2018 John Wiley & Sons Ltd. Published 2018 by John Wiley & Sons Ltd.

## Physiology of Female Genital Arousal Responses

Sexual arousal of genital tissues in women occurs, in part, secondary to the central nervous system processing of both physical and emotional stimuli before and during sexual activity. This enhanced neurological activity in the sympathetic (hypogastric) and parasympathetic (pelvic) autonomic nervous systems results in multiple central and peripheral physiological changes [1–4].

Concerning central changes, increased sympathetic hypogastric efferent activity increases a woman's focus, wakefulness, and concentration. Sympathetic activation is associated with increases in heart rate, respiratory rate, and blood pressure. At the height of sexual arousal in women, just prior to orgasmic release, these physiological parameters may reach values as high as 120 beats/min for heart rate, 40/min for respiratory rate, and 180/120 mmHg for blood pressure [5].

Concerning peripheral changes, the increased parasympathetic nervous system efferent activity leads primarily to vasodilation of baseline arteriolar resistance within genital tissues, resulting in increased blood inflow to genital and some nongenital tissues. Classic, well-documented peripheral genital responses that are associated with sexual arousal in women depend, in part, on the integrity of the hypogastric-cavernosal arterial bed that perfuses the genital tissues to cause tumescence of: (i) the labia minora, (ii) the vaginal introitus, (iii) the glans clitoris and the corpora cavernosa of the clitoral shaft and clitoral crura, (iv) the periurethral glans including the tissue of the urethral meatus, (v) the anterior vaginal wall structures including the periurethral region and prostatic tissue, and (vi) Halban's fascia [3, 4, 6, 7].

Other sexual arousal physiological changes in women include vaginal lubrication, smooth muscle relaxation of the vaginal wall leading to lengthening and widening of the vaginal lumen, increased temperature of the engorged tumescent genitals that can be identified by thermography [8], and increased sensitivity of the genitalia to touch [3, 4, 6].

The increase in lubricating secretions in the vestibule and vagina include a combination of mucin released from androgen dependent minor vestibular glands and major vestibular Bartholin glands, and the prostate in the periurethral region of the anterior vaginal wall. Within the vagina, increased arterial blood flow results in a transudate of plasma that passes through water channels in the vaginal mucosa [3, 4, 6, 7].

During sexual arousal in women, the pelvic floor muscles initially relax but as sexual arousal increase and orgasm approaches, sympathetic hypogastric motor stimulation results in eventual rhythmic contraction of the pelvic floor muscles during orgasm [3, 4].

In addition, there are nongenital changes noted during sexual arousal in women. Extragenital arousal includes erection of the nipples, sensitivity of the skin of the ear lobes, fingers, wrists, thighs, buttocks, and flushing of the facial skin [3, 4].

Several different methodologies have been used to objectively measure the genital changes during sexual arousal in women, including heated oxygen electrode, infrared thermography, impedance plethysmography, vaginal photoplethysmography, color duplex Doppler ultrasonography, and magnetic resonance imaging (MRI) [3, 4].

## Subjective Component of Female Sexual Arousal

Sexual arousal in women may also include a central subjective awareness of the genital and extragenital changes. The presence or absence of genital sexual arousal may be either congruent or incongruent with the perceived subjective awareness of arousal. For example, genital arousal has been documented to occur in situations without any subjective enjoyment, such as in cases of sexual assault. In the context of sexual assault, subjective sexual arousal is not present, yet evidence of peripheral genital arousal may be present [9, 10]. The literature that supports the existence of female sexual arousal being considered as both genital and subjective subtypes is limited. Some investigations consider that vasocongestion and vaginal lubrication are perhaps evolutionary mechanisms, in part, to prevent vaginal injury during sexual activity, including unwanted sexual activities [11, 12].

## Nomenclature – Female Sexual Arousal Disorder (FSAD)

The International Society for the Study of Women's Sexual Health (ISSWSH) has developed new expert consensus definitions of female sexual arousal disorders. Female genital arousal disorder (FGAD) is considered to be the inability to develop or maintain adequate genital responses, including vulvovaginal lubrication, engorgement of the genitalia, and sensitivity of the genitalia, associated with sexual activity and causes distress for a minimum of six months. If the woman's difficulty with genital arousal is due to insufficient stimulation, then female genital arousal disorder should not be diagnosed. Subcategories of female genital arousal disorder are related to: (a) vascular injury or dysfunction and/or (b) neurological injury or dysfunction. Vulvovaginal infection/inflammation, vestibulodynia, and/or clitorodynia should be excluded before the diagnosis of female genital arousal disorder is made. This disorder is most often acquired and generalized, although there are unusual cases of lifelong female genital arousal disorder [13]. Female cognitive arousal disorder (FCAD) is defined as difficulty or inability to attain or maintain adequate mental excitement associated with sexual activity as manifested by problems with feeling turned on, engaged, and/or mentally sexually aroused for a minimum of six months.

Female genital arousal disorder is separate and distinct from other female sexual dysfunctions, such as hypoactive sexual desire disorder (HSDD), orgasm dysfunction, and/or

sexual pain disorders. In 2013, the DSM-5, released by the American Psychiatric Association, combined the diagnoses of the DSM-IV-TR definitions of female sexual arousal disorder (FSAD) with hypoactive sexual desire disorder [14, 15]. There are insufficient scientific data to consider that female genital arousal disorder and hypoactive sexual desire disorder are a single female sexual dysfunction entity. The ISSWSH Consensus definition of hypoactive sexual desire disorder highlights the differences and the interrelations between hypoactive sexual desire disorder and female genital arousal disorder [13].

## Risk Factors for Women with FGAD

Risk factors for female genital arousal disorder are categorized primarily as psychological, cardiovascular, neurological, and other such as anatomical changes that may occur after pelvic radiation and/or surgery [13].

Concerning cardiovascular integrity, the relationship between cardiovascular health and female genital arousal disorder was examined in the summary of the third Princeton Consensus conference [16]. This consensus document provides a review of the literature that shows that cardiovascular conditions, such as hypertension, hyperlipidemia, metabolic syndrome, obesity, diabetes, and coronary artery disease, increase the risk of female genital arousal disorder. Metabolic syndrome is a multifactorial disorder that includes concomitant impaired glucose tolerance/diabetes, central obesity, high triglycerides, low levels of high-density lipoprotein, and hypertension. This group of risk factors increases the relative risk for developing coronary artery disease, diabetes, stroke, and other health problems.

Concerning neurologic integrity, disorders that can adversely affect the central nervous system and peripheral nervous system, such as diabetes and multiple sclerosis, may also affect female sexual arousal. Pudendal neuropathy from multiple causes, such as childbirth or bicycling, can result in female genital arousal disorder [17]. Radiculopathy of the sacral spinal nerve roots from sacral spinal pathology (Tarlov cyst) or lumbar spinal pathology (annular tear, facet cyst, disc impingement, and spinal stenosis) can cause female genital arousal disorder [18].

Research findings suggest that excitation of the sympathetic hypogastric nervous system activation via exercise and sympathetic-activating medications may facilitate the early stages of female sexual arousal, while drugs that cause inhibition of the sympathetic hypogastric nervous system, may inhibit female sexual arousal and contribute to the symptoms of female genital arousal disorder [19, 20].

Anatomical changes associated with pelvic irradiation and/or pelvic surgery may cause damage to both small blood vessels and nerve endings and may result in female genital arousal disorder. Radiation therapy to the cervix can induce vaginal fibrotic anatomical changes that lead to female genital arousal disorder. Pelvic surgeries, including radical hysterectomy with or without irradiation, total abdominal hysterectomy, and pelvic organ prolapse surgery have been reported as causing female genital arousal disorder [21, 22].

## Endocrine Changes and Endocrine Risk Factors in Women with Female Genital Arousal Disorder

Estradiol and progesterone levels fall during perimenopause and menopause when ovulation eventually ceases. In contrast, total and free testosterone levels fall from the third to the fifth decade in premenopausal women. such that women in their 40s have about half the circulating levels of women in their 20s. Furthermore, in the late reproductive years there is failure of the mid-cycle rise in free testosterone that characterizes the menstrual cycle in young ovulating women. The levels of dehydroepiandrosterone sulfate and dehydroepiandrosterone also fall with increasing age. This may contribute significantly to the decline in total and free testosterone level with age, as dehydroepiandrosterone sulfate serves as a prehormone for about half of ovarian testosterone production [23–26].

Hormonal changes may play a pathophysiological role in younger women concerning inadequate sexual arousal based on inadequate blood flow to the sexually responsive organs. Estrogen influences vascular function via genomic and nongenomic mechanisms. Estrogen has direct effects on genital anatomy, enhancing peripheral blood flow and improving vaginal lubrication. Testosterone also appears to be important for vasomotor effects, enhancing vaginal blood flow and lubrication from effects that may be due to direct androgen actions or in part be due to estradiol biosynthesis from testosterone in the vascular bed. Research indicates that vaginal tissue may express a specific nuclear receptor for the androgen, $\Delta$5-androstenediol [27].

As long as women continue to regularly ovulate, estrogen and progesterone levels are maintained until the time of perimenopause. However, factors that interfere with cyclical sex steroid production, such as weight loss and anorexia nervosa, in which estrogen and progesterone levels may fall, will interfere with sex steroid levels. Androgen levels do decline with age from the young reproductive years; therefore, aging contributes to a decline in androgens [25, 26].

Hyperprolactinemia can result in hypogonadotrophic hypogonadism and loss of libido, and distress. Adrenal insufficiency is associated with reductions in dehydroepiandrosterone sulfate and free and total testosterone. Similarly, glucocorticosteroid excess, either endogenous or exogenous, leads to adrenal suppression and androgen insufficiency and, thus, may indirectly inhibit sexual function [26].

Traditionally, hormonal action has been understood as endocrine and paracrine. Labrie described intracrinology as the formation of active hormones that exert their action in the same cells in which synthesis took place without release into the pericellular compartment. Tissue sensitivity to androgens will vary according to the amount and activity of the enzymes 5α-reductase and aromatase that may vary considerably between individuals. Tissue responses may also vary, with subtle differences in individual receptors. Thus, even with highly sensitive assays for sex steroids the measurement of any sex steroids will provide only an indication of deficiency or excess, but not an absolute measure of tissue exposure or tissue sensitivity and responsiveness, and the clinical features will be the mainstay of diagnosis [28].

Because of its high affinity for sex hormone binding globulin, under normal physiological conditions in women only 1–2% of total circulating testosterone is free or biologically available. Elevations in estradiol, as occur during pregnancy, hyperthyroidism, and liver disease, cause a marked increase in sex hormone binding globulin levels, whereas hypothyroidism, obesity, and hyperinsulinemia are associated with decreased sex hormone binding globulin levels. In addition, oral administration of steroid hormones can alter sex hormone binding globulin levels whereas parenteral administration of these compounds, such as topical or intravaginal, typically has a much weaker influence on sex hormone binding globulin [29].

Standard doses of oral nonbiologically identical estrogen as used in the oral contraceptive pill will increase sex hormone binding globulin to values as much as 3–10 times the normal sex hormone binding globulin value. Use of the oral contraceptive pill results in additional hormonal changes, such as suppressed ovarian function, suppressed estradiol and progesterone levels, suppressed ovarian testosterone production, and low pituitary gonadotrophins [30, 31].

## Diagnosis of Women With Female Genital Arousal Disorder

Symptoms of female genital arousal disorder in menopausal women in the vulva, clitoris, vestibule, urethral meatus, and vagina are similar to symptoms of genitourinary syndrome of menopause (GSM or vulvovaginal atrophy). Ideally, adequate management of systemic and local genital sex steroid hormones, such as estradiol and testosterone, in women with genitourinary syndrome of menopause may result in symptom resolution [32].

The diagnosis of female genital arousal disorder is made primarily by history and physical examination. Even after adequate stimulation, women with female genital arousal disorder are distressed or bothered by such complaints as lack of: swelling of the labia and/or clitoral tumescence, vaginal lubrication, and/or increased sensitivity in genital tissues. Physical examination, especially using vulvoscopy, can be used to rule out the exclusionary conditions listed above, such as vulvovaginal infection/inflammation, vestibulodynia, and/or clitorodynia.

Laboratory testing that can be used to help establish a neurologic and/or vascular basis for female genital arousal disorder includes: quantitative sensory testing (biothesiometric, hot and cold perception testing) [18], sacral dermatome testing in the prone position over the gluteal, thigh, and calf regions (Sacral 1–4) using biothesiometry [18], bulbocavernosus reflex latency testing [18], pelvic floor electromyography, vaginal blood flow as measured by color duplex Doppler ultrasonography [33], vaginal blood flow using vaginal pulse amplitude during photoplethysmography [34], vascular resistance using impedance plethysmography, infrared thermography [8, 35], and heated vaginal electrode. The drawback of all these objective tests of neurologic and vascular integrity in women is the limited data on what values constitute absent FGAD and what values are consistent with female genital arousal disorder. In particular, for vaginal plethysmography the correlation between vaginal blood flow measures and verbal reports of arousal is poor.

Diagnostic questionnaires such as the female sexual function inventory (FSFI) have not been validated in this new female genital arousal disorder diagnosis/domain [36].

Women presenting with sexual arousal concerns should have routinely measured hormone blood tests. For example, thyroid stimulating hormone is indicated to assess for hypothyroidism or hyperthyroidism. Measurement of estradiol and follicle stimulating hormone is indicated especially to diagnose premature ovarian failure in amenorrheic women. Prolactin should be measured in the setting of oligomenorrhea, amenorrhea and/or galactorrhea. Free or bioavailable testosterone measures are the most reliable indicators of tissue testosterone exposure. Testosterone levels reach a nadir during the early follicular phase, with small but less significant variation across the rest of the cycle. Thus, blood should be drawn after day 8 of the cycle, and preferably before day 20 [37].

The gold standard methodology for measurement of free testosterone is considered by many investigators to be equilibrium dialysis. The Sodergard equation can be reliably used to calculate free testosterone if total testosterone, albumin and, sex hormone binding globulin are known. Measurement of free testosterone by analogue assays are unreliable and should not be used in clinical practice. The free androgen index [nmol/l total testosterone100/nmol/l sex hormone binding globulin] has been used as a surrogate for free testosterone, but it is unreliable when sex hormone binding globulin levels are low. The measurement of sex hormone binding globulin is relatively simple to perform with good reproducibility. Dehydroepiandrosterone is usually measured in the sulfated form, dehydroepiandrosterone sulfate, because the half-life is much longer, resulting in more stable levels. Dehydroepiandrosterone sulfate does not vary in concentration within the various phases of the menstrual cycle. There are published normal, age-related decline curves for dehydroepiandrosterone sulfate. If low levels are found, a morning cortisol level should be drawn to rule out adrenal insufficiency [38].

# Treatment of Women with Female Genital Arousal Disorder

## Psychological strategies

Concerning women with female genital arousal disorder who have accompanying psychological concerns, psychological management options, such as formal psychotherapy including sensate focus therapy, cognitive behavior therapy, and/or mindfulness therapy, can be considered as part of a broader biopsychosocial approach. Such strategies typically focus on adjusting feelings, attitudes, actions, sentiments, and relationship communication/behaviors that may be interrelated to the female genital arousal disorder state. Alternatively, more conservative approaches to lessen anxiety and improve symptoms if female genital arousal disorder may include yoga, massage therapy, and acupuncture [39–41].

## Vaginal Lubricants and/or Vaginal Moisturizer Strategies

For women with female genital arousal disorder, one treatment strategy is to try vaginal lubricants and/or vaginal moisturizers. Arousal disorder complaints in women with female genital arousal disorder typically include vaginal dryness, itching, irritation, and/or dysuria and are especially common in women with genitourinary symptoms of menopause (GSM) [32]. In women with female genital arousal disorder, the vulva, vestibule, and vagina may be quite sensitive to touch or to pressure application, such that the patient may have varying difficulties with any sexual contact or even with sitting, walking, or running. Specifically, vaginal intercourse or penetration including gynecologic speculum examination in a woman with female genital arousal disorder may become bothersome and uncomfortable.

Menopausal symptoms, especially vaginal dryness, itching, irritation, and dysuria, have traditionally been managed by a regimen of hormone replacement therapy. Hormone replacement therapy is, however, contraindicated with a history of breast cancer or a history of venous thromboembolic disease. In place of traditional hormone replacement therapy, there are several nonhormonal treatment strategies for the woman with female genital arousal disorder, such as nonhormonal moisturizers and lubricants, that can help with distressing symptoms of decreased arousal [42–44]. If use of moisturizers and lubricants does not provide sufficient symptom relief, patients may then consider other nonhormonal strategies, such $CO_2$ fractional lasers [45, 46], or even the use of local hormonal strategies that are not associated with clinically relevant increases in systemic hormone blood levels, such as local, low-dose estradiol (0.03%) and low dose testosterone (0.1%) applied daily directly to the vestibule and vagina.

Concerning the use of vaginal moisturizers as treatment of female genital arousal disorder, these are applied directly to the vaginal epithelium multiple times per week as a regular practice, independent of sexual activity. Vitamin E oil is an example of a vaginal moisturizer; Luvena is another example of a vaginal moisturizer that is free of parabens and glycerin [47]; these latter agents may increase the risk of vaginal Candida infections. Vaginal moisturizers appear to act by trapping moisture, hydrating vaginal tissues, and lowering vaginal pH levels. A lower vaginal pH level is more effective at controlling bacterial growth. Regular use of a vaginal moisturizer may be sufficient to reduce bothersome symptoms of decreased arousal, especially vaginal dryness, itching, and irritation, and enable vaginal intercourse/penetration [42–44].

Concerning the use of vaginal lubricants as treatment of female genital arousal disorder, these are applied as needed to the vaginal introitus to reduce friction and relieve symptoms of dryness and irritation during the sexual event. Vaginal lubricants may be either liquid or gel, and may be either water based or silicone based. Silicone-based lubricants clinically last longer than water-based vaginal lubricants. Silicone lubricants should not be used in conjunction with silicone vibrator or mechanical devices. Petroleum-based vaginal lubricants, such as petroleum jelly or oil-based vaginal lubricants, may damage latex condoms. It is suggested to avoid specific vaginal lubricants with perfumes or flavors, or with actions advertised as causing warmth or tingling, since these have little data concerning safety. It is further suggested to avoid specific vaginal lubricants that have ingredients such as parabens, or propylene glycol, or glycerin, as these may promote yeast infections. The simpler the list of ingredients in a vaginal lubricant, the more it is preferred. Examples of water-based vaginal lubricants intended for vaginal use include Good Clean Love and Slippery Stuff Paraben Free. Examples of silicone-based vaginal lubricants intended for vaginal use include Uberlube and Sliquid. Other options for vaginal lubricants intended for vaginal use include natural oils such as mineral oil, olive oil, emu oil, and coconut oil, but these can degrade the material in condoms [42–44, 48, 49].

## Device Strategies

Concerning the use of vibrator or nonvibrating mechanical devices as treatment of female genital arousal disorder, these have been shown to augment bothersome peripheral arousal symptoms. Vibrator and/or nonvibrating mechanical devices provide a vital nonhormonal, nonpharmacological treatment option and, thus, allow women with female genital arousal disorder to avoid drugs as a first-line strategy.

Herbenick *et al.* found that the more than half of women used vibrator or mechanical devices during sex activity [50, 51]. Vibrator devices generate vibration stimuli, via a series of pulses of electromagnetic waves of variable amplitude and frequency, to the peripheral dorsal, perineal, and/or external hemorrhoidal nerves, branches of the pudendal nerve that pass afferent sensory information to sacral roots S2, 3, 4. A-beta fibers, are the largest fibers within the peripheral nerves that mediate touch, mild pressure, sensation of joint position, and vibration.

Vibrators come in a variety of shapes and sizes, for internal use (typically phallic shaped) or external use (often with a loop attachment for use as a finger toy or mechanical ring). The rabbit vibrator comprises of a penetration shaft with an attached vibrating clitoral stimulator. Vibrator wands, such as the Hitachi Magic Wand, are large powerful vibrators that generally plug into an electrical outlet [52].

There are no safety regulations for the manufacture of vibrator or nonvibrating devices, as these are sold as novelties and do not require manufactures to adhere to regulations reporting the chemicals and materials used in the device. For example, a high level of phthalates, chemical plasticizers that help create the malleable and soft effect, and banned in children's toys, can be often be found in vibrator or nonvibrating devices. Brands that use silicone as their main material, like LELO and We-Vibe, have no phthalates. The patient with female genital arousal disorder should always check the ingredients in a device and avoid devices that contain PVC, vinyl and/or jelly rubber, and/or if the device has a rubber or chemical like odor. These vibrator devices have been shown to increase blood flow to genital tissues and increase temperature in these genital tissues. These vibrator devices also decrease the bothersome peripheral symptoms of low arousal in women with female genital arousal disorder [50–52].

A dildo is a nonvibrating device that is used for sexual stimulation of the vagina and/or anus. Dildos are generally made of silicone but can be made of other body safe materials, such as Titanium or clear medical grade borosilicate hard glass, that is nontoxic, able to withstand high physical forces without structural compromise, nonporous, and can even be put in the dishwasher, making them easy to clean [53].

Clitoral engorgement, which plays a vital function in sexual arousal in many women, can also be facilitated by use of mechanical vacuum clitoral engorgement devices. Such vacuum clitoral engorgement devices provide negative pressure suction to the glans clitoris, acting to enhance clitoral blood inflow and achieve a non-neurogenic mechanical clitoral engorgement. There are several devices that combine both various levels of vibratory stimulation to the clitoris, with vacuum engorgement to the clitoris, and achieve an enhanced clitoral engorgement. We recently investigated the degree of engorgement of the external genitalia, as measured by thermography, to a mechanical device (Fiera) that combined vibration and vacuum suction functions, and found a statistically significant increase in temperature in the labia, vestibule, and clitoris from baseline values. Of the participants, 92% endorsed the development of genital arousal [8].

## Local and Systemic Vasodilation Agents

There are no current government-approved topically applied or systemic arousal drugs for treatment of female genital arousal disorder. All pharmacologic agents, local or systemic, used to induce vasodilation in women with female genital arousal disorder are considered off-label.

Concerning the use of local vasodilating pharmacologic agents as treatment of female genital arousal disorder, the drug most widely studied in women's genital tissues has been prostaglandin $E_1$, a vasodilator that produces a rise in intracellular cyclic adenosine monophosphate (cAMP) and activation of protein kinase A. Prostaglandin $E_1$, unlike orally administered phosphodiesterase type 5 inhibitors, increases blood flow without the requirement for accompanying sexual arousal. Genital smooth muscle relaxation is induced by increased protein kinase A activity, so that in women with FGAD, application of prostaglandin $E_1$ can be predicted to result in local genital vasodilation and enhanced vestibular and vaginal lubrication [35]. Alprostadil, a synthetic form of PGE1, has been approved in men to treat erectile dysfunction using intracavernosal and intraurethral delivery systems, but alprostadil has never been shown to be effective in men as treatment for erectile dysfunction when used locally on penile skin.

Several studies have examined the use of alprostadil in the treatment of female genital arousal disorder. Becher *et al.* studied topical alprostadil on the clitoris using duplex Doppler sonography [54]. We evaluated using thermography as an assessment of genital blood flow the effect of topical alprostadil on the external genitalia compared with an over-the-counter (OTC) marketed lubricant. Compared to placebo, there was a statistically significant increase in temperature recorded in three different genital regions – the vulva, vestibule, and clitoris – in women not subjected to visual sexual stimulation. These differences occurred at different time points, with the most rapid difference occurring in the vulva. The increases in genital temperature and arousal occurred with no reported systemic or local adverse events.

The prime advantage of topical vasodilator vasodilation products is that these are not systemically delivered and, thus, would not be expected to be associated with the usual unwanted systemic side effects of orally administered vasodilator treatments, such as phosphodiesterase type 5 inhibitors. In clinical trials examining the safety of alprostadil in women with female genital arousal disorder, adverse events were classified as mild and were usually transient. These included local, topical reactions, such as vaginal itching and burning, which were likely related to the delivery base compound and not the active drug. Another advantage of topical vasodilatory agents is quick absorption yielding fast onset of action [35, 54, 55].

Concerning the use of systemic vasodilating pharmacologic agents as treatment of female genital arousal disorder, the drug class most widely studied in women has been phosphodiesterase type 5 inhibitors. Use of peripherally acting oral phosphodiesterase type 5 inhibitors has, however, yielded inconsistent results. One study found a significant improvement in arousal sensation and lubrication in women who received the oral phosphodiesterase type 5 inhibitor sildenafil versus placebo, whereas a large randomized double-blinded study of subjects with female genital arousal disorder found no significant responses in patients given the active sildenafil drug. Daily tadalafil, another oral phosphodiesterase type 5 inhibitor, studied in a small group of premenopausal women with type 1 diabetes with arousal difficulty, showed subjective sexual improvement versus placebo. Vardenafil, another oral phosphodiesterase type 5 inhibitor along with systemic testosterone caused an improvement in genital responses, as measured by vaginal photoplethysmography, in women with female genital arousal disorder. Oral phosphodiesterase type 5 inhibitors are associated with systemic side effects that deter treatment continuation, such as headache, flushing, nausea, rhinitis, and visual disturbances [56–60].

On-demand subcutaneously delivered bremelanotide, a centrally acting melanocortin receptor agonist, was used in the treatment of women with female genital arousal disorder and hypoactive sexual desire disorder and demonstrated significantly greater improvement in multiple outcome variables versus placebo. This agent has reported side effects of nausea, flushing, somnolence, and increases in blood pressure [61].

## Local and Systemic Hormone Agents

Concerning the use of local estrogen hormonal agents as treatment of dryness and discomfort, typically associated with genitourinary syndrome of menopause, these have been widely used and have received government approval especially for treatment of menopausal symptoms. Local estrogen hormonal agents should be considered if nonhormonal agents such as moisturizers and lubricants have not shown efficacy, and especially if other vulvar, vestibular, and vaginal pathologic conditions have been ruled out, such as infection, dermatologic conditions, vestibulodynia, or high tone pelvic floor disorders. Local vaginal estrogen therapy may then be considered a reasonable option and involves placing low-dose estrogen directly inside the vagina, to facilitate regrowth of vaginal epithelial lining, reducing the number of para-basal cells, increasing the number of glycogenated epithelial cells, and decreasing the vaginal pH, thus promoting hormonal-based angiogenesis in the lamina propria layer of the vagina and facilitating vaginal lubrication opportunity during sexual arousal [62–64].

There are several widely used, FDA-approved, local estrogen hormonal agent treatment options for patients with dryness associated with genitourinary syndrome menopause. Vaginal estrogen creams with either biological identical estradiol (Estrace), or conjugated equine estrogen (Premarin) are typically applied intravaginally daily for several weeks and then several times a week after that. Intravaginal estradiol rings can be used including Estring, a soft silicone ring that slowly releases estradiol into the local vaginal environment and needs to be replaced every three months. Intravaginal estradiol tablets (Vagifem) 10 mcg are small pills placed via a preloaded applicator, inside the vagina daily for several weeks, and then subsequently several times a week. Systemic estradiol blood test values are not relevantly increased with local cream, ring or pill-based delivery system, especially after the vaginal epithelium has regrown. Women who choose to use local vaginal estrogen therapy do not need to use concomitant progestogen to protect the uterus, as local estrogen does not seem to increase the risk of endometrial cancer. Research on the safety of vaginal estrogen in women with breast cancer is ongoing; studies, however, suggest that the amount of estrogen released is not likely to increase the risk of breast cancer recurrence [62–64].

Concerning the use of local testosterone hormonal agents in combination with local estradiol as treatment of genital discomfort or pain, these agents have been reported as most useful when applied to the vestibule, the site of endodermal embryology that is anatomically located between Hart's line and the hymen. Vestibular tissue has numerous androgen receptors and plays an important role in release of mucous from minor and major vestibular glands during sexual arousal. There are no FDA-approved testosterone products considered safe and effective for women with female genital arousal disorder. All local testosterone products are considered off-label. A typical dose to be applied to the vestibule daily is testosterone 0.1% and estradiol 0.03%, in a hypoallergenic base, in a pea-sized amount [65].

Concerning the use of systemic estrogen hormonal agents as treatment of dryness and discomfort, typically associated with genitourinary syndrome of menopause, there are many FDA-approved delivery systems, including oral pills, patches, gels, vaginal rings, and intramuscular injections. For women with a uterus, those who have not had a hysterectomy, concomitant use of progesterone will act to protect the endometrial lining of unopposed stimulation. The ideal goal of estradiol therapy is a value of approximately 35–50 pg/ml, the usual upper value of normal for many reference laboratories in menopause and values consistent with 8–10% of peak estradiol values in the reproductive years. Follow-up blood tests for estradiol should considered initially at three-month intervals and then as needed, such as every 6–12 months if stable. Side effects of estradiol treatment include breast pain, nipple discharge, and uterine bleeding. Usually, the dose of estradiol is decreased if side effects occur. Other side effects that need to be discussed include breast cancer and thromboembolic disease. If systemic estradiol treatment results in improvement of arousal function in women with female genital arousal disorder, the patient should consider staying on estradiol therapy for 6–12 months and taking a drug holiday from the treatment to see if the treatment is still required. In most cases, estradiol therapy is needed to maintain the arousal function improvement in women with female genital arousal disorder [66–68].

In 2013, the FDA approved ospemifene, a selective estrogen receptior modulator (SERM) as a safe and effective treatment for moderate to severe dyspareunia in menopause [69, 70].

Concerning the use of systemic testosterone hormonal agents as treatment of female genital arousal disorder, discussion should ensue as to the carefully monitored use of biologically-identical testosterone. There are no FDA-approved testosterone products for women, so the choices include off-label use of FDA-approved testosterone products for men dosed at approximately one-tenth of the intended male dose or off-label use of compounded testosterone products. Testosterone values diminish with age and testosterone may yet prove to be a useful therapy for female genital arousal disorder, especially in late premenopausal women. Data addressing systemic testosterone treatment of female genital arousal disorder in premenopausal women have relied primarily on observational data, and *in vitro* and *in vivo* animal models, with few published randomized placebo-controlled trials. Thus, at this time the use of testosterone therapy in premenopausal women with female genital arousal disorder remains controversial, as large multi-institutional placebo-controlled evidence for efficacy and safety in this population is limited at present [25, 71–73].

Potential adverse effects of testosterone therapy need to be considered, including hirsutism and acne, balding, voice deepening, and cliteromegaly. Other symptoms associated with exogenous androgen excess may include menstrual disturbances and polycythemia. There is no evidence that parenteral testosterone therapy has adverse cardiovascular effects. There is no evidence that exogenous testosterone increases the risk of endometrial cancer or endometriosis. Any woman with female genital arousal disorder treated with testosterone therapy needs to thoroughly counseled regarding contraception and risk of adverse effects on a fetus. Ongoing monitoring should include assessment for signs of androgen excess, regular breast and pelvic examination, monitoring of serum testosterone levels and in the presence of abnormal bleeding, endometrial biopsy [73, 74].

An ideal goal of testosterone therapy is a calculated free testosterone value of 0.6–0.8 ng/dl. Follow-up blood tests for total testosterone, sex hormone binding globulin, and dihydrotestoserone should initially be made at three-month intervals and then as needed, such as every 6–12 months if stable. The three choices of testosterone therapy include: daily topical products typically applied to the back of the calf; weekly intramuscular injections of testosterone, typically into the vastus lateralus; and 4–6 monthly testosterone pellets. A 75 mg testosterone pellet product is FDA-approved for men. Side effects of testosterone treatment typically are cosmetic and include increased facial hair, thinning of scalp hair, acne, and oily facial skin. Usually, the dose of testosterone is decreased if side effects occur. If testosterone treatment results in improvement of arousal function, the patient should consider staying on testosterone treatment for 6–12 months and taking a drug holiday from the treatment to see if the treatment is still required. In most cases, testosterone therapy is needed to maintain the arousal function improvement [73, 74].

## Systemic Agonists to Central Nervous System (CNS) Excitatory Neurochemicals and Central Nervous System (CNS) Antagonists to Inhibitory Neurochemicals

All pharmacological strategies for female genital arousal disorder management are considered off-label. Hypothetical off-label pharmacologicl strategies are based on using pharmacologic agents that are agonists to the excitatory neurochemicals of the central nervous system and are antagonists to the inhibitory neurochemicals in critical nuclei [75].

In female genital arousal disorder management, it is hypothesized that increasing central nervous system sexual excitatory processes with agonists of dopamine, oxytocin, and/or norepinephrine, or decreasing central nervous system sexual inhibitory processes with antagonists of opioid and/or serotonin would improve the genital arousal function in women with female genital arousal disorder.

Off-label pharmaceutical agonist agents potentially for female genital arousal disorder that may act on excitatory neurotransmitters in critical nuclei and the doses we recommend initially to women include: bupropion 75 mg/d in the morning; cabergoline 0.5 mg each Monday and each Thursday; ropinirole 0.25 mg one to three times a day; oxytocin lozenges 250 U sublingually – one hour prior to sexual activity; and/or amphetamine, dextroamphetamine mixed salts, 2.5–10 mg taken 30 minutes prior to sexual activity, but if taken after 2:00 p.m., difficulty with sleep should be considered [5].

Off-label pharmaceutical antagonist agents potentially for female genital arousal disorder that may act on inhibitory neurotransmitters in critical nuclei and the doses we recommend initially include: buspirone 10 mg BID, and/or naltexone 50 mg/d [75].

Off-label pharmaceutical agonist and antagonist agents potentially for female genital arousal disorder that may act on both excitatory and inhibitory neurotransmitters in critical nuclei include the use of flibanserin at a dose of 100mg/night. Flibanserin is a nonhormonal, centrally acting, postsynaptic serotonin 1A receptor agonist and a serotonin 2A receptor antagonist; it is classified as a multifunctional serotonin agonist and antagonist. Flibanserin use results in a decrease in serotonin activity and an increase in dopamine and norepinephrine activity. While flibanserin is currently an FDA-approved treatment for generalized acquired hypoactive sexual desire disorder in premenopausal women, studies have reported that all domains in the female sexual function index, including arousal function, are increased. To prescribe flibanserin, the health-care provider needs to be certified in the risk evaluation and mitigation strategy (REMS) program. Efficacy for libido improvement may not develop for up to 8–12 weeks; it is anticipated it is similar for the arousal function improvement.

## Neurologic Interventions

Concerning women with female genital arousal disorder from suspected reduced sensory information, some women state: "I cannot feel my vagina, I cannot feel my clitoris, and I cannot feel my labia when they are being touched". Such women may have a hypofunctioning sacral spinal nerve root (SSNR) radiculopathy within the cauda equina from various sacral and lumbar pathologies. Under such circumstances, neurogenital testing may help establish the loss of neurological integrity, abnormalities may be visualized on sacral and lumbar spine MRIs, and targeted epidural steroid injections show diminished female genital arousal disorder symptoms. It is hypothesized that female genital arousal disorder may occur as a manifestation of mechanical irritation of the genital sensory and possibly autonomic nerve roots, which could result in hypofunction of sacral spinal nerve roots. Our hypothesis is based, in part, on subsequent surgical reduction of the intervertebral discs, or surgical treatment of Tarlov cysts, that successfully alleviates the symptoms. Mechanical impingement of intervertebral discs on the cauda equina seems to be an etiological factor in certain cases of female genital arousal disorder [18].

## Conclusions

This chapter on female sexual arousal disorders first reviewed the physiology of female genital arousal responses and concluded that the peripheral genital arousal occurs secondary to the central nervous system processing of both physical and emotional stimuli before and during sexual activity. Eventually sexual arousal occurs because of enhanced and progressive neurologic activity in the sympathetic (hypogastric) and parasympathetic (pelvic) autonomic nervous systems that results in multiple central and peripheral physiological changes. Based on the current ISSWSH nomenclature, female genital arousal disorder is considered to be the inability to develop or maintain adequate genital responses, including vulvovaginal lubrication, engorgement of the genitalia, and sensitivity of the genitalia, associated with sexual activity, and causes distress, for a minimum of six months. Subcategories of female genital arousal disorder are related to: (i) vascular injury or dysfunction, and/or (ii) neurological injury or dysfunction. Female cognitive arousal disorder is defined as difficulty or inability to attain or maintain adequate mental excitement associated with sexual activity as manifested by problems with feeling turned on, engaged, and/or mentally sexually aroused for a minimum of six months. The risk factors for women with female genital arousal disorder include psychological, cardiovascular, neurological, and other factors such as anatomic changes that may occur after pelvic radiation and/or surgery.

## References

1 Pfaus J. Pathways of sexual desire. *J Sex Med.* 2009;6(6):1506–1533.

2 Holstege G. How the emotional motor system controls the pelvic organs. *Sex Med Rev.* 2016;4(4):303–328.

3 Levin R. VIP, vagina, clitoral and periurethral glans – an update on human female genital arousal. *Exp Clin Endocrinol.* 1991;98(2):61–69.

4 Levin R. Sex and the human female reproductive tract – what really happens during and after coitus. *Int J Impot Res.* 1998;10(Suppl 1):S14–S21.

5 Palmeri T, Kostis JB, Casazza L, *et al.* Heart rate and blood pressure response in adult men and women during exercise and sexual activity. *Am J Cardiiol.* 2007;100(12):1795–1801.

6 Levin R. Female orgasm: correlation of objective physical recordings with subjective experience. *Arch Sex Behav.* 2008;37(6):855.

7 Levin R. The pharmacology of the human female orgasm – its biological and physiological backgrounds. *Pharmacol Biochem Behav.* 2014;121:62–70.

8 Goldstein I, Goldstein S, Millheiser L. The impact of Fiera, a women's personal care device, on genital engorgement as measured by thermography: a proof-of-principle study. *Menopause.* 2017; 24(11):1257–1263. doi: 10.1097/GME.0000000000000912.

9 Laan E, Everaerd W, Evers A. Assessment of female sexual arousal: response specificity and construct validity. *Psychophysiology.* 1995;32:476–485.

10 Both S, Everaerd W, Laan E. Modulation of spinal reflexes by aversive and sexually appetitive stimuli. *Psychophysiology.* 2003;40:174–183.

11 Chivers M, Bailey JM. A sex difference in features that elicit genital response. *Biol Psychiatry.* 2005;70:115–120.

12 Levin R, van Berlo W. Sexual arousal and orgasm in subjects who experience forced or non-consensual sexual stimulation—a review. *J Clin Forensic Med.* 2004;11:82–88.

13 Parish SJ, Goldstein, AT, Goldstein, SW, *et al.* Toward a more evidence-based nosology and nomenclature for female sexual dysfunctions – Part II. *J Sex Med.* 2016;13(12):1888–1906.

14 American Psychiatric Association. Diagnostic and Statistical Manual of Mental Disorders IV, Text Revision (DSM-IV-TR). Washington DC: American Psychiatric Association; 2003.

15 American Psychiatric Association. Diagnostic and Statistical Manual of Mental Disorders, Fifth Edition: DSM-5. Arlington, VA: American Psychological Association.

16 Miner M, Esposito K, Guay A, *et al.* Cardiometabolic risk and female sexual health: the Princeton III summary. *J Sex Med*. 2012;9(3):641–651.

17 Popeney C, Ansell V, Renney K. Pudendal entrapment as an etiology of chronic perineal pain: Diagnosis and treatment. *Neurourol Urodyn*. 2007;26(6):820–827.

18 Goldstein I, Komisaruk BR, Rubin RS, *et al.* A novel collaborative protocol for successful management of penile pain mediated by radiculitis of sacral spinal nerve roots from Tarlov cysts. *Sex Med*. 2017; 5(3):e203–e211. doi: 10.1016/j. esxm.2017.04.001.

19 Meston C, Gorzalka BB. Differential effects of sympathetic activation on sexual arousal in sexually dysfunctional and functional women. *J Abnorm Psychol*. 1996;105(4):582–591.

20 Meston C. Sympathetic nervous system activity and female sexual arousal. *Am J Cardiiol*. 2000;86(2A):30F–4F.

21 Zhou W, Yang X, Dai Y, *et al.* Survey of cervical cancer survivors regarding quality of life and sexual function. *J Cancer Res Ther*. 2016;12(1):938–944.

22 Jensen P, Froeding LP. Pelvic radiotherapy and sexual function in women. *Transl Androl Urol*. 2015;4(2):186–205.

23 Davison S, Bell R, Donath S, *et al.* Androgen levels in adult females: changes with age, menopause, and oophorectomy. *J Clin Endocrinol Metab*. 2005;90(7):3847–3853.

24 Davis S, Davison, SL, Donath, S, Bell, RJ. Circulating androgen levels and self-reported sexual function in women. *JAMA*. 2005;294:91–96.

25 Davison S, Davis SR. Androgenic hormones and aging – the link with female sexual function. *Horm Behav*. 2011;59(5):743–753.

26 Wierman M, Nappi RE, Avis N, *et al.* Endocrine aspects of women's sexual function. *J Sex Med*. 2010;7(1):561–585.

27 Traish A, Huang YH, Min K, *et al.* Binding characteristics of [3H]delta(5)-androstene-3beta,17beta-diol to a nuclear protein in the rabbit vagina. *Steroids*. 2004;69(1):71–78.

28 Labrie F, Bélanger A, Pelletier G, *et al.* Science of intracrinology in postmenopausal women. *Menopause*. 2017;24(6):702–712.

29 Bachmann G, Bancroft J, Braunstein G, *et al.* Female androgen insufficiency: the Princeton consensus statement on definition, classification, and assessment. *Fertil Steril*. 2002;77(4):660–605.

30 Goldstein A, Burrows L, Goldstein I. Can oral contraceptives cause vestibulodynia? *J Sex Med*. 2010;7(4):1585–1587.

31 Panzer C, Wise S, Fantini G, *et al.* Impact of oral contraceptives on sex hormone-binding globulin and androgen levels: a retrospective study in women with sexual dysfunction. *J Sex Med*. 2006;3(1):104–113.

32 Portman D, Gass M, Kingsberg S, *et al.* Genitourinary syndrome of menopause: new terminology for vulvovaginal atrophy from the International Society for the Study of Women's Sexual Health and the North American Menopause Society. *Menopause*. 2014;21(10):1063–1068.

33 Maseroli E, Fanni E, Cipriani S, *et al.* Cardiometabolic risk and female sexuality: focus on clitoral vascular resistance. *J Sex Med*. 2016;13(11):1651–1661.

34 Rellini A, Meston C. The sensitivity of event logs, self-administered questionnaires and photoplethysmography to detect treatment-induced changes in female sexual arousal disorder (FSAD) diagnosis. *J Sex Med*. 2006;3(2):283–291.

35 Goldstein S, Gonzalez JR, Gagnon C, Goldstein I. Peripheral female genital arousal as assessed by thermography following topical genital application of alprostadil vs placebo arousal gel: a proof-of-principle study without visual sexual stimulation. *Sex Med*. 2016;4(3):e166–175.

36 Rosen R, Brown C, Heiman J, *et al.* The female sexual function index (FSFI): a multidimensional self-report instrument for the assessment of female sexual function. *J Sex Marit Ther*. 2000;26(2):191–208.

37 Polyzos N, Davis SR, Drakopoulos P, *et al.* Testosterone for poor ovarian responders: lessons from ovarian physiology. *Reprod Sci.* 2016. Epub Aug 3. doi: 1933719116660849.

38 Davis S, Panjari M, Stanczyk FZ. Clinical review: DHEA replacement for postmenopausal women. *J Clin Endocrinol Metab.* 2011;96(6):1642–1653.

39 Stephenson K, Kerth J. Effects of mindfulness-based therapies for female sexual dysfunction: a meta-analytic review. *J Sex Res.* 2017;15:1–18.

40 Brotto L, Krychman M, Jacobson P. Eastern approaches for enhancing women's sexuality: Mindfulness, acupuncture and yoga. *J Sex Med.* 2008;5(12):2741–2748.

41 Brotto L, Basson, R, Luria, M. A mindfulness-based group psychoeducational intervention targeting sexual arousal disorder in women. *J Sex Med.* 2008;5(7):1646–11659.

42 Stabile C, Goldfarb S, Baser RE, *et al.* Sexual health needs and educational intervention preferences for women with cancer. *Breast Cancer Res Treat.* 2017;165(1):77–84.

43 Edwards D, Panay N. Treating vulvovaginal atrophy/genitourinary syndrome of menopause: how important is vaginal lubricant and moisturizer composition? *Climacteric.* 2016;19(2):151–161.

44 Carter J, Goldfrank D, Schover LR. Simple strategies for vaginal health promotion in cancer survivors. *J Sex Med.* 2011;8(2):549–559.

45 Pitsouni E, Grigoriadis T, Tsiveleka A, *et al.* Microablative fractional $CO_2$-laser therapy and the genitourinary syndrome of menopause: An observational study. *Maturitas.* 2016;94:131–136.

46 Salvatore S, Leone Roberti Maggiore U, *et al.* Histological study on the effects of microablative fractional $CO_2$ laser on atrophic vaginal tissue: an ex vivo study. *Menopause.* 2015;22(8):845–849.

47 Costantino D, Guaraldi C. Preliminary evaluation of a vaginal cream containing lactoferrin in the treatment of vulvovaginal candidosis. *Minerva Ginecol.* 2008;60:121–5.

48 Hickey M, Marino JL, Braat S, Wong S. A randomized, double-blind, crossover trial comparing a silicone- versus water-based lubricant for sexual discomfort after breast cancer. *Breast Cancer Res Treat.* 2016;158(1):79–90.

49 Herbenick D, Reece M, Schick V, *et al.* Women's use and perceptions of commercial lubricants: prevalence and characteristics in a nationally representative sample of American adults. *J Sex Med.* 2014;11(3):642–652.

50 Herbenick D, Reece M, Sanders S, *et al.* Prevalence and characteristics of vibrator use by women in the United States: results from a nationally representative study. *J Sex Med.* 2009;6(7):1857–1866.

51 Leiblum S. Arousal disorders in women: complaints and complexities. *Med J Aust.* 2003;178(12):638–640.

52 Herbenick D, Barnhart KJ, Beavers K, Benge S. Vibrators and other sex toys are commonly recommended to patients, but does size matter? Dimensions of commonly sold products. *J Sex Med.* 2015;12(3): 641–645.

53 Anderson T, Schick V, Herbenick D, *et al.* A study of human papillomavirus on vaginally inserted sex toys, before and after cleaning, among women who have sex with women and men. *Sex Transm Infect.* 2014;90(7):529–531.

54 Becher E, Bechara A, Casabe A. Clitoral hemodynamic changes after a topical application of alprostadil. *J Sex Marit Ther.* 2001;27(5):405–410.

55 Kielbasa L, Daniel KL. Topical alprostadil treatment of female sexual arousal disorder. *Ann Pharmacother.* 2006;40(7–8): 1369–1376.

56 Nurnberg H, Hensley PL, Heiman JR, *et al.* Sildenafil treatment of women with antidepressant-associated sexual dysfunction: a randomized controlled trial. *JAMA.* 2008;300(4):395–404.

57 Gao L, Yang L, Qian S, *et al.* Systematic review and meta-analysis of

phosphodiesterase type 5 inhibitors for the treatment of female sexual dysfunction. *Int J Gynaecol Obstet.* 2016;133(2):139–115.

58 Caruso S, Cicero C, Romano M, *et al.* Tadalafil 5 mg daily treatment for type 1 diabetic premenopausal women affected by sexual genital arousal disorder. *J Sex Med.* 2012;9(8):2057–2065.

59 Brown D, Kyle JA, Ferrill MJ. Assessing the clinical efficacy of sildenafil for the treatment of female sexual dysfunctiob. *Ann Pharmacother.* 2009;43(7):1275–1285.

60 Alexander M, Rosen RC, Steinberg S, *et al.* Sildenafil in women with sexual arousal disorder following spinal cord injury. *Spinal Cord.* 2011;49(2):273–279.

61 Clayton A, Althof,SE, Kingsberg S, *et al.* Bremelanotide for female sexual dysfunctions in premenopausal women: a randomized, placebo-controlled dose-finding trial. *Womens Health.* 2016;12(3):325–337.

62 Simon J, Archer DF, Constantine GD, *et al.* A vaginal estradiol softgel capsule, TX-004HR, has negligible to very low systemic absorption of estradiol: Efficacy and pharmacokinetic data review. *Maturitas.* 2017;99:51–58.

63 Lethaby A, Ayeleke RO, Roberts H. Local oestrogen for vaginal atrophy in postmenopausal women. *Cochrane Database Syst Rev.* 2016;8:CD001500.

64 Santen R. Vaginal administration of estradiol: effects of dose, preparation and timing on plasma estradiol levels. *Climacteric.* 2015;18(2):121–134.

65 Burrows L, Goldstein AT. The treatment of vestibulodynia with topical estradiol and testosterone. *Sex Med.* 2013;1(1):30–33.

66 Rossouw J, Anderson GL, Prentice RL, *et al.* Risks and benefits of estrogen plus progestin in healthy postmenopausal women: principal results From the Women's Health Initiative randomized controlled trial. *JAMA.* 2002;288(3): 321–333.

67 Simon J. Identifying and treating sexual dysfunction in postmenopausal women: the role of estrogen. *J Women's Health.* 2011;20(10):1453–1465.

68 Nappi R, Polatti F. The use of estrogen therapy in women's sexual functioning. *J Sex Med.* 2009;6(3):603–616.

69 Wurz G, Kao CJ, DeGregorio MW. Safety and efficacy of ospemifene for the treatment of dyspareunia associated with vulvar and vaginal atrophy due to menopause. *Clin Interv Aging.* 2014;9:1939–1950.

70 Constantine G, Graham S, Portman DJ, *et al.* Female sexual function improved with ospemifene in postmenopausal women with vulvar and vaginal atrophy: results of a randomized, placebo-controlled trial. *Climacteric.* 2015;18(2):226–232.

71 Achilli C, Pundir J, Ramanathan P, *et al.* Efficacy and safety of transdermal testosterone in postmenopausal women with hypoactive sexual desire disorder: a systematic review and meta-analysis. *Fertil Steril.* 2017;107(2):475–482.

72 Kathryn Korkidakis A, Reid RL. Testosterone in women: measurement and therapeutic use. *J Obstet Gynaecol Can.* 2017;39(3):124–130.

73 Davis S. Androgen therapy in women, beyond libido. *Climacteric.* 2013;16 (Suppl 1):18–24.

74 Davis S, Worsley R, Miller KK, *et al.* Androgen treatment of postmenopausal women. *J Steroid Biochem Mol Biol.* 2014;142.

75 Belkin Z, Krapf JM, Goldstein AT. Drugs in early clinical development for the treatment of female sexual dysfunction. *Expert Opin Investig Drugs.* 2015;24(2):159–167.

11

# Pathophysiology and Medical Management of Persistent Genital Arousal Disorder

*Barry R. Komisaruk and Irwin Goldstein*

### Abstract

Persistent genital arousal disorder (PGAD), first described in 2001, is characterized by persistent or recurrent, unwanted or intrusive, distressing feelings of genital arousal or being in the verge of orgasm not associated with concomitant sexual interest, thoughts or fantasies. Prevalence ranges from about 0.5 to 6.7%. Patients with PGAD often exhibit catastrophizing behavior from the unremitting genital arousal, sometimes resorting to suicide. Treatment strategies focus on either disease modification designed to resolve underlying pathology causing abnormal sensory information passing to the brain, or symptomatic treatments designed to increase inhibition of abnormal information. A common cause of PGAD is sacral spinal nerve radiculopathy, from Tarlov cysts, herniated intervertebral discs or stenosis-induced chronic Cauda Equina Syndrome. It is hypothesized that PGAD might result from hyperactivity of sacral nerve roots. Surgical reduction of the intervertebral discs, or treatment of Tarlov cysts successfully alleviated the PGAD symptoms, supporting this hypothesis.

**Keywords:** *persistent genital arousal disorder (PGAD); unwanted feelings of clitoral engorgement; emotional lability; suicidality; compromised orgasm; overactive bladder; psychological stress; brain neurochemical imbalance; radiculitis of sacral spinal nerve root; Tarlov cyst*

---

Persistent genital arousal disorder is associated with despair, emotional lability, and/or suicidality.

Risk factors include abnormal psychological states, imbalance in brain excitatory and inhibitory neurochemicals; pelvic floor dysfunction; abnormal venous or arterial vascular issues; peripheral neuropathies, genital infections, genital dermatological conditions; radiculopathies of the sacral spinal nerve roots.

Treatments are either "disease modification treatment strategies" designed to resolve underlying pathology passing abnormal information to the brain or "symptomatic strategies" designed to increase central neurochemical inhibition reducing symptoms

---

## Introduction

Persistent genital arousal disorder was first described in 2001 [1] but remains an under-researched sexual medicine condition. The prevalence rate for persistent genital arousal disorder ranges from approximately 0.5 to 6.7% [2]. In a study of 1634 female college students, the prevalence of persistent genital arousal disorder was 1.5% [3]. Thus, hundreds of thousands of women in the United States are predicted to have this disorder. Persistent genital arousal disorder is a symptom-based condition

*Textbook of Female Sexual Function and Dysfunction: Diagnosis and Treatment*, First Edition. Edited by Irwin Goldstein, Anita H. Clayton, Andrew T. Goldstein, Noel N. Kim, and Sheryl A. Kingsberg.
© 2018 John Wiley & Sons Ltd. Published 2018 by John Wiley & Sons Ltd.

characterized by unwanted and intrusive feelings of peripheral sexual arousal that are not usually associated with objective evidence of peripheral sexual arousal [4]. There is a broad spectrum of patient complaints associated with persistent genital arousal disorder. Symptoms may last minutes to hours or days and may be intermittent or persistent. Sometimes the symptoms remit after orgasm(s). Sometimes nothing is associated with symptom relief. Several online questionnaire-based survey studies have confirmed the negative impact of persistent genital arousal disorder on psychological and sexual health [2, 5]. Patients with persistent genital arousal disorder often exhibit catastrophizing behavior from the unwanted and unremitting genital arousal [4], even resorting to suicide in several documented cases [6].

There are no known animal models of persistent genital arousal disorder and much of the knowledge concerning pathophysiology, diagnosis, and treatments of persistent genital arousal disorder in the peer-reviewed literature is in the form of case studies [7–19]. Consequently, researchers and clinicians have a limited understanding of the condition and its medical management. Multiple etiologies of persistent genital arousal disorder have been proposed and, as with many other sexual dysfunctions, it is likely that there are multiple pathophysiological causes that can result in the symptoms typically consistent with the condition.

Since 2001, multiple management strategies for persistent genital arousal disorder have been attempted but the condition has traditionally defied usual psychological and biological strategies for management of sexual dysfunctions. As a result, the focus of management has been on reducing the distressing bothersome and intrusive symptoms through the judicious use of oral medication that induces an increase in brain neurochemical inhibition and/or a reduction in brain neurochemical excitation [12, 17, 20, 21]. Despite continuing challenges, management of persistent genital arousal disorder has improved such that contemporary treatment strategies now more frequently result in the cure of the condition. Consistent with the perspective of multiple and independent etiologies for persistent genital arousal disorder, a wide range of psychological and physical treatments have been investigated with variable success rates, as reported in case studies, including: psychological therapy for persistent genital arousal disorder associated with mood concerns [10], pelvic floor physical therapy for high-tone pelvic floor dysfunction [14], discontinuing certain medications such as trazodone [16], hormone treatment for genitourinary syndrome of menopause (GSM), pudendal nerve blocks or trigger point injections or nerve entrapment surgery for pudendal neuropathy [22, 23], electroconvulsive therapy or transcranial magnetic stimulation [15, 24, 25], spine surgery such as resection of Tarlov cysts [26], endoscopic lumbar discectomy that resolves radiculitis of the sacral spinal nerve root [27], embolization of a pelvic arterial-venous malformation or of pelvic varicose veins for pelvic congestion syndrome [28], dorsal slit surgery and removal of keratin pearls for clitorodynia [29], and vestibulectomy for neuro-proliferative vestibulodynia [30].

## International Society for the Study of Women's Sexual Health (ISSWSH) Consensus Conference Nomenclature – Persistent Genital Arousal Disorder

As in the consensus reached by the ISSWSH Consensus Nomenclature Conference, persistent genital arousal disorder is characterized by persistent or recurrent, unwanted or intrusive, distressing feelings of genital arousal or being in the verge of orgasm (genital dysesthesia) not associated with concomitant sexual interest, thoughts or fantasies [4].

Persistent genital arousal disorder may be associated with:

- limited resolution, no resolution, or aggravation of symptoms by sexual activity with or without aversive and/or compromised orgasm in terms of impaired orgasm frequency, intensity, timing, and/or pleasure;
- aggravation of genital symptoms by certain circumstances (sitting, car driving, listening to music, general anxiety, stress or nervousness;
- despair, emotional lability, catastrophization and/or suicidality;
- inconsistent evidence of genital arousal on physical examination during symptoms (lubrication, swelling of clitoris or labia).

When persistent genital arousal disorder occurs concomitantly with complaints of overactive bladder and/or restless leg syndrome, it may be considered restless genital syndrome [48].

## Risk Factors and Clinical Etiology of Persistent Genital Arousal Disorder

Persistent genital arousal disorder is likely a symptom-based condition in which multiple pathophysiologies can result in the symptoms typically associated with the disorder [4]. Persistent genital arousal disorder may be associated with:

- psychosocial issues resulting in stress, worry, anxiety and/or panic [31]; examples in which psychosocial issues may result in increased persistent genital arousal disorder symptoms include: personal losses, unresolved marital conflict, traumatic relationship experiences, mood disorders, fatigue, emotional concerns, past trauma and abuse history, cultural and religious exclusions;
- psychiatric disorders including anxiety, panic and/or depressive disorders [10, 25, 32],

ingestion of certain medications such as trazodone, or abrupt discontinuation of medications such as selective serotonin reuptake inhibitors [12, 16, 19, 33];
- increased sexual excitatory processes in the central nervous system that involve dopamine, oxytocin, melanocortin, and norepinephrine, as well as decreased sexual inhibitory processes in the central nervous system that involve opioids, endocannabinoids, and serotonin [34];
- pelvic floor dysfunction, specifically high-tone pelvic floor dysfunction [14];
- abnormal venous or arterial vascular issues emanating from large pelvic varices associated with pelvic congestion syndrome [28] or from large pelvic arterio-venous malformations sending unrelenting arterial inflow to the clitoris [35];
- abnormal sensory information (neuropathy) from peripheral genital nerves (dorsal, perineal, inferior hemorrhoidal, pudendal, pelvic) associated with various peripheral pathologies such as: vestibulodynia, clitorodynia or genitourinary syndrome of menopause; injury to or irritation of the pudendal nerves that transmit pain and other sensations; abnormal response of tissues to Candida infection or allergy; dermatologic conditions such as lichen sclerosus or lichen planus; vulvar granuloma fissuratum; pathology of the peri-urethral glans; and bladder or rectal prolapse or rectal diverticulum [14, 22, 23, 29, 30];
- abnormal sensory information (radiculopathy) passing from sacral spinal nerve roots within the cauda equina from various sacral and/or lumbar pathologies such as Tarlov cysts [26, 36], disc impingement from annular tear, facet cyst, and/or spinal stenosis; abnormal sensory information from S2, S3 and S4 may then synapse in the conus medullaris and then ascend to the brain;
- abnormal sensation originating from central spinal cord pathology above the cauda equina that affects genital afferent activity.

Note that "sexual dysfunction" and "altered sensation of the genitals" are major characteristics of the "cauda equina syndrome" [37–39]. The cauda equina consists of the sensory and motor nerve roots of the sacral and lumbar dermatomes. The sacral dermatomes are innervated by the pudendal and pelvic nerves, which convey sensation from the clitoris, vagina, perineum and anal sphincter, and homologous genital components in men, which enter the sacrum at levels S2–S4. These nerves enter the sacrum, pass superiorly as individual nerve roots of the cauda equina and first synapse in the sacral division of the spinal cord proper (i.e. in the "conus medullaris"), which is typically located at vertebral level Thoracic 12, just below the lowest rib [40, 41, 42]. The cauda equina also contains lower lumbar nerve roots, which convey sensation from the feet, legs, and buttocks. Efferent sacral and lumbar nerve roots comprise part of the cauda equina, providing the parasympathetic and somatic motor innervation of the genital region and lower limbs.

As a result of this innervation pattern, irritation of, or damage to, the cauda equina by physical herniation/compression by one or more intervertebral discs (most commonly at L5–S1 or L4–L5) or other pathology such as inflammation, edema, displaced vertebra (spondylolisthesis), or a constellation of one or more of the following symptoms may occur (Figure 11.1): altered genital sensation, dyspareunia, reduced genital arousal, abnormal genital arousal (persistent genital arousal disorder), less intense orgasm, anorgasmia, decreased or absent penile/vaginal sensation, incontinence during intercourse, absent or reduced bulbocavernosus reflex, numbness, perineal ("saddle") burning sensation, sensory deficit or anesthesia, other lumbosacral root sensory deficits, lower extremity weakness, sensory deficit below the knee, leg reflex change, bladder or bowel incontinence or retention), altered urinary sensation, low back pain, and/or sciatica.

It is important to note that the pathology consistent with persistent genital arousal

**Pre-accident condition**

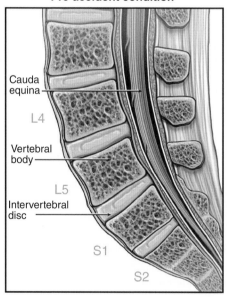

**Pre-operative condition**

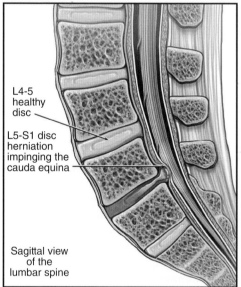

**Figure 11.1** Schematic representation of a herniated intervertebral disc at L5-S1 impinging on, and irritating, the nerve roots of the cauda equina. If the radiculitis affects the sacral spinal nerve roots (SSNR) various neurogenic sexual dysfunctions, such as persistent genital arousal disorder (PGAD), may be experienced. Several cures of men and women with PGAD secondary to radiculitis of the SSNR have been realized with minimally-invasive out-patient lumbar spine surgery. (*See plate section for color representation of the figure*)

disorder includes hyperstimulated sensory and/or motor function. Minimal mechanical irritation can have significant stimulatory effect on sensory nerves, as seen in the case of inducing a chronic pain and allodynia model in rats by placing a ligature of surgical thread loosely around the sciatic nerve. Thus, it seems plausible that even minimal mechanical impingement by a herniated intervertebral disc against the nerve fibers of the cauda equina could generate inflammation and/or edema and, thereby, stimulate genital awareness, hypersensitivity, and even hyperreflexivity, such as can occur in persistent genital arousal disorder [43–48].

## Diagnosis of Women with Persistent Genital Arousal Disorder

Women with persistent genital arousal disorder should undergo a thorough biopsychosocial history and physical examination, and laboratory tests. Diagnostic efforts should be made to identify if there are any reversible causes of persistent genital arousal disorder. In this case, modification of any reversible causes would be recommended prior to focus on the initiation of symptomatic therapeutic interventions for persistent genital arousal disorder. It should be noted that, for various reasons, some women with persistent genital arousal do not wish treatment and prefer to leave the persistent genital arousal condition untreated.

Potential diagnostic strategies for persistent genital arousal disorder symptoms, depending on the types of concerns, are:

- psychological: psychological assessment;
- psychiatric: referral to a psychiatrist or other mental health professional for appropriate psychiatric assessment;
- pelvic floor pathophysiologies: pelvic floor physical therapy assessment; for women with persistent genital arousal disorder who may be considered to have high-tone pelvic floor dysfunction, a diagnostic local

anesthesia nerve block to the specific suspected location (trigger point injection) may result in reduction of the persistent genital arousal disorder symptoms;
- medication-related pathophysiologies: a full history of medication use;
- abnormal sensory information passing from peripheral genital nerves associated with various peripheral pathologies: physical examination, including diagnostic procedures such as vulvoscopy, cotton swab (Q-tip) testing, and vaginal wet mount and smear testing should be performed to assess for such pathologies as lichen planus, lichen sclerosus, vulvar granuloma fissuratum and desquamative inflammatory vaginitis;
- endocrine disorders, such as elevated thyroid hormone: diagnostic blood testing may be performed to obtain baseline and then posttreatment values; these include: thyroid stimulating hormone (TSH), free triiodothyronine (free T3), total triiodothyronine (total T3), free thyroxine (free T4), and total thyroxine (total T4);
- vascular pathophysiologies, such as pelvic varices or pelvic arterio-venous malformations: physical examination may reveal lower extremities with vulvar varicose veins; pelvic ultrasound studies, CT or MRI examinations of the pelvis, and venography or selective arteriography may be considered.

Nerve blocks with steroids and local anesthetics to specific suspected locations may aid in the diagnosis of neuropathy of the dorsal nerve, perineal nerve, inferior hemorrhoidal nerve, or pudendal nerve if the injections result in marked reduction of the persistent genital arousal disorder symptoms. Similarly, diagnostic nerve blocks may also be used to confirm vestibulodynia (hormone-mediated, neuro-proliferative) or urethral meatal pathology (prolapse). Specifically for women with suspected hormone-mediated vestibulodynia or genito-urinary syndrome of menopause (vulvovaginal atrophy), diagnostic hormonal assessment should be considered by measuring serum values of testosterone, sex hormone binding globulin, calculated free testosterone, estradiol, progesterone, luteinizing hormone, follicle stimulating hormone, prolactin, and thyroid stimulating hormone.

Diagnostic neuro-genital tests (e.g. quantitative sensory testing, sacral dermatome testing, bulbocavernosus reflex latency testing, urodynamic testing) may be useful in diagnosing abnormal sensory information (radiculopathy) passing from central sacral spinal nerve roots *within* the cauda equina from various sacral and lumbar pathologies. Diagnostic MRI studies of the sacral and lumbar spine areas should further be considered. If a suspicious lesion is noted on MRI, a diagnostic epidural local steroid/anesthesia injection to the specific lesion that resulted in marked reduction of the persistent genital arousal disorder symptoms would provide evidence that the symptoms result from the lesion. If it is suspected that persistent genital arousal disorder symptoms may be due to abnormal sensory information (radiculopathy) passing from central sacral spinal nerve roots *above* the cauda equina, a reduction in symptoms after a targeted diagnostic epidural injection of analgesic or anesthetic would provide evidence of pathology of the nerve roots in the cauda equina (e.g. impingement by protruding intervertebral discs).

# Treatment of Women with Persistent Genital Arousal Disorder

There are two types of treatment for women with persistent genital arousal disorder. Firstly, disease modification treatment strategies are designed to resolve the underlying pathology or pathologies causing the abnormal sensory information eventually passing to the brain. Alternatively, when no curative strategies are identified or are feasible, symptomatic treatment strategies are considered to increase

inhibition of the abnormal information. This latter strategy can be used to therapeutically intervene in patients with persistent genital arousal disorder toward keeping the condition tolerable.

## Disease Modification Treatment Strategies for Persistent Genital Arousal Disorder

Potential therapeutic strategies for addressing conditions that may be causing or contributing to symptoms of persistent genital arousal disorder are outlined here.

- Psychological concerns: treatment strategies, such as formal psychotherapy, including sensate focus therapy, cognitive behavioral therapy, and/or mindfulness therapy, typically focus on modifying feelings, attitudes, actions, sentiments, and relationship communication/behaviors that may be causally related to the persistent genital arousal disorder condition [10]. More conservative strategies to reduce anxiety may include yoga and acupuncture.
- Psychiatric therapy: judicious use of psychiatric medications may help the persistent genital arousal disorder condition [12, 21]. These include such medications as: antidepressants, which address such different complaints as depression, dysthymia, anxiety disorders, eating disorders, and borderline personality disorder; antipsychotics, which address such psychotic complaints as schizophrenia and psychotic symptoms arising in the setting of other conditions such as mood disorders; anxiolytics, which address anxiety disorders; depressants, which are used as hypnotics and sedatives; and mood stabilizers, which address bipolar disorder and schizoaffective disorder.
- Pelvic floor pathophysiologies: pelvic floor physical therapy should be performed especially for women with high-tone pelvic floor dysfunction [14]. Adjunctive use of trigger point injections, vaginal or rectal

diazepam or baclofen, and/or intramuscular onabotulinum toxin A may result in reduction of the persistent genital arousal disorder symptoms.

- Medication-related pathophysiologies (e.g. trazodone): consider identifying strategies to eliminate the suspected medication [16].
- Endocrine pathophysiologies: for conditions such as hyperthyroidism, therapeutic methimazole should be considered.
- Vascular pathophysiologies: for pelvic varices or pelvic arterio-venous malformations, therapeutic embolization strategies by a vascular interventionalist should be considered [28, 35].
- Abnormal sensory information passing from peripheral genital nerves associated with various peripheral pathologies: consider therapeutic strategies related to the diagnosis.
- Clitorodynia: consider therapeutic release of clitoral adhesions or dorsal slit surgery with removal of keratin pearls [30].
- Neuropathy of the dorsal, perineal, inferior hemorrhoidal nerves and/or pudendal nerves: consider therapeutic local anesthesia combined with steroid blocks to the specific suspected location, therapeutic strategies such as transcutaneous electrical nerve stimulation (TENS) or neuromodulation through inferential stimulation (InterStim™, Medtronic) of the sacral nerves or specific targeting of the pudendal nerves [22, 49, 50].
- Hormonally-mediated vestibulodynia: consider therapeutic hormonal intervention such as systemic testosterone and/or local administration of testosterone/estradiol cream to the vestibule.
- Neuro-proliferative vestibulodynia: consider therapeutic complete vestibulectomy with vaginal advancement flap.
- Vestibulodynia related to suspected dermatologic conditions such as lichen sclerosus or lichen planus: consider therapeutic use of ultrapotent steroids.
- Prolapse of the urethral meatus: therapeutic reconstructive urethral prolapse repair.
- Vulvar granuloma fissuratum: consider therapeutic reconstructive posterior vestibulectomy with vaginal advancement flap.
- High-tone pelvic floor dysfunction: consider therapeutic pelvic floor physical therapy strategies with or without local skeletal muscle relaxants or onabotulinum toxin A injections.
- Abnormal sensory information passing from suspected central nervous system pathology *above* the cauda equina: consider neurosurgery strategies or electroconvulsive therapy.
- Abnormal sensory information (radiculopathy) passing from sacral spinal nerve roots *within* the cauda equina from various sacral and lumbar pathologies: consider minimally invasive endoscopic and navigational spine surgery [26].

In clinical experience, sacral spinal nerve radiculopathy is being increasingly appreciated as a common cause of persistent genital arousal disorder. More specifically, radiculopathy may result from Tarlov cysts and/or herniated intervertebral discs or stenosis-induced chronic cauda equina syndrome. It is hypothesized that persistent genital arousal disorder may occur as a manifestation of mechanical irritation of the genital sensory (and possibly autonomic) nerve roots, which could stimulate hyperactivity of sacral nerve roots. Our hypothesis is based in part on the attenuation of symptoms upon administration of epidural anesthesia within the spinal canal at the site of genital sensory nerve roots that are affected (e.g. impingement by intervertebral discs), as determined by MRI findings. Our hypothesis is also based on our experience of attenuation of symptoms by morphine-induced analgesia produced by intrathecal (i.e. direct subdural) injection at the conus medullaris (site of the first synapse of the genital sensory nerve roots). Further support of our hypothesis is provided by the attenuation of symptoms by subsequent surgical reduction of the intervertebral discs, or surgical treatment of

Tarlov cysts, which successfully alleviated the persistent genital arousal disorder symptoms.

Thus, we believe that persistent genital arousal disorder is a form of genital radiculopathy due to stimulatory irritation of the genital sensory nerve roots. We suggest that persistent genital arousal disorder be included as a subtype of the chronic form of cauda equina syndrome on the basis that mechanical impingement of intervertebral discs on the cauda equina seems to be a clear etiological factor in certain cases of persistent genital arousal disorder. Furthermore, "sacral spinal nerve radiculopathy" would seem to be a more general and inclusive terminology to characterize both Tarlov cyst-induced persistent genital arousal disorder and cauda equina irritation-induced persistent genital arousal disorder. This perspective is consistent with reports that surgical removal of the clitoris or uterus as a presumptive treatment for persistent genital arousal disorder did not result in relief of the disorder, and that this was incorrectly perceived as persistent arousal originating in the "phantom" organ [50]. Evidently, the phenomenon would be better explained, in those cases, by recognition that the pathology was "upstream", affecting the sensory nerves proximal to the genitals *per se*, and only perceived by the patient as originating in the genitals. The present clinical experience provides an hypothesis that for effective curative treatment of persistent genital arousal disorder, "sacral spinal nerve radiculopathy" should be considered as a specific neuropathic etiology [36–41, 43–48].

### Symptomatic Treatment Strategies for Persistent Genital Arousal Disorder

Symptomatic therapeutic strategies for persistent genital arousal disorder are based on pharmacologic agents that can increase inhibition of the response to the abnormal sensory activity. This option can be used to therapeutically intervene toward keeping the condition manageable and tolerable. To achieve increased inhibition of abnormal sensory information, pharmacologic agents that decrease neurotransmission should be considered. These agents may include tricyclic antidepressants, calcium channel blocking agents, and anticonvulsants. Also, pharmacologic agents that decrease dopamine action, such as vareniclene tartrate [17], or that potentiate the action of serotonin, should be considered. These agents may include selective serotonin reuptake inhibitors and/or serotonin and norepinephrine reuptake inhibitors. Opioid agonist pharmacologic agents should also be considered. We recently reported that zolpidem, a nonbenzodiazepine indirect gamma-aminobutyric acidA receptor agonist that potentiates GABA release by modifying the benzodiazepine binding site, can be effective in reducing persistent genital arousal disorder symptoms [20].

### Conclusion

Persistent genital arousal disorder is an uncommon sexual pathology that has been recognized for the first time in the ISSWSH Nomenclature for Female Sexual Dysfunctions. Persistent genital arousal disorder may be caused by numerous underlying pathological conditions, which may be unraveled by multiple diagnostic procedures. Therapies include disease modification strategies directed at curing the persistent genital arousal disorder condition and symptomatic therapies to reduce the persistent genital arousal disorder symptoms so that the condition is manageable and tolerable. In several cases where persistent genital arousal disorder may have been caused by sacral spinal nerve radiculopathy, minimally-invasive spine surgery may be helpful. While more research is needed in this area, detailed and systematic diagnostic investigation by a dedicated health-care provider can greatly inform therapeutic approaches to assist patients in alleviating symptoms or even curing this debilitating condition.

# References

1 Leiblum S, Nathan SG. Persistent sexual arousal syndrome: a newly discovered pattern of female sexuality. *J Sex Marit Ther.* 2001;27(4):365–380.

2 Jackowich R, Pink L, Gordon A, Pukall CF. Persistent genital arousal disorder: a review of its conceptualizations, potential origins, impact, and treatment. *Sex Med Rev.* 2016;4(4):329–342.

3 Jackowich R, Pukall CF. Prevalence of persistent genital arousal disorder criteria in a sample of Canadian undergraduate students. *J Sex Med.* 2017;14(6):e368–e369.

4 Parish SJ, Goldstein AT, Goldstein SW, *et al.* Toward a more evidence-based nosology and nomenclature for female sexual dysfunctions – Part II. *J Sex Med.* 2016;13(12):1888–1906.

5 Jackowich R, Pink L, Gordon A, *et al.* Symptom characteristics and medical history of an online sample of women who experience symptoms of persistent genital arousal. *J Sex Marit Ther.* 2017. doi: 10.1080/0092623X.2017.1321598.

6 Jaslow R. Gretchen Molannen's suicide spotlights debilitating effects of persistent genital arousal disorder. CBS Interactive Inc.; 2012. http://www.cbsnews.com/news/gretchen-molannens-suicide-spotlights-debilitating-effects-of-persistent-genital-arousal-disorder/; last accessed 23 December 2017.

7 Hrynko M, Kotas R, Pokryszko-Dragan A, *et al.* Persistent genital arousal disorder – a case report. *Psychiatr Pol.* 2017;51(1):117–124.

8 Sawamura M, Toma K, Unai Y, *et al.* A case of Parkinson's disease following restless genial sensation. *Rinsho Shinkeigak.* 2015;55(4):266–268.

9 Erős E, Brockhauser I, Pólyán E. Symptomatology and treatment of persistent genital arousal disorder. *Orv Hetil.* 2015;156(15):614–618.

10 Elkins G, Ramsey D, Yu Y. Hypnotherapy for persistent genital arousal disorder: a case study. *Int J Clin Exp Hypn.* 2014;62(2):215–223.

11 Bedell S, Goldstein AT, Burrows L. A periclitoral mass as a cause of persistent genital arousal disorder. *J Sex Med.* 2014;11(1):136–139.

12 Philippsohn S, Kruger TH. Persistent genital arousal disorder: successful treatment with duloxetine and pregabalin in two cases. *J Sex Med.* 2012;9(1):213–217.

13 Anzellotti F, Franciotti R, Bonanni L, *et al.* Persistent genital arousal disorder associated with functional hyperconnectivity of an epileptic focus. *Neuroscience.* 2010;167(1):88–96.

14 Rosenbaum T. Physical therapy treatment of persistent genital arousal disorder during pregnancy: a case report. *J Sex Med.* 2010;7(3):1306–1310.

15 Korda J, Pfaus JG, Kellner CH, Goldstein I. Persistent genital arousal disorder (PGAD): case report of long-term symptomatic management with electroconvulsive therapy. *J Sex Med.* 2009;6(10):2901–2909.

16 Battaglia C, Venturoli S. Persistent genital arousal disorder and trazodone. Morphometric and vascular modifications of the clitoris. A case report. *J Sex Med.* 2009;6(10):2896–2900.

17 Korda J, Pfaus JG, Goldstein I. Persistent genital arousal disorder: a case report in a woman with lifelong PGAD where serendipitous administration of varenicline tartrate resulted in symptomatic improvement. *J Sex Med.* 2009;6(5):1479–1486.

18 Goldmeier D, Leiblum S. Interaction of organic and psychological factors in persistent genital arousal disorder in women: a report of six cases. *Int J STD AIDS.* 2008;19(7):488–490.

19 Leiblum S, Goldmeier D. Persistent genital arousal disorder in women: case reports of association with anti-depressant usage and withdrawal. *J Sex Marit Ther.* 2008;34(2):150–159.

20 King S, Goldstein I, Pfaus JG. Mechanism of action and pre-liminary clinical experience with zolpidem, a non-benzodiazepine indirect GABA A receptor agonist, for symptomatic treatment of persistent genital arousal disorder (PGAD). *J Sex Med.* 2016;13(6):S247–S248.

21 Yildirim E, Hacioglu Yildirim M, Carpar E, Sarac I. Clomipramine trial for treatment-resistant persistent genital arousal disorder: a case series. *J Psychosom Obstet Gynaecol.* 2017;38(4):260–267. doi: 10.1080/0167482X.2017.1296427.

22 Gaines N, Odom BD, Killinger KA, Peters KM. Pudendal neuromodulation as a treatment for persistent genital arousal disorder – a case series. *Female Pelvic Med Reconstr Surg.* 2017. Epub Jun 27. doi: 10.1097/SPV.0000000000000435.

23 Pink L, Rancourt V, Gordon A. Persistent genital arousal in women with pelvic and genital pain. *J Obstet Gynaecol Can.* 2014;36(4):324–230.

24 Yero S, McKinney T, Petrides G, *et al.* Successful use of electroconvulsive therapy in 2 cases of persistent sexual arousal syndrome and bipolar disorder. *J ECT.* 2006;22(4):274–275.

25 McMullen R, Agarwal S. Persistent genital arousal disorder – case report of symptomatic relief of symptoms with transcranial magnetic stimulation. *J ECT.* 2016;32(3):e9–e10.

26 Feigenbaum F, Boone K. Persistent genital arousal disorder caused by spinal meningeal cysts in the sacrum; successful neurosurgical treatment. *Obst Gynecol.* 2016;126:839–843.

27 Goldstein I, Komisaruk BR, Rubin RS, *et al.* A novel collaborative protocol for successful management of penile pain mediated by radiculitis of sacral spinal nerve roots from Tarlov cysts. *Sex Med.* 2017; 5(3):e203–e211. doi: 10.1016/j.esxm.2017.04.001.

28 Thorne C, Stuckey B. Pelvic congestion syndrome presenting as persistent genital arousal: a case report. *J Sex Med.* 2008;5(2):504–508.

29 Aerts L. Successful management of PGAD and clitorodynia caused by a closed compartment syndrome. *J Sex Med.* 2016;13(5):S205–S206.

30 King S, Espenschied C, Gagnon C, *et al.* Lifetime persistent genital arousal disorder: management of PGAD in an adolescent. *J Sex Med.* 2016;12(6):S260–S261.

31 Carvalho J, Veríssimo A, Nobre PJ. Cognitive and emotional determinants characterizing women with persistent genital arousal disorder. *J Sex Med.* 2013;10(6):1549–1558.

32 Eibye S, Jensen HM. Persistent genital arousal disorder: confluent patient history of agitated depression, paroxetine cessation, and a tarlov cyst. *Case Rep Psychiatry.* 2014. doi: 10.1155/2014/529052.

33 de Magalhães F, Kumar MT. Persistent genital arousal disorder following selective serotonin reuptake inhibitor cessation. *J Clin Psychopharmacol.* 2015;35(3):352–354.

34 Pfaus J. Persistent genital arousal disorder – fact or fiction? *J Sex Med.* 2017;14(3):318–319.

35 Goldstein I, De EJB, Johnson J. Persistent sexual arousal syndrome and clitoral priapism. In: Goldstein I, Meston C, Davis S, Traish A (eds) *Women's Sexual Function and Dysfunction: Study, Diagnosis and Treatment.* London: Taylor and Francis; 2006, pp. 674–685.

36 Komisaruk B, Lee HJ. Prevalence of sacral spinal (Tarlov) cysts in persistent genital arousal disorder. *J Sex Med.* 2012;9:2047–2056.

37 Korse N, Pijpers JA, van Zwet E, *et al.* Cauda Equina Syndrome: presentation, outcome, and predictors with focus on micturition, defecation, and sexual dysfunction. *Euro Spine J.* 2017;26:894–904.

38 Ahad A, Elsayed M, Tohid H. The accuracy of clinical symptoms in detecting cauda equina syndrome in patients undergoing acute MRI of the spine. *Neuroradiol J.* 2015;28:438–442.

39 Orlin J, Klevmark B. Successful disc surgery after 17 years of erectile dysfunction caused by a "silent" disc protrusion. *Scan J Urol Nephr.* 2008;42:91–93.

40 Mauffrey C, Randhawa K, Lewis C, *et al.* Cauda equina syndrome: an anatomically driven review. *Br J Hosp Med.* 2005;69:344–347.

41 Petrasic J, Chhabra A, Scott KM. Impact of MR neurography in patients with chronic Cauda Equina Syndrome presenting as chronic pelvic pain and dysfunction. *AJNR.* 2017;38:418–422.

42 McNamee J, Flynn P, O'Leary S, *et al.* Imaging in cauda equina syndrome – a pictorial review. *Ulster Med J.* 2013;82:100–108.

43 Maurice-Williams R, Marsh HT. Priapism as a feature of claudication of the cauda equina. *Surg Neurol.* 1985;23:626–628.

44 Ravindran M. Cauda equina compression presenting as spontaneous priapism. *J Neurol Neurosug Psychiatry.* 1979;42: 280–282.

45 Akbas N, Dalbayrak S, Kulcu DG, *et al.* Assessment of sexual dysfunction before and after surgery for lumbar disc herniation. *J Neurosurg Spine.* 2010;13:581–586.

46 Korse N, Jacobs WC, Elzevier HW, Vleggeert-Lankamp CL. Complaints of micturition, defecation and sexual function in cauda equina syndrome due to lumbar disk herniation: a systematic review. *Euro Spine J.* 2013;22:1019–1029.

47 Kingery W, Castellote JM, Wang EE. A loose ligature-induced mononeuropathy produces hyperalgesias mediated by both the injured sciatic nerve and the adjacent saphenous nerve. *Pain.* 1993;55:297–304.

48 Choy D. Early relief of erectile dysfunction after laser decompression of herniated lumbar disc. *J Clin Laser Med Surg.* 1999;17:25–27.

49 Waldinger M, de Lint GJ, Venema PL, *et al.* Successful transcutaneous electrical nerve stimulation in two women with restless genital syndrome: the role of adelta- and C-nerve fibers. *J Sex Med.* 2010;7(3):1190–1199.

50 Waldinger M, Venema PL, van Gils AP, *et al.* Stronger evidence for small fiber sensory neuropathy in restless genital syndrome: two case reports in males. *J Sex Med.* 2011;8(1):325–330.

**Part III**

**Orgasm Disorders**

# 12

# Nosology and Epidemiology of Female Orgasm Disorder

*Leonard R. Derogatis*

## Abstract

This chapter reviews the history and development of the diagnosis female orgasmic disorder (FOD) and discusses its close ties to the evolution of the diagnostic system of the American Psychiatric Association (i.e. DSM-I to DSM-5). It reviews the principal criteria underlying the diagnosis and their underlying significance. The chapter also discusses the widespread dissatisfaction with the current DSM-5 system and the development, in response, of the new ISSWSH diagnostic system for female sexual dysfunctions. Diagnostic standards for the FOD diagnosis in the ISSWSH system are described and elucidated as an alternative to the DSM-5 system. In addition, the chapter also provides a brief review of the current status of epidemiological research focused on the prevalence of FOD as defined in contemporary nosological systems.

**Keywords:** *diagnosis; prevalence; nosology; nomenclature; FSD; FOD*

## Nosology

In the first half of the twentieth century, a broad spectrum of orgasmic disorders were loosely categorized under the term "frigidity", most centrally defined as the inability of a woman to achieve vaginal orgasm [1]. Although numerous possible causes were advanced, the condition was perceived primarily as a psychological problem. Consistent with the thinking of the times, when the first edition of the Diagnostic and Statistical Manual of Mental Disorders (DSM) [2] was published in 1952, problems with orgasm (specified as "frigidity") were included under a category of "Psychophysiological Autonomic and Visceral Disorders" catalogued under a broader category of "Disorders of Psychogenic Origin".

There was little change to this section of the DSM until the publication of the innovative DSM-III [3] in 1980 when female sexual dysfunctions were categorized under the heading of "Sexual Dysfunctions" and problems with orgasm were labeled "Inhibited Female Orgasm". The core definition focused on the delay or absence of an orgasmic response following a "normal sexual excitement phase". The central focus on "delay or absence of orgasm after a normal sexual excitement phase" continued through the DSM-III-Revised and DSM-IV [4], with the addition of the distress criterion as a pivotal requirement for diagnosis in the DSM-IV.

In the DSM-5 [5], the requirements of key symptoms being present in the majority (≥75%) of sexual encounters was introduced, as was a ≥6 month duration criterion.

*Textbook of Female Sexual Function and Dysfunction: Diagnosis and Treatment*, First Edition. Edited by Irwin Goldstein, Anita H. Clayton, Andrew T. Goldstein, Noel N. Kim, and Sheryl A. Kingsberg.
© 2018 John Wiley & Sons Ltd. Published 2018 by John Wiley & Sons Ltd.

The distress criterion (i.e. the condition causing "clinically significant distress") was retained as a standard feature of the diagnosis. In the DSM-5, "marked reduced intensity of orgasmic sensations" was added to the list of possible symptoms of orgasmic dysfunction. The general admonition to insure that symptoms were not due to another DSM or medical disorder or exclusively due to the physiological effects of another substance or medication was retained in the DSM-5.

The Nomenclature Committee of the International Society for the Study of Women's Sexual Health (ISSWSH), based on its collective clinical deliberations and research review, concluded that while the above criteria for female orgasmic disorder were appropriate and valid, additional features of the orgasm experience (disturbances in *orgasmic pleasure* and *orgasmic timing*) qualified as sufficient to meet the requirements as dysfunctions. The omission of decreased or absent pleasure and the inability to control timing of orgasm in previous definitions of female orgasmic disorder was felt to be a significant oversight and one that should be rectified in a new nomenclature system [6].

In the ISSWSH nomenclature, female orgasmic disorder is defined as "…a persistent or recurrent, distressing compromise of orgasmic frequency, intensity, timing and/or pleasure associated with sexual activity for a minimum of 6 months" [6]. Specific criteria defining female orgasmic disorder are:

- frequency: orgasm occurs with decreased frequency or is absent (anorgasmia);
- intensity: orgasm occurs with decreased intensity (muted orgasm);
- timing: orgasm occurs too early (premature orgasm) or too late (delayed orgasm) than is desired by the woman;
- pleasure: orgasm occurs with absent or diminished pleasure (anhedonic orgasm).

The traditional specifiers of *lifelong/acquired* and *generalized/situational* are retained in the ISSWSH definition.

## Epidemiology

The epidemiology of female orgasmic disorders, like the other categories of female sexual dysfunction, suffers from numerous problems and shortcomings. Firstly, the failure of studies to include a distress criterion until recently represents a major problem that has resulted in a large body of prevalence data no longer relevant to contemporary nomenclatures. Secondly, the restricted historical definitions of orgasmic disorder, which focused heavily on "the delay or absence of an orgasmic response after sufficient stimulation" as a central criterion, have led to a constricted and limited definition of orgasmic disorder to support prevalence data. Nonetheless, there are a small group of studies that have achieved a certain level of acceptable rigor and the prevalence rates from these studies are provided here.

Investigators in the PRESIDE study [7] also collected data on female orgasmic disorder. Importantly, the PRESIDE study also included a distress criterion. The unadjusted prevalence of problems with orgasm in the PRESIDE sample was 20.5%. When the distress criterion was added, the rate fell to 4.7%. When data were analyzed by age group, rates were higher for the older groups, at 5.7% and 5.8% for women aged 45–64 years and ≥65 years, respectively, and lower (3.4%) for women aged 18–44 years. Unlike the data for hypoactive sexual desire and sexual arousal disorders, there was a direct relationship between distressing orgasmic problems and age. A higher rate of female orgasmic disorder was associated with surgical menopause, current depression, anxiety problems, arthritis and urinary incontinence. Interestingly, heart disease and diabetes were not significantly related to any of the sexual problems in the study.

Hayes and his associates published a comprehensive review of prevalence studies of female sexual dysfunctions in 2006 [8]. They reviewed 1248 separate studies but found that only 11 studies met their criteria for inclusion. Of those, only two employed a distress criterion, and the proportions of distressed women in those studies with orgasm problems ranged widely from 21 to 67%. Orgasm difficulty had an unadjusted overall rate of 35% across studies.

Graziottin reported on data from 2467 women from four European countries who participated in the WISHeS study, which also included data on the presence of psychological distress along with orgasmic difficulty [9]. While the main focus was on hypoactive sexual desire disorder, rates of orgasmic difficulty were reported to be almost equivalent across samples from the four countries involved: France, 20%; Italy, 18%; Germany, 21%; United Kingdom, 18%. These rates are highly consistent considering the cultural distinctions across these populations.

In 2001, Simon and Carey published a review of the previous decade of prevalence research on sexual dysfunctions [10]. They reported that 51 studies had been published in the previous decade as compared to 47 studies published in the 50 years preceding that time, suggesting a significant increase in the volume of research in the field. However, research in the field was highly unstandardized during this period. Different nomenclatures were used, diverse operational definitions were employed, distinct prevalence periods (6 months versus 1 year, versus lifetime) were involved, and distress criteria were rarely used, all of which led to extremely uneven methodology in study designs. It is anticipated that the recent development of a rigorous new nomenclature for female sexual dysfunctions by ISSWSH will ensure a more positive assessment of the status of the field a decade from now.

# References

1 Angel, K. The history of 'Female Sexual Dysfunction' as a mental disorder in the 20th century. *Curr Opin Psychiatry.* 2010;23:536–541.

2 American Psychiatric Association. *The Diagnostic and Statistical Manual of Mental Disorders.* Washington, DC: American Psychiatric Association; 1952.

3 American Psychiatric Association. *DSM-III: Diagnostic and Statistical Manual of Mental Disorders*, 3rd edn. Washington, DC: American Psychiatric Association; 1980.

4 American Psychiatric Association. *DSM-IV: Diagnostic and Statistical Manual of Mental Disorders*, 4th edn. Washington, DC: American Psychiatric Association; 1994.

5 American Psychiatric Association. *DSM-5: Diagnostic and Statistical Manual of Mental Disorders*, 5th edn. Washington, DC: American Psychiatric Association; 2013.

6 Parish SJ, Goldstein AT, Goldstein SW, *et al.* Toward a more evidence-based nosology and nomenclature for female sexual dysfunctions – Part II. *J Sex Med.* 2016;13:1888–1906.

7 Shifren JL, Monz BU, Russo PA, *et al.* Sexual problems and distress in United States women: prevalence and correlates. *Obstet Gynecol.* 2008;112(5):970–978.

8 Hayes RD, Bennett CM, Fairly, CK, *et al.* What can prevalence studies tell us about female sexual difficulty and dysfunction. *J Sex Med.* 2006;3:589–595.

9 Graziottin A. Prevalence and evaluation of sexual health problems. *J Sex Med.* 2007;4:211–219.

10 Simon J, Carey JP. Prevalence of sexual dysfunctions: Results from a decade of research. *Arch Sex. Behav.* 2001;30:177–219.

# 13

# Peripheral and Central Neural Bases of Orgasm

*Emmanuele A. Jannini, Nan Wise, Eleni Frangos, and Barry R. Komisaruk*

### Abstract

The clitoris and the clito-urethro-vaginal complex are responsive to ovarian hormones and are the main peripheral structures that, with significant individual differences, provide the genital peripheral afferent component of female sexual pleasure. In the central nervous system during orgasm, essentially all of the major brain systems are activated, including the brainstem, limbic system, cerebellum, and cortex. In a symphony of integration, these peripheral and central systems mediate the sensory, cognitive, autonomic, and motor events of orgasm.

**Keywords:** *autonomic; brain; cervix; clitoris; clito-urethro-vaginal complex; G spot; limbic; neurotransmitters; orgasm; vagina*

> The hormone-dependent clitoris and the clito-urethro-vaginal complex are the main peripheral structures triggering, in an exquisitely individual manner, the genital part of female sexual pleasure.
>
> Centrally, women's orgasm entails activation of essentially all the major brain systems, including brainstem, limbic system, cerebellum and cortex.
>
> These central and peripheral systems mediate the sensory, autonomic, and motor events of orgasm.

## Functional Anatomy

Adult female genital tissues are hormone dependent in their histology, gross anatomy and functionality. This partly can account for the considerable individual variability of the female genitalia (e.g. clitoris and periurethral erectile tissue), which corresponds to evident inter- and intra-individual variability in female sexual response. Female sexual pleasure is a broader term than female orgasm. The absence of a full orgasm in a woman without distress does not always prevent the pleasure of sexual activity [1]. Furthermore, we will distinguish clitoral orgasm from vaginally-activated orgasm (i.e. orgasm elicited with versus orgasm elicited without direct stimulation of the external clitoris, respectively) and from orgasm elicited by stimulation of other anatomical structures (uterus, nipple, brain, etc.) [2]. The stimulated clitoris is the primary anatomical source of clitoral orgasm, while the penetrated vagina is the source of female sexual pleasure in a woman without distress and, probably in a lower number of women, of vaginally-activated orgasm.

### Histology of the Clitoris

The clitoris shares with the penis, in their embryonic derivation, certain macro-anatomical aspects and histologic structure.

*Textbook of Female Sexual Function and Dysfunction: Diagnosis and Treatment*, First Edition. Edited by Irwin Goldstein, Anita H. Clayton, Andrew T. Goldstein, Noel N. Kim, and Sheryl A. Kingsberg.
© 2018 John Wiley & Sons Ltd. Published 2018 by John Wiley & Sons Ltd.

However, it is reductive, both conceptually and ontogenetically, to consider it as an embryological hypo-developed penis.

The microscopic anatomy consists of cavernous tissue encircled by a thin fibrous capsule surrounded by large nerve trunks. This cavernous tissue consists of trabecular smooth muscle and connective tissue, which encase the cavernous sinusoidal spaces. The ultrastructure of the female erectile tissue within the clitoris is comparable to that of the penis, but with some important differences [3]. The nerve network distribution pattern has been studied, using the neuro-marker S-100 and neuron specific enolase-immunoreactivity, demonstrating that tissue organization in the corpora cavernosa of the clitoris is essentially similar to that of the penis, except for the absence of the subalbugineal layer interposed between the tunica albuginea and the erectile tissue [4]. This has functional implications, suggesting that the clitoral erection physiology differs from that of the penis.

The histology of the clitoris is not constant; with increasing age there is a decrease in clitoral cavernous smooth muscle fibers with a relative increase of cavernous connective tissue, as measured by histomorphometry [5]. Clitoral corpora cavernosa are well stained by antibodies against steroid hormone receptors; the biochemical physiology of erection will be described in the next section on vaginal histology [6]. Although it is well known that the clitoris is responsive to androgens, as demonstrated by clitoromegaly in female virilization [7], surprisingly, well-mapped distribution and characterization of sex hormone receptors in the clitoris is currently lacking. Table 13.1 shows the substances found in the genitalia of animals and women, based on immunohistochemistry.

## Histology of the Vagina

To understand the role of the vagina in female orgasm and female sexual pleasure, three basic concepts should be considered: (i) the morphological variability in individuals; (ii) the presence of some structural differences between the anterior and posterior walls; (iii) the histological changes due to hormonal and life cycle.

The vagina in reproductive life is lined by a stratified squamous epithelium organized into rugal folds that enable vaginal distensability (compliance) without the risk of laceration. Beneath the epithelium there is a dense, thin layer of elastic fibers and then the robust fibromuscular layer. The fibrous capsule external to this muscular coat is rich in elastic fibers and large venous plexuses. The vaginal wall contains an innermost layer, the *tunica mucosa*, and an intermediate layer, the *tunica adventitia*.

The immunohistochemical analysis of the vaginal wall (Table 13.1) shows the presence of the nitric oxide–cyclic GMP–type 5 phosphodiesterase (NO-cGMP-PDE5) biochemical machinery and a series of several other substances also involved in female arousal and pleasure. Immunohistochemical studies have demonstrated the presence of a large number of nerve fibers stained for NO synthase (NOS) in the environment of smooth muscle tissue and below the Malpighian vaginal epithelium. The different isoforms of NOS also have a complex pattern of distribution in the human vagina: the constitutive enzyme isoforms (neuronal and endothelial) are expressed in the nerve fiber layer, in the vascular endothelium, and in the smooth muscle fibers of the cavernous erectile tissue of the vaginal wall, and in the Malpighian epithelium of the mucosa. The Malpighian epithelium also expresses the inducible isoform, iNOS. The colocalization of NOS isoforms and PDE5 in the context of the cavernous structures of the anterior vaginal wall is related to the production and catabolism of cGMP produced locally during sexual stimulation [21].

## Gross Anatomy of the Clitoris

The clitoris is an erectile organ located medial and inferior to the pubic arch and symphysis [39], which, due to its multifaceted structure, has been named the "clitoral

**Table 13.1** Histological findings in clitoris and vagina [8].

| Factor | Tissue | Animal | Function/Localization | Reference |
|---|---|---|---|---|
| NOS | Clitoris<br>Vagina | Human<br>Rabbit<br>Mouse<br>Pig<br>Cow | Neurotransmission, blood flow control and capillary permeability | 9, 10, 11, 12, 13 |
| nNOS | Clitoris<br>Vagina | Human<br>Rat<br>Rabbit | Nerve fibers supplying smooth muscle, perivascular nerve plexuses, lamina propria | 14, 15, 16, 17, 18 |
| eNOS | Clitoris<br>Vagina | Human<br>Rat<br>Rabbit | Vascular endothelium, perivascular smooth muscle. | 3, 14, 15, 19<br>17, 18 |
| iNOS | Vagina | Human | Production of NO under certain conditions | 15 |
| PDE5 | Clitoris<br>Vagina<br>Skene's gland | Human<br>Rabbit | Breakdown of cGMP. Decrease of sexual arousal | 15, 20, 21, 22, 23 |
| CGRP | Vagina<br>Clitoris | Human<br>Pig | Neurotransmission, blood flow control and capillary permeability, involved in sensation | 9, 11, 24, 25 |
| SP | Clitoris<br>Vagina | Human<br>Pig<br>Cow | Neurotransmission, blood flow control and capillary permeability | 10, 11, 24 |
| NPY | Clitoris<br>Vagina | Human<br>Pig | Neurotransmission, blood flow control and capillary permeability | 9, 11, 24, 26 |
| Oxytocin | Clitoris<br>Vagina | Rat | efferent neuronal control | 27 |
| Estrogen receptors | Distal vagina | Rabbit | Down-regulation of NOS | 28 |
| Androgen receptors | Proximal Vagina | Rabbit | Facilitation of vaginal smooth muscle relaxation | 28 |
| TGF$\beta$1 | Vagina | Diabetic rat | Fibrosis | 29 |
| VIP | Clitoris<br>Vagina | Human<br>Cat<br>Rat<br>Guinea pig<br>Goat<br>Hen<br>Pig | Smooth muscle relaxation, neurotransmission, blood flow control and capillary permeability | 9, 10, 11, 24, 30, 31, 32, 33 |
| PSA | Skene's gland | Human | Prostatic marker | 34, 35 |
| PAP | Skene's gland | Human | Prostatic marker | 35, 36 |
| UP1 | Skene's gland | Human | Protection of uroepithelium? | 37 |
| Chromogranin | Skene's gland | Human<br>Pig | Marker of neurosecretion | 15, 38 |

complex" [40] (see Tables 13.2 and 13.3 for innervation and vascularization, respectively). In the clitoris, several structures are identified. The external clitoris consists of the *glans* (the visible portions of the clitoral complex), *prepuce* (the skin likened to penile foreskin), and *frenulum* (a posterior fold). The internal clitoris, containing most of the erectile tissue, consists of the *body* (paired corpora, diverging to form the crura), the *bulbs* (comparable to the corpus spongiosum of the penis) [41], and the *crura* (surrounding the urethra and attaching to the ischiopubic rami). The corpora and the bulbs communicate through the venous *plexus of Kobelt*. The suspensory ligaments secure the clitoris to the labia, the mons pubis, and the pubic symphysis, which prevents the straightening of the clitoris. The tunica albuginea is a dense connective tissue sheath covering the body of the clitoris [42].

Some anatomical aspects have been related to clitoral function. While the os penis is widely represented in mammals, with the unique exception of humans and rabbit [43], the occurrence of the os clitoridis is variable. Mice, but not rats, have a small os clitoridis corresponding to the intramembranous part of the proximal element of the os penis. Neonatal treatment with androgens, but not estrogens, stimulates the growth of the os clitoridis [44]. At birth, clitoral size may be related to ethnicity [45, 46]. The following average values have been reported: 5.9 mm in newborns of Jewish origin and 6.6 mm in Bedouin babies [47], which is almost twice

**Table 13.2** Innervation of female sexual organs.

| Nerve | Role | Innervated region |
|---|---|---|
| Dorsal nerve of the clitoris (from the pudendal nerve) | Somatic innervation | Clitoris complex |
| Cavernous nerves (from the inferior hypogastric plexus) | Supply the erectile tissue arteries through visceral fibers | Corpora cavernosa of the clitoris |
| Vaginal plexus | Visceral innervation | Vagina |
| Pelvic splanchnic nerves | Visceral innervation | Vagina |
| Pudendal nerve | Visceral innervation | Lower third of the vagina |

**Table 13.3** Vascularization of female sexual organs.

| Vessel | Role | Vascularized region |
|---|---|---|
| Dorsal clitoral arteries, perineal arteries, and deep arteries | Arterial supply | Erectile tissue of glans and body |
| External pudendal | Arterial supply | Prepuce |
| Dorsal vein | Venous drainage to the vesical venous plexus | Clitoris |
| Kobelt Plexus | Venous drainage | Communication between bulbs and corpora cavernosa of citoris |
| Vaginal arteries and their anastomoses with branches of the uterine, inferior vesical and internal pudendal arteries | Arterial supply | Vagina |
| Internal pudendal artery | Arterial supply | Vaginal walls |

that of the 3.27 mm in white and the 3.66 mm measured in black neonates [48]. There are reports of a negative correlation between birth weight and clitoral length [49] but not with gestational age [50]. Women with anorgasmia were reported to have a smaller clitoral glans and clitoral components farther from the vaginal lumen than women with normal orgasmic function [51].

The anogenital distance is also related to female orgasm and female sexual pleasure. It is considered a biomarker for the prenatal hormonal environment, in particular to the exposure to androgens. Perineum length was reported, on average, to be half that of males [52]. The anogenital distance measurement immediately after birth has been suggested as a noninvasive method to assess uterine exposure to sexual hormones [53]. A greater anogenital distance was associated with higher testosterone levels in women [54]. Another anatomical aspect that may account for the variation in ability to experience orgasm is the distance between the glans clitoris and the urethra. With a distance less than 2.5 cm, vaginally-activated orgasm may more easily occur [55].

## Gross Anatomy of the Vagina

The vagina, too often considered primarily as just a part of the birth canal, is more appropriately defined as the female organ of copulation. It consists of a tubular fibromuscular structure that extends in the direction posterosuperior from the vestibule between the labia minora to the cervix, at a right angle to the long axis of the uterus (see Tables 13.2 and 13.3 for innervation and vascularization, respectively). The vagina can be considered to consist of a posterior wall and an anterior wall, in continuity with each other, with an H-shape when seen in cross-section in the relaxed state.

The vagina is attached laterally to the pelvic sidewalls and caudally to the uterus, thus, further permitting distensability and adaptation to changes in pressure. The connective tissue of the vaginal walls is attached to the pubococcygeal muscle and fixed to the perineal membrane, with individual variation. The posterior wall is separated from the rectum by the rectovaginal septum and from the anus by the perineal fibromuscular tissue.

The vagina, and in particular the anterior vaginal wall, is richly innervated. Microdissection reveals that the distal anterior vaginal wall is significantly thicker than the proximal anterior vaginal wall and that this region is the most densely innervated area, suggesting regional differences in the ability to trigger the erotic stimuli [56].

The female prostate (*prostata foemina*), previously termed Skene glands or periurethral glands, surrounds the urethra within the anterior vaginal wall, with a microscopic structure similar to its male counterpart, albeit with some important differences that underlie functional diversity. The glandular component of the female prostate consists predominantly of ductal structures that open independently into the lumen of the urethra, while the acinar secretory component is relatively less well developed. The female prostate is considered the main source of prostate-specific antigen present in the fluid emitted from the urethra (the "female ejaculate") resulting from direct stimulation of the anterior vaginal wall [57]. The stromal component that surrounds the glands is much more developed in the female prostate than in the male, and is formed by a fibromuscular connective tissue rich in nerve and blood vessel terminations.

## Functional Changes During Arousal and Orgasm

Modern imaging techniques allow visualization of the dynamic interactions of the female genitals during sexual self-stimulation and penetration [58–60]. Although the search for the "mythical" G-spot was unsuccessful in finding a unique structure, it had the merit to have highlighted the dramatic role for female orgasm and female sexual pleasure of the vagina in general, and anterior vaginal wall in particular, and to provide the anatomical basis for vaginally-activated orgasm [61, 62]. The anatomical relationships and the dynamic interaction among clitoris, urethra, and anterior vaginal wall, as evidenced through ultrasound imaging during coitus, made evident the need of an improvement in the nomenclature.

The term clito-urethro-vaginal complex was coined to identify a multifaceted morpho-functional area (Figure 13.1), which, when properly stimulated during penetration, can induce vaginally-activated orgasm in some women [2, 63]. Vaginally-activated orgasm involves the pumping effect on the Kobelt plexus, while the root of the clitoris is particularly stretched by the penis and compressed against the anterior vaginal wall, the pubic symphysis and the urethra with the surrounding exocrine glands and erectile tissue. The anatomical structures that participate in the clito-urethro-vaginal complex formation are exquisitely hormone-sensitive and, hence, different from subject to subject, even possibly changing within the same subject in relation to the different phases of life. Understanding the anatomy and the physiology of the clito-urethro-vaginal complex will help to prevent damage to the neural, muscular and vascular components during surgical procedures of this essential body component.

## Brain Activity and Correlates of Orgasm

While there are many brain imaging studies of sexual arousal [64–74], those of orgasm are fewer and more variable. During orgasm in women, the brain regions reported to be activated include the amygdala and hippocampus [64, 66, 75–77], hypothalamus [64, 65, 72, 73], the dopaminergic system from ventral tegmentum [78] to nucleus accumbens [76, 77], anterior cingulate [76–79], frontal cortices [76, 77], and the cerebellum [76–79]. As yet unresolved is a discrepancy in the literature

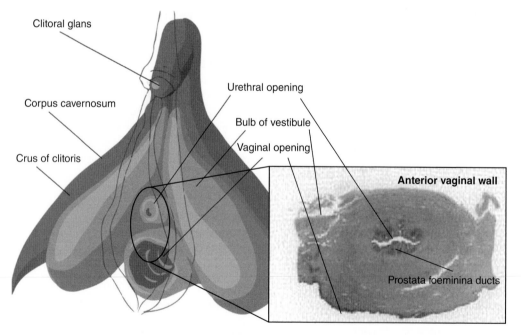

**Figure 13.1** Anatomy of the CUV complex. Schematic representation of the external and internal clitoris and the vaginal opening. The insert, an anterior vaginal wall obtained from a cadaver [15, 21], represent the intimate relationships between all the different anatomical structures involved in the female sexual pleasure. (*See plate section for color representation of the figure*)

as to whether the frontal and temporal cortical regions become activated (based on fMRI) during orgasm [76, 80] or deactivated (based on PET) [81, 82]. The overall similarities in brain activity during orgasm between men and women are greater than the differences, with some exceptions in the amygdala, temporal lobe, lower brainstem [78, 83] and during the post-orgasm refractory period [84].

## Genital Sensation and Projections to the Brain

Orgasm reported as being elicited by stimulation of the clitoris, vagina, and/or cervix has been described as having different qualities. Clitoral orgasm has been characterized as more localized than vaginally-activated orgasm, which has been described as deeper and more whole-body, while cervical orgasm has been described in more abstract terms (e.g. a "shower of stars" or "images of universal spaciousness"). Combining the genital stimulation sites was described as "mixed" orgasms [61, 85]. In a study of 128 women, 95% of the women claimed that clitoral stimulation contributed to their orgasm, while 65% said vaginal stimulation, and 35% said cervical [86].

By selective self-stimulation of the clitoris, vagina or cervix, different, but overlapping, regions of the genital sensory cortex (i.e. the paracentral lobule) were activated, most likely corresponding to the differential but overlapping innervation by pudendal, pelvic, and hypogastric nerves, respectively [79]. On the basis that stimulation of each of these genital components can elicit orgasm and the observation that a larger brain region is activated by the combination of stimulation of these genital components, representing a larger population of genitally-activated neurons, this implies that combined stimulation of these genital components could generate orgasms that are more intense, sensually complex, and pleasurable than if stimulated by more limited genital components. Nipple self-stimulation also activated the paracentral lobule, overlapping with the regions activated

by genital self-stimulation [79, 84, 87, 88]. This could be a basis for anecdotal reports that nipple stimulation may elicit orgasm [89]. Evidently, a complex brain system becomes activated incrementally, leading up to an orgasmic crescendo that involves widespread brain activation, and then "cooling down" as shown in Figures 13.2 and 13.3.

## Brain Activity Related to Orgasm

To characterize the change from high arousal just prior to orgasm in comparison with orgasm *per se*, we electronically subtracted the activity during the 10 seconds just prior to the onset of orgasm (indicated by the women pressing a button at the onset of orgasm) from the 10-s activity during orgasm. The differentially activated brain regions were amygdala, hippocampus, nucleus accumbens, hypothalamus, septum, anterior cingulate and insular cortices, and lower brainstem regions including ventral tegmental area, periaqueductal gray, and dorsal raphe (Figure 13.4).

## Role of Different Brain Components in Orgasm

The nucleus accumbens and the ventral tegmental area were both activated at orgasm.

The ventral tegmental area is a major source of the neurons of the mesolimbic system, which project to the nucleus accumbens where they release dopamine. Dopaminergic antagonists can attenuate, and dopaminergic agonists promote, sexual response and orgasm [61]. In rats, dopamine was released during mating behavior [90].

One of the salient features of orgasm in women is a marked elevation of the pain threshold [91]. We observed an activation of the periaqueductal gray and the dorsal raphe during orgasm. These two brain regions play a significant role in the descending brainstem-spinal cord pain-attenuating system [92] in which serotonin produced by the raphe neurons activates the "pain gate" control mechanism in the spinal cord.

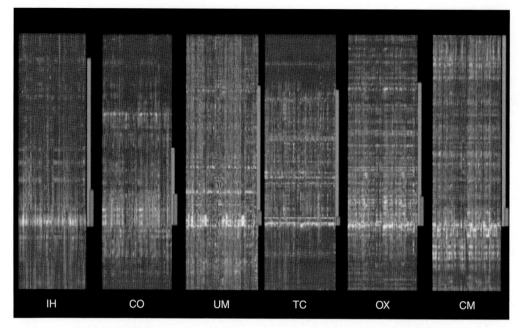

**Figure 13.2** Descriptive "tapestry" representation of brain activity in response to clitoral self-stimulation leading up to, during, and after orgasm in each of six women. Each woman's tapestry consists of 80 columns, each column representing a Brodmann area. Each row represents a successive two-second sample of functional MRI activity, starting at the top. The relative magnitude of brain activity in each region at each time period is represented as brightness. The shorter vertical bars to the right of each tapestry represents the onset and duration of orgasm; the longer bars represent the onset and duration of clitoral self-stimulation. Note the maximum activation in widespread brain regions during orgasm, in contrast to the variable patterns of regional brain activity leading up to, and after, orgasm. These descriptive data and those in the subsequent figures comprise part of the doctoral dissertation of Dr Nan Wise at Rutgers University. Dr Eleni Frangos collaborated in portions of the research. (*See plate section for color representation of the figure*)

This descending system was shown to be activated by vaginal stimulation in rats [93]. The anterior cingulate and insular cortices activated at orgasm have also been shown to be activated by painful stimuli [94–96]. There is a curious similarity between the facial grimaces of women and men during orgasm and pain – labeled on a website as the face of "sweet agony", perhaps related to evidence that the afferent spinal cord pathway for pain and orgasm apparently both use the spinothalamic pathway [97, 98].

The amygdala and posterior hypothalamus are activated at orgasm (Figure 13.4). These two regions may be involved in the sympathetic autonomic division that induces the increased heart rate and blood pressure characteristic of orgasm [99]. The amygdala is also probably involved in the emotional [100] correlates of orgasm.

Penfield showed that electrical stimulation of the hippocampus elicited dreamlike imagery [101]. Perhaps the activation of the hippocampus at orgasm plays a significant role in fantasy generation during orgasm. How may nucleus accumbens, cingulate cortex, insular cortex, amygdala, hippocampus, and paraventricular nucleus of the hypothalamus (PVN) contribute to the characteristics of orgasm? The PVN neurons produce oxytocin and become activated during orgasm, releasing oxytocin into the bloodstream from the posterior pituitary gland [102, 103]. In response to this oxytocin, the uterus contracts vigorously, generating sensations that women claim intensify the pleasure of orgasm [61].

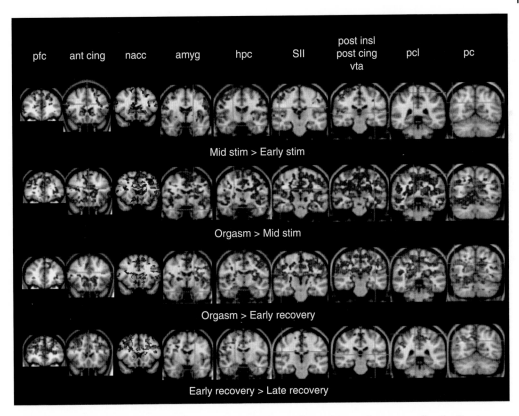

| pfc | ant cing | nacc | amyg | hpc | SII | post insl<br>post cing<br>vta | pcl | pc |

Mid stim > Early stim

Orgasm > Mid stim

Orgasm > Early recovery

Early recovery > Late recovery

**Figure 13.3** Preliminary group fMRI data (N = 10) providing evidence that maximum overall activation in widespread regions of the brain was observed at orgasm. Multiple brain "sections" are shown, representing the regions identified by the labels above them. The data were generated by subtracting one 10-second epoch from another. Thus, activity during the first 10 s of stimulation ("Early stim") was subtracted from the 10-s activity midway between the start of stimulation and the start of orgasm ("Mid stim"). The activity at mid-stim was subtracted from the 10-s epoch starting when the women pressed a button indicating initiation of orgasm. The subsequent postorgasm responses were comparably subtracted as indicated ("recovery" refers to the phase after the women pressed the button to indicate the end of their orgasm). Abbreviations: amyg: amygdala; ant cing: anterior cingulate cortex; hpc: hippocampus; nacc: nucleus accumbens; pc: parietal cortex; pcl: paracentral lobule; pfc: prefrontal cortex; post cing: posterior cingulate cortex; post insl: posterior insula; SII: Supplementary sensory cortex (operculum); vta: ventral tegmental area. (*See plate section for color representation of the figure*)

The PVN also plays an essential role in ejaculation. In rats, these neurons are stimulated by dopamine (at $D_4$ receptors) [104], some of which project to the posterior pituitary and bifurcate. The other oxytocin-containing axons project down through the spinal cord and synapse on neurons at the lumbar to sacral levels that control erection and ejaculation [105], with oxytocin acting as a sympathetic division preganglionic stimulatory neurotransmitter [106, 107]. Thus, oxytocin serves both as a hormone in orgasm in women and men and as a neurotransmitter in ejaculation in males [108].

The nucleus accumbens is activated at orgasm in women [76] (Figure 13.4) and receives a significant dopaminergic input from neurons in the ventral tegmental area. The ventral tegmental area is also activated during orgasm in men [78]. Thus, this dopaminergic system is evidently activated during orgasm in women and men. Pharmacological

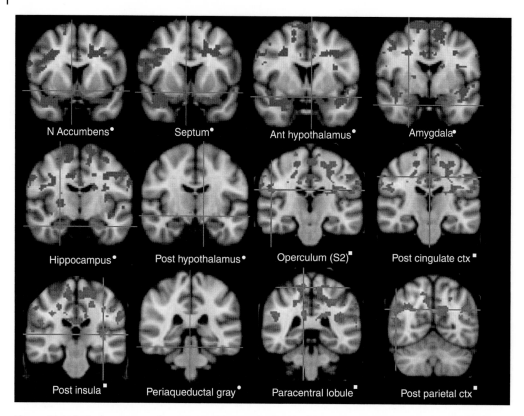

**Figure 13.4** Preliminary group data providing evidence of regional activation pattern "going over" into orgasm. The group activity in each region during the 10 seconds immediately prior to the button press was subtracted from the 10 seconds immediately after the button press, by which the women indicated the start of their orgasm. Brain areas activated at criterion of $z = 1.65$ are labeled by a square; those at a criterion of $z = 1.55$ are labeled by a circle. Brain areas from the brain stem analysis are labeled by an asterisk and are activated at a criterion of $z = 1.0$. While the latter two z criteria are lower than customary, the data are shown in order to represent activity in brainstem regions represented by very few voxels, which might otherwise be subject to a type 2 error. (*See plate section for color representation of the figure*)

studies provide evidence that dopaminergic blockade attenuates orgasmic intensity, and dopaminergic stimulation intensifies it [61]. The nucleus accumbens is activated during cocaine or nicotine-induced euphoric "rush" [75, 109], which share characteristics of orgasm [110].

The cerebellum becomes activated at orgasm in women and men [76, 78, 82, 83]. Increased muscle tension, which can reach peak levels at orgasm [111], is regulated by the cerebellum via proprioception and the gamma efferent system [112]. Since muscle tension contributes to the sensory pleasure of orgasm [110], it is likely that the cerebel-

lum plays not only a motoric, but also a significant perceptual/cognitive-hedonic, role in orgasm.

The cingulate cortex, which is strongly activated at orgasm, likely plays a dual role of stimulating the output of the sympathetic division of the autonomic system and generating the intense feelings of orgasm. At orgasm in women, the heart rate, blood pressure, pupil diameter, and pain thresholds each approximately double in magnitude [99], all of which indicate a net intense activation of sympathetic output. The observations that the cingulate cortex also responds to "... pleasant touch, taste and olfactory stimuli suggests that this region is not only involved in the processing of affectively negative stimuli such as pain and aversive taste" [113], but rather more generally to intense emotion-provoking feelings [114, 115].

The insular cortex, which is also reliably and strongly activated during orgasm, mediates visceral feelings, especially pleasure and pain [116, 117]. Activation of both the amygdala and the hippocampus occurs during orgasm (Figure 13.4). Consistent with this finding is that both the amygdala and the hippocampus are susceptible to temporal lobe or psychomotor epilepsy [118], which may generate orgasmic feelings, and pre-seizure "orgasmic aura" [119–122].

## Corollary Animal Studies

Consistent with the brain regions that are activated during orgasm in humans, studies in the laboratory rat report activation of many of the same-named brain components in response to genital stimulation. Thus, based on the indicator c-fos, activation was reported in the amygdala [123–128] and par-aventricular nucleus of the hypothalamus [124]. Furthermore, dopamine is released in the nucleus accumbens [90]. More precise understanding of the anatomy and functional neurophysiology of orgasm should facilitate in improving current therapeutic strategies and in developing novel treatments for orgasmic dysfunction.

# References

1 Basson R, Brotto LA, Laan E, *et al.* Assessment and management of women's sexual dysfunctions: problematic desire and arousal. *J Sex Med.* 2005;2:291–300.

2 Jannini EA, Rubio-Casillas A, Whipple B, *et al.* Female orgasm(s): one, two, several. *J Sex Med.* 2012;9:956–965.

3 Burnett AL, Calvin DC, Silver RI, *et al.* Immunohistochemical description of nitric oxide synthase isoforms in human clitoris. *J Urol.* 1997;158:75–78.

4 Toesca A, Stolfi VM, Cocchia D. Immunohistochemical study of the corpora cavernosa of the human clitoris. *J Anat.* 1996;188 (Pt 3):513–520.

5 Tarcan T, Park K, Goldstein I, *et al.* Histomorphometric analysis of age-related structural changes in human clitoral cavernosal tissue. *J Urol.* 1999;161:940–944.

6 Giraldi A, Marson L, Nappi R, *et al.* Physiology of female sexual function: animal models. *J Sex Med.* 2004;1:237–253.

7 Martin KA, Chang RJ, Ehrmann DA, *et al.* Evaluation and treatment of hirsutism in premenopausal women: an endocrine society clinical practice guideline. *J Clin Endocrinol Metab.* 2008;93:1105–1120.

8 Jannini E, d'Amati G and Lenzi A. Histology and immunohistochemical studies of female genital tissue. In: Goldstein I, Meston CM, Davis SR, Traish AM (eds) *Women's Sexual Function and Dysfunction: Study, Diagnosis and Treatment.* London: Taylor and Francis; 2006, pp. 125–133.

9 Lakomy M, Happola O, Majewski M, Kaleczyc J. Immunohistochemical localization of neuropeptides in nerve fibers of the porcine vagina and uterine cervix. *Folia Histochem Cytobiol.* 1994;32:167–175.

10 Majewski M, Sienkiewicz W, Kaleczyc J, *et al.* The distribution and co-localization of immunoreactivity to nitric oxide synthase, vasoactive intestinal polypeptide and substance P within nerve fibres supplying bovine and porcine female genital organs. *Cell Tissue Res.* 1995;281:445–464.

11 Hoyle CH, Stones RW, Robson T, *et al.* Innervation of vasculature and microvasculature of the human vagina by NOS and neuropeptide-containing nerves. *J Anat.* 1996;188 (Pt 3):633–644.

12 Al-Hijji J, Batra S. Downregulation by estrogen of nitric oxide synthase activity in the female rabbit lower urinary tract. *Urology.* 1999;53:637–641.

13 Batra S, Al-Hijji J. Characterization of nitric oxide synthase activity in rabbit uterus and vagina: downregulation by estrogen. *Life Sci.* 1998;62:2093–2100.

14 Giraldi A, Persson K, Werkstrom V, *et al.* Effects of diabetes on neurotransmission in rat vaginal smooth muscle. *Int J Impot Res.* 2001;13:58–66.

15 D'Amati G, di Gioia CR, Proietti Pannunzi L, *et al.* Functional anatomy of the human vagina. *J Endocrinol Invest.* 2003;26:92–96.

16 Al-Hijji J, Larsson B, Batra S. Nitric oxide synthase in the rabbit uterus and vagina: hormonal regulation and functional significance. *Biol Reprod.* 2000;62:1387–1392.

17 Berman JR, McCarthy MM, Kyprianou N. Effect of estrogen withdrawal on nitric oxide synthase expression and apoptosis in the rat vagina. *Urology.* 1998;51:650–656.

18 Yoon HN, Chung WS, Park YY, *et al.* Effects of estrogen on nitric oxide synthase and histological composition in the rabbit clitoris and vagina. *Int J Impot Res.* 2001;13:205–211.

19 Chatterjee S, Gangula PR, Dong YL, Yallampalli C. Immunocytochemical localization of nitric oxide synthase-III in reproductive organs of female rats during the oestrous cycle. *Histochem J.* 1996;28:715–723.

20 Park K, Moreland RB, Goldstein I, *et al.* Sildenafil inhibits phosphodiesterase type 5 in human clitoral corpus cavernosum smooth muscle. *Biochem Biophys Res Commun.* 1998;249:612–617.

21 D'Amati G, di Gioia CR, Bologna M, *et al.* Type 5 phosphodiesterase expression in the human vagina. *Urology.* 2002;60:191–195.

22 Morelli A, Filippi S, Mancina R, *et al.* Androgens regulate phosphodiesterase type 5 expression and functional activity in corpora cavernosa. *Endocrinology.* 2004;145:2253–2263.

23 Uckert S, Oelke M, Albrecht K, *et al.* Expression and distribution of key enzymes of the cyclic GMP signaling in the human clitoris: relation to phosphodiesterase type 5 (PDE5). *Int J Impot Res.* 2011;23:206–212.

24 Hauser-Kronberger C, Cheung A, Hacker GW, *et al.* Peptidergic innervation of the human clitoris. *Peptides.* 1999;20:539–543.

25 Yucel S, De Souza A Jr, Baskin LS. Neuroanatomy of the human female lower urogenital tract. *J Urol.* 2004;172:191–195.

26 Cocchia D, Rende M, Toesca A, *et al.* Immunohistochemical study of neuropeptide Y-containing nerve fibers in the human clitoris and penis. *Cell Biol Int Rep.* 1990;14:865–875.

27 Gelez H, Poirier S, Facchinetti P, *et al.* Neuroanatomical evidence for a role of central melanocortin-4 receptors and oxytocin in the efferent control of the rodent clitoris and vagina. *J Sex Med.* 2010;7:2056–2067.

28 Traish AM, Kim N, Min K, *et al.* Role of androgens in female genital sexual arousal: receptor expression, structure, and function. *Fertil Steril.* 2002;77(Suppl 4): S11–18.

29 Park K, Ryu SB, Park YI, *et al.* Diabetes mellitus induces vaginal tissue fibrosis by TGF-beta 1 expression in the rat model. *J Sex Marital Ther.* 2001;27:577–587.

30 Larsson LI, Fahrenkrug J, Schaffalitzky de Muckadell OB. Vasoactive intestinal polypeptide occurs in nerves of the female genitourinary tract. *Science.* 1977;197:1374–1375.

31 Levin RJ. VIP, vagina, clitoral and periurethral glans – an update on human female genital arousal. *Exp Clin Endocrinol.* 1991;98:61–69.

32 Ottesen B, Fahrenkrug J. Vasoactive intestinal polypeptide and other preprovasoactive intestinal polypeptide-derived peptides in the female and male genital tract: localization, biosynthesis, and functional and clinical significance. *Am J Obstet Gynecol.* 1995;172:1615–1631.

33 Costagliola A, Mayer B, Vittoria A, *et al.* NADPH-diaphorase-, nitric oxide synthase- and VIP-containing nerve structures in the hen oviduct: a histochemical and immunohistochemical study. *Arch Histol Cytol.* 1997;60:245–256.

34 Pollen JJ, Dreilinger A. Immunohistochemical identification of prostatic acid phosphatase and prostate specific antigen in female periurethral glands. *Urology.* 1984;23:303–304.

35 Tepper SL, Jagirdar J, Heath D, Geller SA. Homology between the female paraurethral (Skene's) glands and the prostate. *Immunohistochemical demonstration. Arch Pathol Lab Med.* 1984;108:423–425.

36 Zaviacic M. Enzyme histochemistry of the adult human female prostate: acid phosphatase distribution. *Cell Mol Biol.* 1984;30:545–551.

37 Zaviacic M, Danihel L, Ruzickova M, *et al.* Immunohistochemical localization of human protein 1 in the female prostate (Skene's gland) and the male prostate. *Histochem J.* 1997;29:219–227.

38 Czaja K, Sienkiewicz W, Vittoria A, *et al.* Neuroendocrine cells in the female urogenital tract of the pig, and their immunohistochemical characterization. *Acta Anat (Basel).* 1996;157:11–19.

39 Bekker MD, Hogewoning CR, Wallner C, *et al.* The somatic and autonomic innervation of the clitoris; preliminary evidence of sexual dysfunction after minimally invasive slings. *J Sex Med.* 2012;9:1566–1578.

40 O'Connell HE, Sanjeevan KV, Hutson JM. Anatomy of the clitoris. *J Urol.* 2005;174:1189–1195.

41 O'Connell HE, Hutson JM, Anderson CR, Plenter RJ. Anatomical relationship between urethra and clitoris. *J Urol.* 1998;159:1892–1897.

42 Mazloomdoost D, Pauls RN. A comprehensive review of the clitoris and its role in female sexual function. *Sex Med Rev.* 2015;3:245–263.

43 Cellerino A, Jannini EA. Male reproductive physiology as a sexually selected handicap? Erectile dysfunction is correlated with general health and health prognosis and may have evolved as a marker of poor phenotypic quality. *Med Hypotheses.* 2005;65:179–184.

44 Glucksmann A, Ooka-Souda S, Miura-Yasugi E, Mizuno T. The effect of neonatal treatment of male mice with antiandrogens and of females with androgens on the development of the os penis and os clitoridis. *J Anat.* 1976;121:363–370.

45 Callegari C, Everett S, Ross M, Brasel JA. Anogenital ratio: measure of fetal virilization in premature and full-term newborn infants. *J Pediatr.* 1987;111:240–243.

46 Arbuckle TE, Hauser R, Swan SH, *et al.* Meeting report: measuring endocrine-sensitive endpoints within the first years of life. *Environ Health Perspect.* 2008;116:948–951.

47 Phillip M, De Boer C, Pilpel D, *et al.* Clitoral and penile sizes of full term newborns in two different ethnic groups. *J Pediatr Endocrinol Metab.* 1996;9:175–179.

48 Riley WJ, Rosenbloom AL. Clitoral size in infancy. *J Pediatr.* 1980;96:918–919.

49 Litwin A, Aitkin I, Merlob P. Clitoral length assessment in newborn infants of 30 to 41 weeks gestational age. *Eur J Obstet Gynecol Reprod Biol.* 1991;38:209–212.

50 Mondal R, Chatterjee K, Samanta M, *et al.* Clitoral length and anogenital ratio in indian newborn girls. *Indian Pediatr.* 2016;53:299–303.

51 Oakley SH, Vaccaro CM, Crisp CC, *et al.* Clitoral size and location in relation to sexual function using pelvic MRI. *J Sex Med.* 2014;11:1013–1022.

52 McEwen GN Jr, Renner G. Validity of anogenital distance as a marker of in utero phthalate exposure. *Environ Health Perspect.* 2006;114:A19–20; author reply A20-1.

53 Wu Y, Zhong G, Chen S, *et al.* Polycystic ovary syndrome is associated with anogenital distance, a marker of prenatal androgen exposure. *Hum Reprod.* 2017:1–7.

54 Mira-Escolano MP, Mendiola J, Minguez-Alarcon L, *et al*. Longer anogenital distance is associated with higher testosterone levels in women: a cross-sectional study. *Bjog*. 2014;121:1359–1364.

55 Wallen K, Lloyd EA. Female sexual arousal: genital anatomy and orgasm in intercourse. *Horm Behav*. 2011;59:780–792.

56 Song YB, Hwang K, Kim DJ, Han SH. Innervation of vagina: microdissection and immunohistochemical study. *J Sex Marital Ther*. 2009;35:144–153.

57 Rubio-Casillas A, Jannini EA. New insights from one case of female ejaculation. *J Sex Med*. 2011;8:3500–3504.

58 Gravina GL, Brandetti F, Martini P, *et al*. Measurement of the thickness of the urethrovaginal space in women with or without vaginal orgasm. *J Sex Med*. 2008;5:610–618.

59 Maravilla KR, Cao Y, Heiman JR, *et al*. Noncontrast dynamic magnetic resonance imaging for quantitative assessment of female sexual arousal. *J Urol*. 2005;173:162–166.

60 Buisson O, Foldes P, Jannini E, Mimoun S. Coitus as revealed by ultrasound in one volunteer couple. *J Sex Med*. 2010;7:2750–2754.

61 Komisaruk BR, Beyer C, Whipple B. *The Science of Orgasm*. Baltimore: The Johns Hopkins University Press; 2006.

62 Jannini EA, Whipple B, Kingsberg SA, *et al*. Who's afraid of the G-spot? *J Sex Med*. 2010;7:25–34.

63 Jannini EA, Buisson O, Rubio-Casillas A. Beyond the G-spot: clitourethrovaginal complex anatomy in female orgasm. *Nat Rev Urol*. 2014;11:531–538.

64 Hamann S, Herman RA, Nolan CL, Wallen K. Men and women differ in amygdala response to visual sexual stimuli. *Nat Neurosci*. 2004;7:411–416.

65 Karama S, Lecours AR, Leroux JM, *et al* Areas of brain activation in males and females during viewing of erotic film excerpts. *Hum Brain Mapp*. 2002;16:1–13.

66 Rupp HA, James TW, Ketterson ED, *et al*. Lower sexual interest in postpartum women: relationship to amygdala activation and intranasal oxytocin. *Horm Behav*. 2013;63:114–121.

67 Spinella M. The role of prefrontal systems in sexual behavior. *Int J Neurosci*. 2007;117:369–385.

68 Leon-Carrion J, Martin-Rodriguez JF, Damas-Lopez J, *et al*. Does dorsolateral prefrontal cortex (DLPFC) activation return to baseline when sexual stimuli cease? The role of DLPFC in visual sexual stimulation. *Neurosci Lett*. 2007;416:55–60.

69 Huynh HK, Beers C, Willemsen A, *et al*. High-intensity erotic visual stimuli de-activate the primary visual cortex in women. *J Sex Med*. 2012;9:1579–1587.

70 Cera N, Di Pierro ED, Sepede G, *et al*. The role of left superior parietal lobe in male sexual behavior: dynamics of distinct components revealed by FMRI. *J Sex Med*. 2012;9:1602–1612.

71 Wise NJ, Frangos E, Komisaruk BR. Activation of sensory cortex by imagined genital stimulation: an fMRI analysis. *Socioaffect Neurosci Psychol*. 2016;6:31481.

72 Ferretti A, Caulo M, Del Gratta C, *et al*. Dynamics of male sexual arousal: distinct components of brain activation revealed by fMRI. *Neuroimage*. 2005;26:1086–1096.

73 Kuhn S, Gallinat J. A quantitative meta-analysis on cue-induced male sexual arousal. *J Sex Med*. 2011;8:2269–2275.

74 Oei NY, Rombouts SA, Soeter RP, *et al*. Dopamine modulates reward system activity during subconscious processing of sexual stimuli. *Neuropsychopharmacology*. 2012;37:1729–1737.

75 Breiter HC, Gollub RL, Weisskoff RM, *et al*. Acute effects of cocaine on human brain activity and emotion. *Neuron*. 1997;19:591–611.

76 Komisaruk BR, Whipple B, Crawford A, *et al*. Brain activation during vaginocervical self-stimulation and orgasm in women with complete spinal cord injury: fMRI evidence of mediation by the vagus nerves. *Brain Res*. 2004;1024:77–88.

77 Komisaruk BR, Wise, N, Frangos, E, Allen, K. An fMRI timecourse analysis of brain regions activated during self-stimulation to orgasm in women. *Society for Neuroscience Annual Conference.* 2010:285.6.

78 Holstege G, Georgiadis JR, Paans AM, *et al.* Brain activation during human male ejaculation. *J Neurosci.* 2003;23: 9185–9193.

79 Komisaruk BR, Wise, N, Frangos, E, *et al.* An fMRI video animation time-course analysis of regions activated during selfstimulation to orgasm in women. *Society for Neuroscience Annual Conference.* 2011:495.03.

80 Komisaruk BR, Whipple B. Functional MRI of the brain during orgasm in women. *Annu Rev Sex Res.* 2005;16:62–86.

81 Georgiadis JR, Kortekaas R, Kuipers R, *et al.* Regional cerebral blood flow changes associated with clitorally induced orgasm in healthy women. *Eur J Neurosci.* 2006;24:3305–3316.

82 Georgiadis JR, Reinders AA, Paans AM, *et al.* Men versus women on sexual brain function: prominent differences during tactile genital stimulation, but not during orgasm. *Hum Brain Mapp.* 2009;30:3089–3101.

83 Holstege G. How the emotional motor system controls the pelvic organs. *Sex Med Rev.* 2016;4:303–328.

84 Allen K, Komisaruk B. fMRI representation of erotic vs. non-erotic genital self-stimulation; attenuation during the post-orgasmic refractory period in men. *Society for Neuroscience Annual Conference.* 2016:235.06.

85 Ladas A, Whipple B, Perry J. *The G Spot and Other Recent Discoveries about Human Sexuality.* New York: Holt, Rinehart and Winston; 1982.

86 Cutler WB, Zacker M, McCoy N, *et al.* Sexual response in women. *Obstet Gynecol.* 2000;95:S19.

87 Di Noto PM, Newman L, Wall S, Einstein G. The hermunculus: what is known about the representation of the female body in the brain? *Cereb Cortex.* 2013;23:1005–1013.

88 Komisaruk B, Allen K, Wise N, *et al.* Men's genital structures mapped on the sensory cortex: fMRI evidence. *Society for Neuroscience Annual Conference.* 2013.

89 Komisaruk BR, Whipple B. Non-genital orgasms. *Sex Relation Ther.* 2011;26:356–372.

90 Pfaus JG, Damsma G, Wenkstern D, Fibiger HC. Sexual activity increases dopamine transmission in the nucleus accumbens and striatum of female rats. *Brain Res.* 1995;693:21–30.

91 Whipple B, Komisaruk BR. Elevation of pain threshold by vaginal stimulation in women. *Pain.* 1985;21:357–367.

92 Basbaum AI, Fields HL. Endogenous pain control systems: brainstem spinal pathways and endorphin circuitry. *Annu Rev Neurosci.* 1984;7:309–338.

93 Steinman JL, Komisaruk BR, Yaksh TL, Tyce GM. Spinal cord monoamines modulate the antinociceptive effects of vaginal stimulation in rats. *Pain.* 1983;16:155–166.

94 Casey KL, Minoshima S, Berger KL, *et al.* Positron emission tomographic analysis of cerebral structures activated specifically by repetitive noxious heat stimuli. *J Neurophysiol.* 1994;71:802–807.

95 Casey KL, Morrow TJ, Lorenz J, Minoshima S. Temporal and spatial dynamics of human forebrain activity during heat pain: analysis by positron emission tomography. *J Neurophysiol.* 2001;85:951–959.

96 Pukall CF, Strigo IA, Binik YM, *et al.* Neural correlates of painful genital touch in women with vulvar vestibulitis syndrome. *Pain.* 2005;115:118–127.

97 Monnier M. *Functions of the Nervous System.* New York: Elsevier; 1968.

98 Elliott H. *Textbook of Neuroanatomy.* Philadelphia: J.B. Lippincott; 1969.

99 Whipple B, Ogden G, Komisaruk BR. Physiological correlates of imagery-induced orgasm in women. *Arch Sex Behav.* 1992;21:121–133.

100 Phelps E, LeDoux J. Contributions of the amygdala to emotion processing: from animal models to human behavior. *Neuron* 2005;48:175–187.

101 Penfield W. Functional localization in temporal and deep sylvian areas. *Res Publ Assoc Res Nerv Ment Dis.* 1958;36:210–226.

102 Carmichael MS, Humbert R, Dixen J, *et al.* Plasma oxytocin increases in the human sexual response. *J Clin Endocrinol Metab.* 1987;64:27–31.

103 Carmichael MS, Warburton VL, Dixen J, Davidson JM. Relationships among cardiovascular, muscular, and oxytocin responses during human sexual activity. *Arch Sex Behav.* 1994;23:59–79.

104 Melis MR, Succu S, Mascia MS, Argiolas A. PD-168077, a selective dopamine D4 receptor agonist, induces penile erection when injected into the paraventricular nucleus of male rats. *Neurosci Lett.* 2005;379:59–62.

105 Veronneau-Longueville F, Rampin O, Freund-Mercier MJ, *et al.* Oxytocinergic innervation of autonomic nuclei controlling penile erection in the rat. *Neuroscience.* 1999;93:1437–1447.

106 Sansone GR, Gerdes CA, Steinman JL, *et al.* Vaginocervical stimulation releases oxytocin within the spinal cord in rats. *Neuroendocrinology.* 2002;75:306–315.

107 Sansone GR, Komisaruk BR. Evidence that oxytocin is an endogenous stimulator of autonomic sympathetic preganglionics: the pupillary dilatation response to vaginocervical stimulation in the rat. *Brain Res.* 2001;898:265–271.

108 Argiolas A, Melis MR. Central control of penile erection: role of the paraventricular nucleus of the hypothalamus. *Prog Neurobiol.* 2005;76:1–21.

109 Stein EA, Pankiewicz J, Harsch HH, *et al.* Nicotine-induced limbic cortical activation in the human brain: a functional MRI study. *Am J Psychiatry.* 1998;155:1009–1015.

110 Komisaruk BR, Whipple B, Beye, C. Sexual Pleasure. In: Berridge K, Kringelbach M (eds) *Pleasures of the Brain: Neural Bases of Sensory Pleasure.* New York: Oxford University Press; 2009, pp. 169–177.

111 Masters W, Johnson V. *Human Sexual Response.* Boston, MA: Little, Brown; 1966.

112 Mould D. Neuromuscular aspects of women's orgasms. *J Sex Res.* 1980;16:193–201.

113 Francis S, Rolls ET, Bowtell R, *et al.* The representation of pleasant touch in the brain and its relationship with taste and olfactory areas. *Neuroreport.* 1999;10:453–459.

114 Bush G, Luu P, Posner MI. Cognitive and emotional influences in anterior cingulate cortex. *Trends Cogn Sci.* 2000;4:215–222.

115 Vogt B. Cingulate cortex. In: Adelman G, Smith B (eds) *Encyclopedia of Neuroscience.* New York: Elsevier; 1999.

116 Penfield W, Faulk ME, Jr. The insula; further observations on its function. *Brain.* 1955;78:445–470.

117 Small DM, Zatorre RJ, Dagher A, *et al.* Changes in brain activity related to eating chocolate: from pleasure to aversion. *Brain.* 2001;124:1720–1733.

118 Nauta WJ. Neural associations of the frontal cortex. *Acta Neurobiol Exp (Wars).* 1972;32:125–140.

119 Calleja J, Carpizo R, Berciano J. Orgasmic epilepsy. *Epilepsia.* 1988;29:635–639.

120 Janszky J, Szucs A, Halasz P, *et al.* Orgasmic aura originates from the right hemisphere. *Neurology.* 2002;58:302–304.

121 Janszky J, Ebner A, Szupera Z, *et al.* Orgasmic aura – a report of seven cases. *Seizure.* 2004;13:441–444.

122 Reading PJ, Will RG. Unwelcome orgasms. *Lancet.* 1997;350:1746.

123 Erskine MS, Hanrahan SB. Effects of paced mating on c-fos gene expression in the female rat brain. *J Neuroendocrinol.* 1997;9:903–912.

124 Rowe DW, Erskine MS. c-Fos proto-oncogene activity induced by mating in

the preoptic area, hypothalamus and amygdala in the female rat: role of afferent input via the pelvic nerve. *Brain Res.* 1993;621:25–34.

125 Tetel MJ, Getzinger MJ, Blaustein JD. Fos expression in the rat brain following vaginal-cervical stimulation by mating and manual probing. *J Neuroendocrinol.* 1993;5:397–404.

126 Wersinger SR, Baum MJ, Erskine MS. Mating-induced FOS-like immunoreactivity in the rat forebrain: a sex comparison and a dimorphic effect of pelvic nerve transection. *J Neuroendocrinol.* 1993;5:557–568.

127 Pfaus JG, Heeb MM. Implications of immediate-early gene induction in the brain following sexual stimulation of female and male rodents. *Brain Res Bull.* 1997;44:397–407.

128 Veening JG, Coolen LM. Neural activation following sexual behavior in the male and female rat brain. *Behav Brain Res.* 1998;92:181–193.

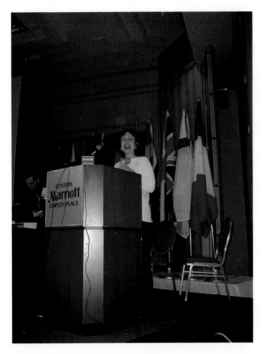

**Figure 1.1** Sandra Leiblum, PhD, first president of the International Society for the Study of Women's Sexual Health, presiding over the business meeting.

*Textbook of Female Sexual Function and Dysfunction: Diagnosis and Treatment*, First Edition. Edited by Irwin Goldstein, Anita H. Clayton, Andrew T. Goldstein, Noel N. Kim, and Sheryl A. Kingsberg.
© 2018 John Wiley & Sons Ltd. Published 2018 by John Wiley & Sons Ltd.

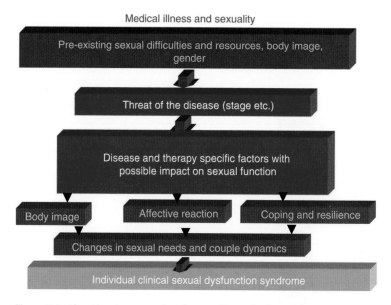

**Figure 2.1** Algorithm incorporating the specific medical condition.

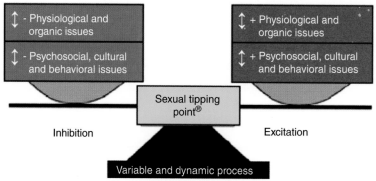

**Figure 4.1** Sexual tipping point model of sexual excitation and inhibition. Cultural, psychological, and physiological factors conspire to tip the balance either toward excitation or inhibition. Sexually functional individuals maintain a degree of lability in the balance, and an ability to have it tipped toward either excitation or inhibition. Persons with hypoactive sexual desire disorder are likely to have the balance weighed down by inhibition. This can occur because of hypofunctional excitation, hyperfunction inhibition, or a combination of the two. After Perelman [67].

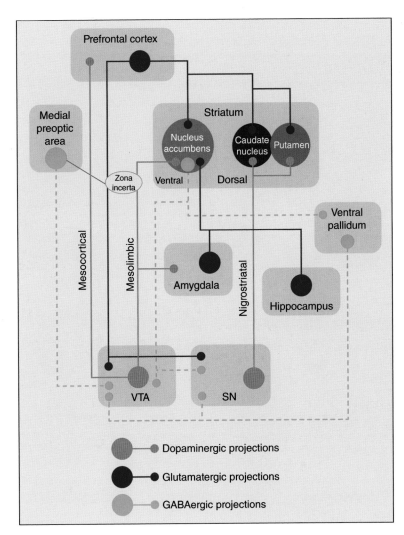

**Figure 4.2** A wiring diagram of sexual excitation and inhibition in the mammalian brain that reflects current understanding of neuroanatomical and neurochemical pathways. VTA: Ventral tegmental area; SN: substantia nigra. Modified from Kingsberg *et al.* [119].

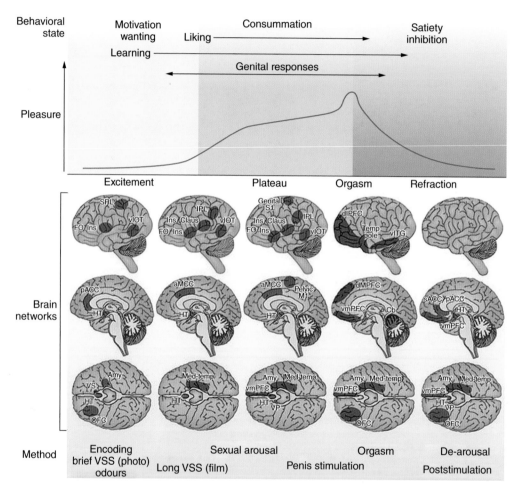

**Figure 4.6** Patterns of brain activation in response to sexual stimulation as a function of the EPOR stages of sexual response. From Georgiadis *et al.* [23].

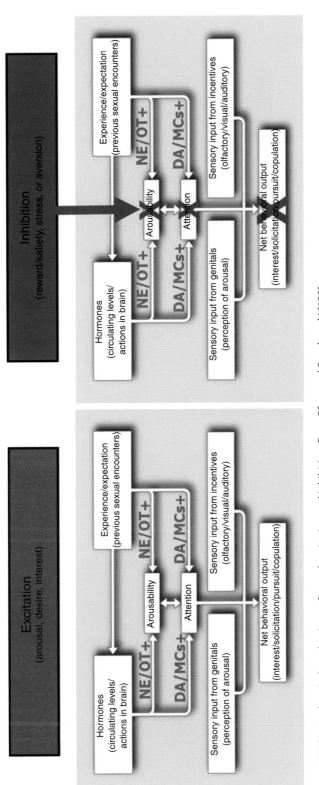

**Figure 4.7** Neurochemical mechanisms of sexual excitation and inhibition. From Pfaus and Scepkowski [120].

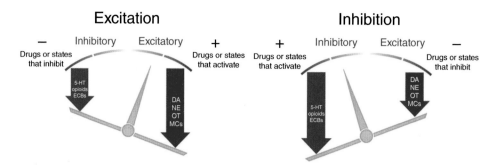

**Figure 4.8** Neurochemical mechanisms of sexual excitation within a tipping point model. Left: sexual excitation. Right: Sexual inhibition. From Pfaus [6].

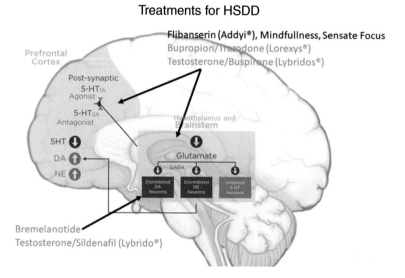

**Figure 4.9** Treatments for sexual desire disorders and their potential mechanisms of action in the brain. From Pfaus [121].

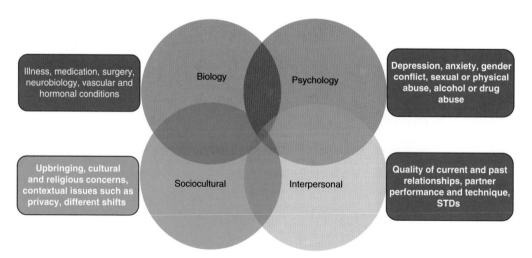

**Figure 5.1** Biopsychosocial model of sexual response.

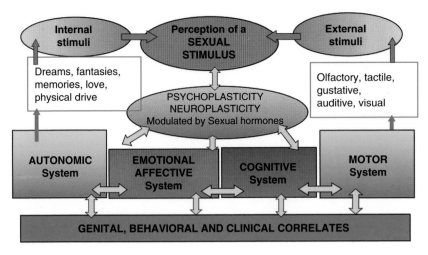

**Figure 8.1** Physiology of sexual desire/interest and central arousal. (Adapted from [6].)

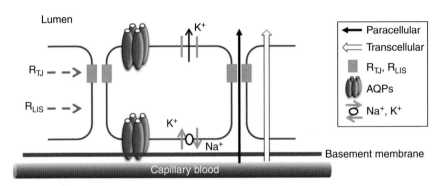

**Figure 8.3** Mechanisms of transvaginal epithelial permeability.

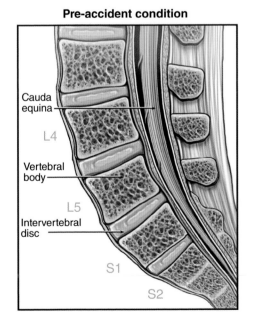

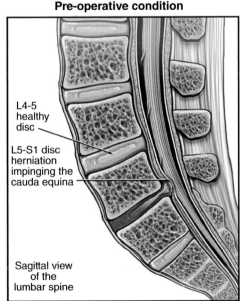

**Figure 11.1** Schematic representation of a herniated intervertebral disc at L5-S1 impinging on, and irritating, the nerve roots of the cauda equina. If the radiculitis affects the sacral spinal nerve roots (SSNR) various neurogenic sexual dysfunctions, such as persistent genital arousal disorder (PGAD), may be experienced. Several cures of men and women with PGAD secondary to radiculitis of the SSNR have been realized with minimally-invasive out-patient lumbar spine surgery.

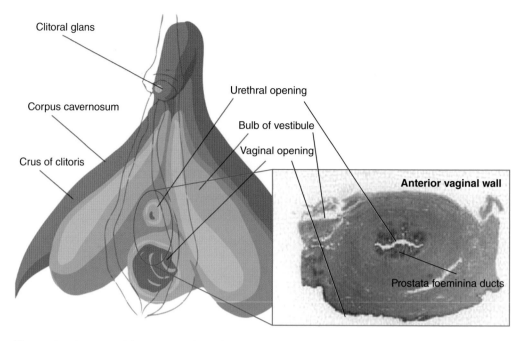

**Figure 13.1** Anatomy of the CUV complex. Schematic representation of the external and internal clitoris and the vaginal opening. The insert, an anterior vaginal wall obtained from a cadaver [15, 21], represent the intimate relationships between all the different anatomical structures involved in the female sexual pleasure.

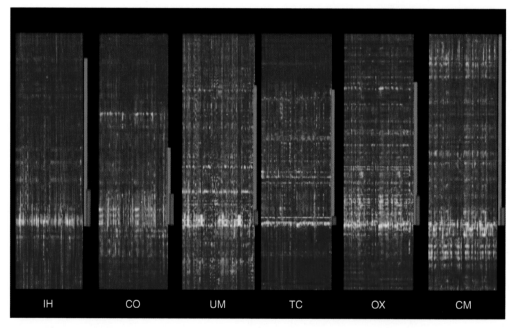

**Figure 13.2** Descriptive "tapestry" representation of brain activity in response to clitoral self-stimulation leading up to, during, and after orgasm in each of six women. Each woman's tapestry consists of 80 columns, each column representing a Brodmann area. Each row represents a successive two-second sample of functional MRI activity, starting at the top. The relative magnitude of brain activity in each region at each time period is represented as brightness. The shorter vertical bars to the right of each tapestry represents the onset and duration of orgasm; the longer bars represent the onset and duration of clitoral self-stimulation. Note the maximum activation in widespread brain regions during orgasm, in contrast to the variable patterns of regional brain activity leading up to, and after, orgasm. These descriptive data and those in the subsequent figures comprise part of the doctoral dissertation of Dr Nan Wise at Rutgers University. Dr Eleni Frangos collaborated in portions of the research.

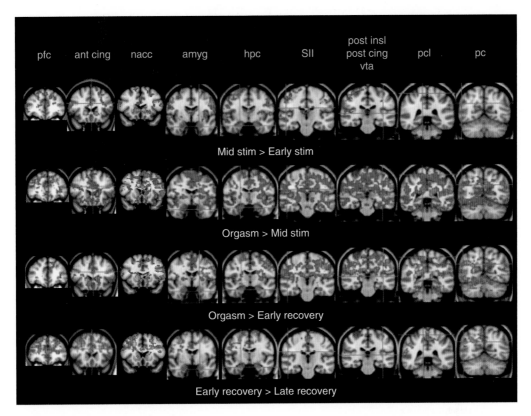

**Figure 13.3** Preliminary group fMRI data (N = 10) providing evidence that maximum overall activation in widespread regions of the brain was observed at orgasm. Multiple brain "sections" are shown, representing the regions identified by the labels above them. The data were generated by subtracting one 10-second epoch from another. Thus, activity during the first 10s of stimulation ("Early stim") was subtracted from the 10-s activity midway between the start of stimulation and the start of orgasm ("Mid stim"). The activity at mid-stim was subtracted from the 10-s epoch starting when the women pressed a button indicating initiation of orgasm. The subsequent postorgasm responses were comparably subtracted as indicated ("recovery" refers to the phase after the women pressed the button to indicate the end of their orgasm). Abbreviations: amyg: amygdala; ant cing: anterior cingulate cortex; hpc: hippocampus; nacc: nucleus accumbens; pc: parietal cortex; pcl: paracentral lobule; pfc: prefrontal cortex; post cing: posterior cingulate cortex; post insl: posterior insula; SII: Supplementary sensory cortex (operculum); vta: ventral tegmental area.

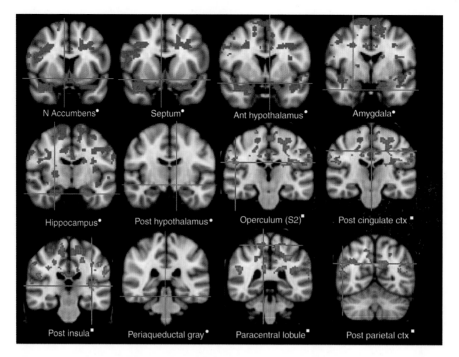

**Figure 13.4** Preliminary group data providing evidence of regional activation pattern "going over" into orgasm. The group activity in each region during the 10 seconds immediately prior to the button press was subtracted from the 10 seconds immediately after the button press, by which the women indicated the start of their orgasm. Brain areas activated at criterion of $z = 1.65$ are labeled by a square; those at a criterion of $z = 1.55$ are labeled by a circle. Brain areas from the brain stem analysis are labeled by an asterisk and are activated at a criterion of $z = 1.0$. While the latter two z criteria are lower than customary, the data are shown in order to represent activity in brainstem regions represented by very few voxels, which might otherwise be subject to a type 2 error.

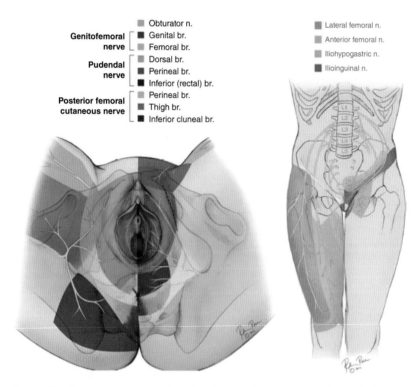

**Figure 21.4** Cutaneous nerves of the vulva, thigh, and groin. Used with permission from A. Lee Dellon, MD, PhD, from www.Dellon.com.

# 14

# Psychological Management of Orgasm Disorders

*Sara Nasserzadeh*

### Abstract

Psychological factors involve in facilitating or hindering the experience of orgasm are still under study. This chapter discusses orgasm as an element in the human sexual response cycle as we understand to date. It provides a summary of the most common predisposing, precipitating, and maintaining factors known to be underlying orgasmic disorders. It then discusses various models, ideas, and techniques that were proposed by clinicians and researches to assess, manage or treat these problems including the Holistic Assessment and Therapies Model (HAT). Definition and expression of orgasm related problems and their clinical implications are discussed.

**Keywords:** *orgasm; psychological; orgasmic; sexual response; social; cultural; language; holistic; assessment; treatment; diagnosis; disorder*

> The linear model of sexual response has evolved over the years to a more circular model which is much more aligned with what an individual might experience.
>
> Psychosocial and psychological factors can predispose a person to orgasmic dysfunction, precipitate an episode of concerning experience, or contribute to the perpetuation of the condition.
>
> Definition and expression of orgasm related problems vary across cultures, which could have clinical implications.

## Introduction

This chapter focuses on optimizing clinical success with women presenting with orgasm disorders where underlying psychological factors are at play. It will provide an overview of some of the psychosocial and psychological factors that could predispose a woman to orgasm dysfunction, precipitate an episode of dysfunction, or contribute to the perpetuation of the orgasm condition.

## Orgasm

This simple word could be a reminder of pleasure or pain, grief or gain for many women and couples. Orgasms have been defined and redefined throughout history. The word itself derives from the ancient Greek *orgasmos*, which means, "to swell as with moisture, be excited or eager" (Oxford Dictionary). One of the most quoted definitions today belongs to John Money and

*Textbook of Female Sexual Function and Dysfunction: Diagnosis and Treatment*, First Edition. Edited by Irwin Goldstein, Anita H. Clayton, Andrew T. Goldstein, Noel N. Kim, and Sheryl A. Kingsberg.
© 2018 John Wiley & Sons Ltd. Published 2018 by John Wiley & Sons Ltd.

colleagues (1991) "The zenith of sexuoerotic experience that men and women characterize subjectively as voluptuous rapture or ecstasy. It occurs simultaneously in the brain/mind and pelvic genitalia. ..." [1].

This conceptualization of orgasm as a measure of the success of any sex-related behavior or activity also stems, in part, from the significance sexual pleasure has within a specific cultural context. Is sexuality seen as an integral part of overall health and well-being or is it linked to a certain stage of life such as puberty or marriage? [2]. Is sexual pleasure seen as part of every healthy sexual relationship or is it considered as a luxury? Is orgasm an entity that only one of the partners is permitted, expected to have or believed to experience? Who, within a culture, is expected to receive sexual pleasure? Is sexual pleasure seen as a component of overall health or a luxury men enjoy, or something that is given to certain people by certain others?

We could dedicate a whole book to definitions of orgasm, as it is such an individualistic and subjective experience. Barry Komisaruk at Rutgers University explains: "It is like asking someone to describe how something tastes!" To have a baseline, though, this chapter defines orgasms as a buildup of pleasurable sensations and excitement to a peak intensity that releases tension and creates a feeling of satisfaction and relaxation [2].

## Orgasms and the Sexual Response Cycle

There is still much debate around whether female orgasm is necessary, unnecessary, fictional, a luxury, how it should feel and how frequently. In a study of heterosexual couples King and Belsky from University of East London, report that women experience two types of orgasms which they call Surface and Deep orgasms. According to King and colleagues, Deep orgasms are associated with internal feelings like floating and internal pulsing. Surface orgasms

are described as more intense, but located in the outer region of the vagina. They further report that deep orgasms with internal sensation were linked to male partners who were perceived to be considerate, dominant, with a noticeably attractive smell, and providing firm penetration [3]. However, it is also important to note that some hypothesized reproductively significant characteristics, such as being muscular, masculine, and aggressive, were not differentially associated with women experiencing deep orgasms. According to Gallup and colleagues, orgasm frequency was highly correlated with orgasm intensity but intensity was found to be a better predictor of sexual satisfaction than orgasm frequency [4]. In the same research, frequency of orgasms for heterosexual female college students was found to be dependent on three factors: partner's family income, his self-confidence, and how attractive he was. Orgasm intensity, on the other hand, was found to depend on how attracted women felt toward their male partners, the number of times they had sex per week, and ratings of sexual satisfaction. Gallup and colleagues also found that women who had started having sex at a younger age reported being more satisfied with their sex lives in general. Men's sense of humor was also reported to enhance orgasm frequency in the 54 women who were included [4].

In criticizing evolutionary explanations of female orgasms (i.e. the idea that female orgasms had a purpose for the sake of reproduction), Elizabeth Lloyd in The Case of the Female Orgasm takes on questions of how data on female sexuality and orgasms were obtained and debunks explanations that she believes to be inadequate [5]. For the sake of providing context for this chapter, it is worthwhile to consider an overview of the evolution of sexual response models since the linear model was introduced by Masters and Johnson in 1966 [6]. In the linear model of sexual response, both men and women thought to undergo four stages, beginning with excitement/arousal and proceeding to

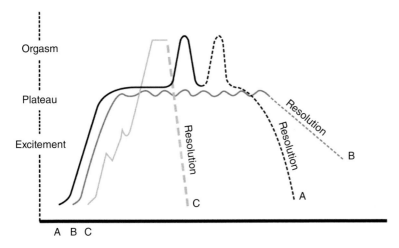

**Figure 14.1** Female sexual response model developed by Masters and Johnson, 1966 [6].

**Figure 14.2** Circular model of female sexual response developed by Whipple and Brash-McGreer, 1997 [8].

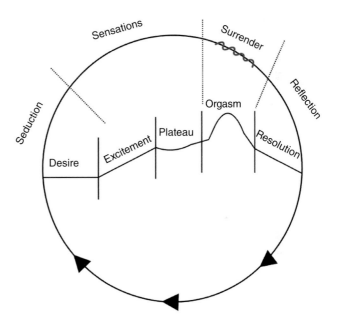

plateau, orgasm, and resolution (Figure 14.1). Helen Kaplan added the concept of desire to the model and presented the model in three phases: desire, arousal, and orgasm [7]. While this model was more generally applicable, as the science of sexology and empirical cases of psychosexual therapy accumulated, the model needed some further revisions to fit the evolving understanding around women's sexual response.

Both Masters and Johnson, as well as Kaplan, assumed that men and women have similar sexual responses, which then could lead to unnecessary pathologization of normal behavior in women [6, 7]. Whipple and Brash-McGreer then argued that many women do not move progressively and sequentially through the phases as described [8]. This gave birth to the circular model of sexual response. This new model was based on David Reed's Erotic Stimulus Pathway (published for the first time by William Stayton in 1998) [9], which comprises four stages (Figure 14.2): seduction (encompassing desire), sensations (excitement and plateau), surrender (orgasm), and reflection (resolution). The main insight of this model was that women may not experience all of the phases introduced in previous models. For example, they may move from sexual arousal to orgasm and satisfaction without experiencing sexual desire or they can experience desire, arousal, and satisfaction but not orgasm. The pleasant and satisfying sexual experiences may have a reinforcing effect on a woman, leading to the seduction phase of the next sexual experience. If, during reflection, the sexual experience did not provide pleasure and satisfaction, the woman may not have a desire to repeat the experience, based on the reward-seeking tendency of the brain. The circle is a pleasure oriented, not a goal oriented model, where any activity can lead to pleasure and there is not a goal of orgasm.

This thinking was then further developed by Dr. Rosemary Basson within the context of the responsive nature of women's sexual desire [10]. According to Basson, women have many reasons to engage in sexual activity other than sexual drive. The Basson model clarifies that the goal of sexual activity for women is not necessarily orgasm but rather personal satisfaction, which can manifest as physical satisfaction (could be orgasm) and/or emotional satisfaction (a feeling of intimacy and connection with a partner) [10]. This could be an important piece of information we could share with clients who feel the pressure of experiencing a certain outcome from their sexual engagement. As it is presented in Figure 14.3, this model incorporates the importance of emotional intimacy, sexual stimuli, and relationship satisfaction. It further acknowledges that female sexual functioning can proceed in a complex and circuitous manner, and is dramatically and significantly affected by numerous psychosocial issues (e.g. satisfaction with the relationship, self-image, previous negative sexual experiences).

## Orgasms within the Cultural Framework

Does one *have* an orgasm, or *experience* one? Is an orgasm like an object, something one can own, give and take? Or is it an experience, a journey, something that is subjectively felt and described rather than being witnessed or confirmed by others? Should it be treated differently when it comes to existence in solitude or amongst partners?

Defining issues around pleasure and orgasm outside of the clinical diagnostic definitions will rely heavily on culture, gender roles, and the public's level of awareness and knowledge around sexuality, sexual health, and the functioning of the human body. When assessing a

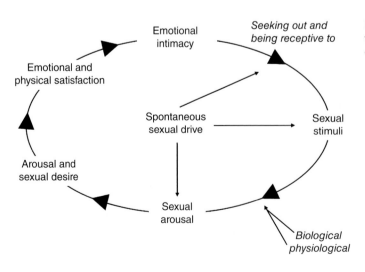

**Figure 14.3** Nonlinear model of female sexual response developed by Basson, 2000 [10].

woman, it is important to consider how sexual acts are perceived within that person's culture. Who is expected to receive pleasure and who is expected/deserves to give it? Traditional cultures do not see all types of pleasure, sexual experience, and sexual expressions through the same lens as more egalitarian and goal-focused cultures.

Today, in our current sociopsychological context, sexual desire, sexual fulfillment, love, and happiness are seen as closely related. Pleasure and orgasms are considered to be critical parts of adult sexuality and, as such, are necessary to maintaining a healthy lifestyle and healthy romantic/sexual relationship [11]. Simply put, orgasms are seen as being a part of healthy adult sexuality, which is, in turn, part of a healthy adult lifestyle. Therefore, the Basson model, which does not present orgasm as a necessary phase in sexual response for women, may be a relief for women but is not always as acceptable or appealing to some male partners, as they expect reactions and gratifications for their loved ones similar to what they experience.

In fact, the experience of orgasm for many couples seems to be so central to their idea of sexuality that it is often used as a measurement of the success of any given sexual activity, of the compatibility of partners, and of the pleasure experienced [4]. This mostly stems from the way in which sexuality is conceptualized in the western world. When *sexuality* is equated to, or synonymous with, *sexual activity* it becomes measurable like any other individual achievements. It is seen as a physical response (mainly erection, lubrication) followed by the individual's ability to experience orgasms as a result of that performance. Compatibility, additionally is measured more so from an evolutionary perspective, focusing on reproduction and success of reproduction, as outlined by Gallup and colleagues [4].

This is to the extent that the whole issue of pretending or faking orgasm has become a point of conversation and research on its own. Muehlenhard and Shippe reported that in a study with 180 male and 101 female college students, 85% of the men and 68% of the

women had experienced penile-vaginal intercourse, out of which 25% of men and 50% of women reported pretending orgasm [12]. This might not seem a problem at face value; however, some of these students might go on to shape long-term relationships in which at some point they do not wish to "fake" their orgasms anymore, which could cause their partners to develop a sense of betrayal, humiliation, and distrust. The fact that there is a way to "imitate" or "fake" an orgasm tells us a lot about an unspoken normative construct that exists around what orgasms should look like. On the other hand, struggling individuals might be in search of reassurance to become certain that what they or their partners feel is, in fact, orgasm.

In another study which looked at linguistic representation and definition of orgasm across 27 languages, Chiang and Chiang categorized orgasm into three groups: orgasm as a physiological response, orgasm as a psychological state, and orgasm as an ideal goal [11]. The terminology in Bengali (anonndo kora, "enjoy oneself"), French (Je jouis, "I enjoy"), Persian (Farsi) (lezat bordan, "Enjoying"), and Portuguese (Brazilian) (Eu estou gozando, "I'm enjoying") can be translated and understood as the English concept of "I'm enjoying". It has been mentioned that orgasm consists of related concepts such as (feeling of) satisfaction and (feeling of) pleasure. In French (la petite mort), an orgasm directly translates to something that refers to the altered state of consciousness and the feeling experienced during orgasm of not having control over the body [13–15].

Taking a closer look at the ways in which orgasms were defined across cultures, a significant deal of crossover between the psychical state and feelings became apparent. In Bengali, as in Persian (Farsi), "satisfaction is happening" and in Vietnamese "extreme pleasure" all denote a certain type of feeling [11]. The way orgasms were articulated within the linguistic analysis, 16 languages had adapted a version of or a meaning similar to "I'm coming," three languages used endings "I'm ending". Wilkins and Hill note that the motion verbs "come" and "go" vary from culture to culture as to "whom the deictic center can be shifted, how far the deictic center can grow to include other places/peoples, and what metaphorical extensions are possible" [16]. Location, direction of movement, the number of speakers involved, and the context determine whether going or coming is used when linguistically conceptualizing orgasms. "When the 'reaching' of an orgasm is being conceptualized as 'coming', it may be implying that orgasm is a process of reaching a certain destination" [11]. Out of all the orgasm terminologies collected, linguistic expressions with the meaning "I'm discharging" have the most gender-specific usages out of all the other categories. Specifically, for Mandarin Chinese, Indonesian, and Turkish, the terminology used for orgasm in males are "I'm shooting", "about to shoot", and "discharge", respectively. In these linguistic expressions, it seems that the focus is on the physiological response of an ejaculation during a male orgasmic experience [15, 17, 18]. In Vietnamese, both genders can use "to (get) out" to announce an orgasm. All of the linguistic expressions used in these languages appear to be indicating that an orgasm is a physiological experience of discharging fluid or releasing tension out of the body depending on the gender specific experiences of a male or female orgasm. In other words, it is predominantly conceptualized as a physical response.

The overview just provided should form our basic tools for assessment, the way we word our history-taking questions, and the way we formulate and present our treatment plans to the clients. This will also help with our understanding regarding the client's presentation of their issue area of emphasis and concern.

## Orgasm Dysfunctions

### Cultural Context

For any physical or psychological condition to be perceived as an issue worthy of attention, it first must be acknowledged as a "problem" – something that is not within the range of normal. But what is normal will depend in large part on the context within which the "problem" is embedded. Thus, the overall culture and, more specifically, the sexual culture in which we are immersed can sometimes contribute to the existence or prevalence of a certain disorder, as culture affects human psychology, values, attitudes, and behaviors.

Today, in the West, many people experience significant pressure not only to perform sexually but to "dangle from the chandeliers". Women's partners are expected to "give", and women are expected to "have", earth-shattering orgasmic experiences. This pressure, along with many others, remains as a shadow of expectation that haunts many women who may struggle to experience something (an orgasm) that they are taught to believe should be effortless. Both men and women are expected to have satisfying sex lives (while their idea of it is very much tainted) and if they do not then they begin to look for the "problem".

At the opposite end of the spectrum, consider a more traditional culture where women's sexuality is equated with reproduction and wifely duty. Orgasms are perceived as something meant for men to enjoy; not for women. In this case, the lack of female orgasms will not be addressed as issues, since it is simply the way things are in their natural state. Sexual pain disorders can also be viewed in a similar light, especially in cultures where pain is taught to be an expected outcome of sexual intercourse for women. Pain, in such cases, will less likely be perceived as something that is problematic since it is considered normal and even expected.

### Clinical Context

According to the fifth edition of the *Diagnostic and Statistical Manual for Mental Disorders* (DSM-5), female orgasm disorder is characterized by a significant change in orgasm, such as delay, reduction of intensity, or cessation, that has been present for at least six months and that causes significant distress for the woman

[19]. Although no single cause has been identified, female orgasm disorder has been associated with relational problems, stress, depression, anxiety, the use of medication, and the existence of chronic underlying medical conditions. (Ironically, orgasms are also known to reduce physiological and psychological stress.) For some women, the condition is lifelong and has persisted since the first sexual encounter, which makes it a primary disorder. For others, the problematic change in orgasm might occur after a period of satisfying sexual activity and enjoyment and, as such, it is considered to be a secondary disorder. In some cases, the disturbance may only happen with some sexual activities or partners but not persist in other situations (situational versus lifelong disorder). In other cases, the condition persists in all sexual encounters.

When it comes to orgasm disorders, women are overrepresented as compared to men, which adds to our responsibility to assess this condition in an accurate and timely manner. Male orgasm disorder was changed to delayed ejaculation in DSM-5, which arguably has its pros and cons and is beyond the scope of this chapter [19]. However, it is wise to keep the partner's sexual profile and problems in mind when assessing a female client. Laan and colleagues found that more than half of married women report arousal or orgasm problems. Of these, more than three quarters reported they were otherwise satisfied with their sexual relationships [20]. Hopefully, the long-standing myth that if you fix the relationships, your sexual problem will be gone, can be dispelled right here and now, and for good. Also, referring to Basson's model and her argument that orgasm is not necessarily what women are after in any given sexual encounter, we, as clinicians, have to be conscious of not using these statistics to frame a problem that is not seen as such by clients.

Not all women experiencing difficulty with orgasms would come in to our offices with similar concerns or expectations. Some women experience high levels of distress, while others are only mildly bothered [19].

The presence of distress is one of the main criterion that differentiates a clinically significant orgasm disorder from other complaints. Kluck and colleagues found that while high standards directed toward sexual partners caused few problems sexually, an individual's perception that her partner expects her to be the "perfect sexual partner" had a much more serious and at times deleterious effect on individuals [21]. It could almost be the equivalent of performance anxiety in a male who presents with ejaculatory or erectile difficulty due to the heightened pressure they perceive from their partners or themselves to perform in an ideal way. The fact that we use the language of "achieving or reaching orgasm" should be reconsidered since, for many women, an orgasm is not the chief end. As discussed in a previous publication, "experiencing orgasm" may be more appropriate [2].

In a clinical setting, it becomes important to study and analyze not only the ways in which orgasms are experienced but also how they are thought about, expressed, and discussed. The way an individual conceptualizes "orgasm" plays a critical role in understanding the sociocultural nuances around his or her perceptions, attitudes, and values surrounding sexuality, sexual well-being, and sexual health. The language used to describe what an orgasm is to the client gives critical insight into what meaning is loaded on to "orgasm" as a word, idea, and ideal. An orgasm is only one part of the entire human sexual experience, and only one of a number of ways in which an individual might experience sexuality and pleasure throughout the life course.

## Clinical Considerations

The clinical suggestions provided in this chapter are based on the Holistic Assessment and Therapies (HAT) model for the assessment, diagnosis, and management/treatment of sexual dysfunctions [22]. HAT encourages practitioners to work holistically and as a part of a team to conduct a thorough investigation of the client's sexual concern by taking the overall well-being and context of the life of the client into account. It also stands for the various "hats" that a practitioner wears during the whole process of working with clients through the five stages of the clinical journey. This takes the previously suggested bio-psycho-social model [23, 24] and adds five practical dimensions to it: addressing, assessment, diagnosis, management/treatment, and follow-up [22].

A significant aspect of addressing sexuality-related issues or sexual dysfunctions with clients is the healing power that is offered by being able to express what previously may not have been expressible due to relational, cultural or interpersonal barriers. Keeping the PLISSIT Model [Permission (P), Limited information (LI), Specific Suggestions (SS), and Intensive Therapy (IT)] in mind [25], even in cases when the clinicians expertise may not be psychosexual therapy, giving permission to the client to talk about his or her sexuality, sexual experiences (or lack thereof), worries, needs, fears, and desires can be a significant stepping stone toward healing. In cases like this, the assessment is part of the treatment.

After (or if needed) in parallel to these stages, the author would like to suggest an added element to the original PLISSIT model [Referral (R)], to encourage the clinicians to make a referral to an appropriate colleague if that is necessary. This practice is not thought about by some and frowned upon by others who equate making referrals to firing a client or giving up. [22].

There are other factors that will impact the assessment, management and, in general, the outcome of our work with a client. Psychosexual therapists do not have the same privileges as a medical professional who can examine the client physically; therefore, the importance of a thorough history taking questionnaire is paramount. For example, there are genital practices by various cultural groups that could impact their experience and expressions of orgasm, lack of awareness about them could hinder or even mislead our treatment process [26, 27].

## Common Beliefs/Myths that Perpetuate Orgasm Dysfunction

In addition to examining an individual's socio-cultural beliefs, biases, thoughts, and feelings around sexuality, it is also important to address any points of misinformation that could be perpetuating the client's distress. For example, some common misconceptions include:

- women fear that if they experience orgasm while pregnant – or even if they have sexual encounter while pregnant – it could harm the baby;
- if a woman does not have an orgasm during intercourse she will not get pregnant;
- if a woman does not experience orgasms through vaginal intercourse, there must be something wrong with her;
- if a woman is unable to experience an orgasm with a partner but has no problem experiencing one through masturbation, it will mean that her partner is not a compatible one;
- if a woman has an orgasm it will be embarrassing because she will lose control;
- intersex individuals have less capability to experience orgasm and sexual pleasure;
- lesbian women are attracted to women because they have never experienced "real pleasure" with a man;
- asexual people are told that if they had ever experienced an orgasm then they would have changed their minds.

Finally, one of the most common beliefs about female orgasms is that they are given to women by their partners. This perception can go both ways in further creating complications around what it means to experience orgasm. On one hand women may feel as if they are not in control of their pleasure, since orgasms are given and, therefore, passively received. On the other hand, if a woman does not experience orgasm while with a partner, her perception of her partner may shift negatively. Also, it may create feelings of dissatisfaction and anxiety in their partners, as they may feel they are unable to pleasure their female partners.

---

**Box 14.1 First point of contact.**

- Sex therapists
- Sex coaches
- Physical therapists
- Medical professionals and surgeons
- Spiritual guides
- Body workers
- Somatic coaches
- Psychoanalysts
- Surrogates.

---

The help-seeking behavior of the client and the first point of contact for each individual might be different (Box 14.1), depending on their exposure to resources, their information and knowledge regarding their condition, as well as what is available to them personally and socially, including insurance coverage. Also, the purpose of seeking help for various individuals might differ. For the majority, it might be to see if they are normal, why they are experiencing (or not) what they do, how to compensate for their shortcoming in their relationship or how to fix themselves and the issue. For others, it might be to receive a label and put themselves and their partners at ease or even make a legal case for divorce. All of these will inform the client's decision on where to seek help. For example, in countries such as Turkey and Iran that recognize sexual dysfunction as grounds for divorce, diagnosis has a completely different purpose and outcome. Sexual incompatibility between spouses is one of the most frequently cited grounds for divorce in these countries [28, 29].

## Assessment

When assessing for orgasm disorder it is recommended to start by establishing a baseline by administering the female sexual function index (FSFI) [30]. The female sexual distress scale (FSDS) is subsequently used to determine the level of impact that the current condition has on the individual [31]. This would offer an overall picture of the woman's sexual life and will provide the opportunity to discuss various aspects in more detail. It is important to make note of any significant transitions that have occurred in the woman's life. Has there been a chronic or life-threatening medical condition such as surgery, cancer, a heart attack or a spinal cord injury? What are the individual's concerns about re-engaging in sex? Is sexuality seen as a quality of life issue and, therefore, less important than other, life-or-death concerns? It is important to look at body image issues, particularly around surgeries.

Another line of questioning regarding transitions refers to recent changes in the family structure. For some women, after childbirth they feel guilty experiencing pleasure for themselves, or they feel that sexuality is somehow less appropriate after one has become a mother [32]. There could also be issues related to painful intercourse [33]. Alternatively, have there been any recent additions to the family in terms of elderly parents who now require care?

It is important for therapists to have the basic knowledge to rule out medical, physiological, pharmacological, and physical comorbidities. For example, for women whose sexual dysfunction developed during or after menopause, hormonal treatment is often useful in conjunction with behavioral treatments. Just having such basic knowledge, the therapist could make a suggestion to the client to go for an assessment by her obstetrician/gynecologist to determine if it is safe for her to go on hormone therapy [34].

In our Western goal-oriented, egalitarian culture it is important to pay attention to the language that women use. When someone expresses distress, is it her own distress or her partner's distress? At least theoretically, a woman who no longer wishes to have sex with her partner might not be experiencing "clinically significant distress" though her partner might be.

Understanding the client's expectations around sex and sexuality is another area for assessment. Perhaps she thought she was satisfied but now her friends think her orgasm should be more intense and she is missing out. Given the media's fixation on sex and sexuality, many individuals and couples might need to manage their expectations of what is desirable and even possible for them.

Of course, as mentioned above, throughout the assessment the clinician must pay close attention to the language the client uses. Experiencing fears may play a significant role in orgasm dysfunction (Box 14.2). She might have an underlying fear of being considered loose or overexperienced if she shows that she is enjoying sexual acts or experiencing orgasm. If she fears she will lose control and be embarrassed she might altogether ignore or prevent any act that may lead to an orgasm. She could be worried about the mess that lubrication or emission may create or, alternatively, she could be worried about not "ejaculating", which is increasingly expected from women by partners who are influenced by commercial videos and pornography (personal clinical observations).

I personally have seen women who were caught by the myth of "when you have an orgasm you will know" and, therefore, were worried that they might have never experienced orgasm (especially through intravaginal stimulation). When I give them and their partners stimulatory exercises, I ask the partners to insert a finger or two inside the vaginal canal while stimulating the clitoris and report any contractions after. In six cases that presented with anorgasmia with penile-vaginal intercourse, the report was that at a certain point the woman was experiencing some contractions that were similar to orgasm contractions but the feeling was not reported by the woman as orgasm "like how it feels with clitoral stimulation". This might be an interesting area for further research to see if there is any nerve block, dissociation of sensation or mental block that prevents certain women from feeling the pleasure of orgasm while their body reportedly has gone through the physical expressions of it. Another possibility is that if the clitoral orgasm has been experienced by these women long before they experienced penetrative sex then the primary feeling they associate with orgasm might be the one they know from this experience. They might not recognize the sensation created via intravaginal stimulation as it is not as intense as they are used to experiencing (described as Deep and Surface orgasm [3]).

## Diagnosis

Taking into account the previous discussion on the importance of cultural and clinical context, and after thorough assessment, the diagnosis phase (see DSM-5 definition in the *Clinical Context* section) is inevitable for some clients. To some, this might come as a relief, while to others, it might add to the burden [35]. Box 14.3 summarizes the common pros and cons that are partially reported by King and Nazareth [36].

## Management/Treatment

Several psychological treatment options are available to address the complex components of female orgasm disorder. Couples therapy is reported to be an effective intervention for couples whose relationship issues are contributing factors to the orgasm disorder [20]. Pereira and colleagues suggest that

---

**Box 14.2 Fears experienced.**

- Fear of losing control
- Fear of not ejaculating
- Fear of being embarrassed
- Fear of being considered loose
- Fear of being considered overexperienced
- Fear of lubricating too much and creating a mess.

---

**Box 14.3 Pros and cons of giving a diagnosis.**

**Pros**

- She is not alone
- There is an explanation
- There is the possibility of a treatment
- Opportunity for education as a part of the treatment process
- Opening communication between the couple.

**Cons**

- High expectations from the medical treatment
- Medicalization
- Labeling
- Polarizing the sexual relationship.

---

during couples therapy, the woman and her partner have an opportunity to improve on their communication skills, listening, reflection, emotional expression, and conflict resolution [37]. In cases where the woman is treated individually, cooperation from the sexual partner is recommended and encouraged. It is important for this inclusion to happen in a delicate manner and in consideration of the client's and the couple's cultural context. This is particularly important around issues of gender roles and also around what is permissible or allowed in terms of sexual encounters (e.g. certain kinds of touching, the inclusion of assisted devices and toys, and certain positions). When distressing and conflicting thoughts and emotions are present in a women diagnosed with female orgasm disorder, cognitive behavioral therapy (CBT) can effectively address these concerns to reduce symptoms [20].

In cases where sexual inexperience or discomfort is involved, self-stimulation training is recommended. Again considering the cultural background and the context of the couple, the therapist might want to consider giving these trainings in individual sessions.

For example, if the couple does not disclose their self-stimulation habits in front of each other for any given reason, it would not be wise to bring this up in a conjoint session.

The CBT approaches usually are short and do not go beyond 12–14 weeks. During these self-exploration and stimulation trainings, clients are gradually exposed to genital stimulation and may incorporate role play, sexual fantasy, and vibrators to facilitate orgasm. There are a number of workshops and trainings that might be recommended to the clients depending on the ease of the clinician in making these referrals, the code of ethics and conduct within the licensure body of the place of practice, and the willingness of the client to take part in such workshops. Meston and colleagues suggest that CBT that focuses on promoting changes in attitudes and sexually relevant thoughts, decreasing anxiety, and increasing orgasm ability and satisfaction could be beneficial for clients presented with orgasm dysfunctions [38, 39].

Laan, Rellini, and Barnes report that "direct masturbation training" can take place in individual therapy, when sexual inexperience or discomfort is present [20]. It is reported that this technique is extremely effective, resulting in 90% of women becoming orgasmic during treatment. For women whose sexual dysfunction stems from inability to focus or remain "in the moment" during sexual activity, yoga practice and mindfulness training were reported to be effective interventions [40]. In general, Barker shares that existential therapy could move the couple's thinking beyond orgasm and, with this easing of pressure, their overall sexual encounters would be more pleasurable [41].

In a recent article, Safron introduced "the rhythmic entrainment" model wherein sexual stimulation induces entrainment of coupling mechanical and neuronal oscillatory systems, thus creating synchronized functional networks within which multiple positive feedback processes intersect synergistically to contribute to sexual experience [42]. Safron explains that: These processes generate states of deepening sensory absorption and trance, potentially culminating in orgasm if critical thresholds are surpassed. The centrality of rhythmic stimulation (and its modulation by salience) for surpassing these thresholds suggests ways in which differential orgasmic responding between individuals (or with different partners) may serve as a mechanism for ensuring adaptive mate choice. Being aware of all these techniques will help add to the therapist's toolbox.

Education and a bibliography could be an impactful part of addressing any sexual issue. What we learn from media and popular culture about orgasms sometimes assists in making the subject less of a taboo; however, at times it also creates or strengthens myths about anatomy, functioning, pleasure, and orgasms. In cases where sexuality education is not commonplace (either not accessible or not permitted), the sources of these myths, whether media or porn, also become the source of sexuality education.

Lack of literacy in sexual health, anatomy and sexual function is common. Even intercourse is challenging for some couples, let alone experiencing pleasure. Relationship stress also was found to be highly associated with female sexual dysfunction [43]. These factors are further complicated by the couples' lack of information regarding sexual organs, their function, and ingrained misconceptions regarding what the outcome of any sexual encounter should be [22].

Educating clients about their sexuality in general will go a long way toward dispelling myths and this is true specifically after a life-altering event, such as being diagnosed with cancer and going through treatments, having a child, miscarriage, starting menopause, having a heart attack, or having experienced or living with severe injuries. Each of these events may have individual as well as relational consequences. For example, the woman who has survived a heart attack, or her partner, might fear that she will be too excited by orgasm and, therefore, more prone to another heart attack. Some cancer survivors report that they feel estranged by their bodies or feel anger as if their bodies have failed them. Therefore, there is a psychological block to experiencing pleasure [44]. These clients need to be instructed to give themselves time and try not to pressure themselves or push away their partners out of fear of disappointing the partner if the client doesn't experience orgasm. They can be encouraged to find enjoyment in reconnecting with their bodies and their partner's and gradually widen their experience of pleasure. Giving reassurance, along with accurate medical and scientific information to the woman and her partner of any gender, will go a long way.

## Follow-Up and Referral

Due to the multidimensional nature of any sexual dysfunction, including orgasm disorders, it is extremely important to have an effective, accessible, and expert network for referral and support. Not only for the client but also for the clinicians. Within the community of mental health practitioners, by large, it is frowned upon to refer a client to another provider (before they form their detachment with the therapist), which sometimes has its merit. However, due to lack of comprehensive education and training of practitioners within the field of psychosexual therapy, at times, it seems that keeping the clients in one's care would be an ethical dilemma of its own [45]. Thankfully, this is a bit less stigmatized when working with professionals across disciplines. The importance of having a referral network and knowing how to refer and when is pivotal.

## Acknowledgements

The author would like to thank Rayka Kumru for her dedicated assistance with research, and formatting of the content provided in this chapter.

# References

1 Money J, Wainwright G, Hingsburger D. *The Breathless Orgasm*, 1st edn. Buffalo, NY: Prometheus Books; 1991.

2 Komisaruk BR, Whipple B, Nasserzadeh S, Beyer-Flores C. *Orgasm Answer Guide*, 1st edn. Baltimore, MA: Johns Hopkins University Press; 2009.

3 King R, Belsky J. A Typological approach to testing the evolutionary functions of human female orgasm. *Arch Sex Behav*. 2012;41(5): 1145–1160.

4 Gallup GG, Ampel BC. Wedberg N, Pogosjan A. (2014). Do orgasms give women feedback about mate choice? *Evol Psychol*. 2014;12(5):958–978.

5 Lloyd EA. *The Case Of The Female Orgasm*, 1st edn. Cambridge, MA: Harvard University Press; 2005.

6 Masters WH, Johnson VE. *Human Sexual Response*, 1st edn. New York: Bantam Books; 1966.

7 Kaplan HS. *Disorders of Sexual Desire and Other New Concepts and Techniques in Sex Therapy*. New York: Simon and Schuster; 1979.

8 Whipple B, Brash-McGreer K. Management of female sexual dysfunction. In: Sipski ML, Alexander CJ (eds) *Sexual Function in People with Disability and Chronic Illness. A Health Professional's Guide*. Gaithersburg, MD: Aspen Publishers, Inc.; 1997, pp 509–534.

9 Stayton WR. A theology of sexual pleasure. *Am Baptist Q*. 1989;8(2):1–15.

10 Stehle B. *Incurably Romantic*. Philadelphia, PA: Temple University Press; 1985. Basson R. Human sex-response cycles. *J Sex Marital Ther*. 2001;27(1):33–43.

11 Chiang AY, Chiang W-Y.(2016) Behold, I am coming soon! A study on the conceptualization of sexual orgasm in 27 languages. *Metaphor and Symbol*. 2016;31(3):131–147.

12 Muehlenhard CL, Shippee SK. Men's and women's reports of pretending orgasm. *J Sex Res*. 2010;47(6):552–567.

13 Bancroft, J. *Human Sexuality and its Problems*, 1st edn. London: Churchill Livingstone; 1989.

14 Davidson JM. (1980). The psychobiology of sexual experience. In Davidson JM, Davidson R J (eds) *The Psychobiology of Consciousness*. New York: Plenum Press; 1980, pp. 271–332.

15 Mah K, Binik YM. The nature of human orgasm: a critical review of major trends. *Clin Psychol Rev*. 2001;21(6) 823–856.

16 Wilkins DP, Hill D. (1995). When "go" means "come": Questioning the basicness of basic motion verbs. *Cogn Linguist*. 1995;6:209–259

17 Newman HF, Reiss H, Northup JD. Physical basis of emission, ejaculation and orgasm in the male. *Urology*. 1982;19:341–350

18 Tuckwell HC. A neurophysiological theory of a reproductive process. *Int J Neurosci*. 1989;44:143–148.

19 American Psychiatric Association. *Diagnostic and Statistical Manual of Mental Disorders*, 1st edn. Washington, DC: American Psychiatric Publishing, 2013.

20 Laan E, Rellini AH, Barnes T. (2013), Standard Operating Procedures for Female Orgasmic Disorder: Consensus of the International Society for Sexual Medicine. *J Sex Med*. 2013;10:74–82.

21 Kluck AS, Zhuzha K, Hughes K. Sexual perfectionism in women: not as simple as adaptive or maladaptive. *Arch Sex Behav*. 2016;45(8):2015–2027.

22 Nasserzadeh S. Practical recommendation to work with couples presenting with unconsummated marriages in any healthcare setting. *Middle Eastern Society for Sexual Medicine*. 2014;6.

23 Rosen RC, Barsky J. Normal sexual response in women. *Obstet Gynecol Clin North Am*. 2006;33(4):515–526.

24 Althof SE, Leiblum SR, Chevret-Measson M, *et al*. Original research—psychology: psychological and interpersonal dimensions of sexual function and dysfunction. *J Sex Med*. 2005;2(6):793–800.

25 Annon JS. The PLISSIT model: a proposed conceptual scheme for the behavioral treatment of sexual problems. *J Sex Educ Ther.* 1976;2(1):1–15.

26 Nasserzadeh S. Ethnic and cultural aspects of sexuality. In: Wylie K (ed) *ABC of Sexual Health*, 3rd edn. Chichester, UK: Wiley Blackwell; 2015, pp. 101–103.

27 Nasserzadeh S. Genital practices around the world and implications for policy and practice. Plenary address, World Congress of Sexology, Prague, Czech Republic, May 2017.

28 Barikani A, Ebrahim SM, Navid M. The cause of divorce among men and women referred to marriage and legal office in Qazvin, *Iran. Glob J Health Sci.* 2012;4(5):184–191.

29 Aker S, Böke Ö. The effect of education on the sexual beliefs of family physicians. *Int J Sex Health.* 2016;28(1): 111–116.

30 Rosen R, Brown C, Heiman J, *et al.* The Female Sexual Function Index (FSFI): a multidimensional self-report instrument for the assessment of female sexual function. *J Sex Marit Ther.* 2000;26:191–208

31 Derogatis LR, Rosen R, Leiblum S, *et al.* The Female Sexual Distress Scale (FSDS): Initial Validation Of A Standardized Scale For Assessment Of Sexually Related Personal Distress In Women". *J Sex Marit Ther.* 2002;28(4):317–330.

32 Kenny JA. Sexuality in pregnant and breastfeeding women. *Arch Sex Behav.* 1973;2:215–229.

33 Leeman LM, Rogers RG. Sex after childbirth: postpartum sexual function. *Obstet Gynecol.* 2012;119(3):647–655.

34 Basson R, Wierman ME, van Lankveld J, and Brotto L. Summary of the recommendations on sexual dysfunctions in women. *J Sex Med.* 2010;7:314–326.

35 Shifren JL, Monz BU, Russo PA, Segreti A, Johannes CB. Sexual problems and distress in United States women: prevalence and correlates. *Obstet Gynecol.* 2008; 112(5):970–978.

36 King M, Holt V, Nazareth I. Women's views of their sexual difficulties: agreement and disagreement with clinical diagnoses. *Arch Sex Behav.* 2007;36(2):281–288.

37 Pereira VM, Arias-Carrión O, Machado S, *et al.* Sex therapy for female sexual dysfunction. *Int Arch Med.* 2013;6(1):37.

38 Meston CM. Hull E, Levin RJ, Sipski M. Disorders of orgasm in women. *J Sex Med.* 2004;1(1):66–68.

39 Meston CM, Levin RJ, Sipski ML, *et al.* Women's orgasm. *Annu Rev Sex Res.* 2004;15:173–257.

40 Brotto LA, Barker M. *Mindfulness in Sexual and Relationship Therapy*, 1st edn. London: Routledge: 2014.

41 Barker M. Existential sex therapy. *Sex Relation Ther.* 2001;26(1):33–47.

42 Safron A. What is orgasm? A model of sexual trance and climax via rhythmic entrainment. *Socioaffect Neurosci Psychol.* 2016;6:3163.

43 McCabe MP, Connaughton C. Sexual dysfunction and relationship stress: how does this association vary for men and women? *Curr Opin Psychol.* 2017;13:81–84.

44 Lindwall L, Bergbom I. The altered body after breast cancer surgery. *Int J Qual Stud Health Well-being.* 2009;4(4):280–287.

45 Nasserzadeh S. Sex therapy: a marginalized specialization. *Arch Sex Behav.* 2009;38(6): 1037–1038.

# 15

## Musculoskeletal Management of Orgasm Disorders

*Karen Brandon*

### Abstract

Understanding the role of contractile and noncontractile tissue in different phases of the sexual response cycle is a key to determining impairment in the myofascial and musculoskeletal systems in orgasm disorder. The continuum from attenuating arousal and peak sexual tension, and spasms occurring afterwards, lends to multiple points of dysfunction. Diagnosis starts with history and physical examination including overall observation and focused examination of the genitalia. The clinician should request a pelvic floor volitional contraction, relaxation and elongation, and observe the correctness, timing, and excursion of the muscle unit. Other assessments include electromyography and 4D transperineal ultrasound. Orgasmic disorder can be the result of overactivity or underactivity of the pelvic floor muscles, or noncontractile connective tissue restriction. Treatments include myofascial, musculoskeletal, and neuromotor interventions. Clinicians should screen for alterations in musculoskeletal structures after surgery or parity that cause change in sexual function related to orgasm.

**Keywords:**   *hypertonus; hypotonus; musculoskeletal; myofascial; pelvic floor; orgasm; ischiocavernosus muscle; bulbospongiosus muscle; rehabilitation; physical therapy*

---

Orgasmic disorder may result from dysfunctional (hypertonic or hypotonic) muscles intimately associated with genital organs or within the surrounding pelvic floor, as well as noncontractile elements like the viscerofascia.

Diagnostic efforts should assess connective tissue and muscular units of the pelvic floor, as well as the related skeletal elements of the trunk, pelvic girdle, and hips to identify any pain or issues with muscle mobility, stability, and strength.

Identifying incidents/events (e.g. surgery or local trauma) that would change the myofascial structures or chemical/hormonal changes or stressors/neural changes that might cause changes in orgasmic function are critical to formulating successful treatment or management strategies.

---

## Introduction

Understanding the role of contractile and noncontractile tissue in different phases of the sexual response cycle is key to determining if there is an impairment in the myofascial and musculoskeletal systems in sexual dysfunction. In orgasm, which has been believed to be an automated (fixed) response cycle to particular stimuli, pathology models have been challenged by new research in functional neuroimaging of the mechanisms of orgasm

*Textbook of Female Sexual Function and Dysfunction: Diagnosis and Treatment*, First Edition. Edited by Irwin Goldstein, Anita H. Clayton, Andrew T. Goldstein, Noel N. Kim, and Sheryl A. Kingsberg.
© 2018 John Wiley & Sons Ltd. Published 2018 by John Wiley & Sons Ltd.

[1–3]. The significance of a healthy, functioning myofascial and musculoskeletal system as a responder and attenuator to the arousal experienced as the woman approaches orgasm is often overlooked in clinical practice. This chapter focuses on describing assessment of these systems and interventions for addressing relative dysfunctions.

## Diagnosis

Excluding pain, the conditions that may involve a mechanical dysfunction of the structural tissues (end organ or peripheral) could include female orgasmic disorder as defined by the ISSWSH Nomenclature Consensus panel [4]. This definition includes conditions that adversely affect orgasm after normal sexual excitement, such as clitoral phimosis, scar/contraction, connective tissue restriction or pelvic floor muscular underactivity, overactivity, or incoordination of pelvic floor muscles.

The basis for female orgasm has been extensively studied [5–7]. From a neuromotor perspective, a thorough description of the clonic nature of the reflexive response has been linked to the need for sufficient arousal. The increasing vasocongestion in the pelvic muscles triggers the muscle spindle stretch reflex and, therefore, overcomes the gamma bias to produce a rhythmic contraction. These contractions serve to reduce the pressure that the excess fluid is creating and these contractions continue until the spindle bias afferents determine the resistance is back to baseline [8]. This brief description does not exclude the influence of higher neural centers and recognizes that an orgasm is a multisystem expression, but this description attempts to explain the mechanisms of the local contractile tissue.

Pathophysiologic factors of the local genital structures, therefore, would include any restriction that prevents arterial filling, vasoconstriction maintenance, trigger of the afferent response at the clitoris, and muscles that will not respond to slight stretch or do not coordinate well to contract [9].

Conditions that affect physiologic achievement and maintenance of arousal may overlap with orgasmic potential in the musculoskeletal domain. The ischiocavernosus and bulbospongiosus muscles are primarily responsible for maintaining pressure on the dorsal vein of the clitoris but the role this has in the physiology of clitoral engorgement is unclear. The clitoral hood must be mobile enough to allow for the examination of the glans clitoris and to ensure there are no underlying clitoral adhesions. Clitoral adhesions may permit the presence of keratin pearls and balanitis that may interfere and cause discomfort and hypersensitivity with orgasm. The levator ani muscles reduce the vasocongestion by rhythmic contractions [8]. In addition, noncontractile elements like the viscerofascia surrounding the lower third of the vaginal canal and the vestibule and vulva must have mobility free of restrictions. Arguably the continuum between the attenuating arousal, peak sexual tension, and spasms occurring afterwards [5] lends itself to multiple points of dysfunction that must be clarified with clinical assessment. The subcategories previously described by earlier versions of classification models include a breakdown of the symptoms and signs [10].

## Evaluation of Musculoskeletal Function

### History taking

A comprehensive history should be taken to determine if there are any red-flags that would explain changes in sexual function that need immediate medical management (i.e. signs and symptoms of cancer, new neurological symptoms, or acute pain/blood loss). Secondly, a detailed medical history would identify comorbidities that may impact orgasmic sexual function, including a list of current medications and surgical procedures. Screening for other conditions that impact the musculoskeletal system is imperative as changes in bowel, bladder [11], and lower quarter mobility through lumbar spine, pelvic girdle, and hips could highlight impairments in the pelvic musculature. It is important to ask for current or historic neural signs including numbness, weakness, or any alteration that may warrant further neurological assessment of the cauda equina.

After a detailed history is taken, the clinician asks for further clarification of the onset of the orgasmic dysfunction and includes overview of a brief sexual history to screen for other sexual domain dysfunction. Sexual function questionnaires, such as the Female Sexual Function Index (FSFI) items 11–13 [12], the Female Sexual Function Questionnaire (SFQ-28) items 22-24 [13], and the Changes in Sexual Functioning Questionnaire (CSFQ-FC) items 11–14 [14], cover orgasm conditions. A previous reported baseline for orgasm function is established (if possible) and conditions under which the problem occurs (i.e. specific partner, self-stimulation with or without tools/toys, under stressful circumstance) are noted.

Special attention is also paid to changes in orgasmic function after incidents that would change the myofascial structures via surgery or local trauma and those that would affect tissue directly (chemical/hormonal changes) or indirectly (stressors/neural changes). If pain is identified, preventing orgasm, or during or afterwards, reclassification of condition is made to address multifactorial pain etiology.

## Physical Examination

After history is taken, gross observation is used for screening functional mobility for trunk, pelvic girdle (Figure 15.1), and the hip. Coordination of trunk and extremity muscles to meet demand of required postures and positions is tested against gravity and resistance, inclusive of desired sexual positions. (Figures 15.2 and 15.3). Restrictions in breathing pattern and availability of lumbopelvic-hip movement should be assessed (Figure 15.4), as well as palpation of the rectus abdominus and evaluation of length and strength (Figure 15.5). Any abnormal

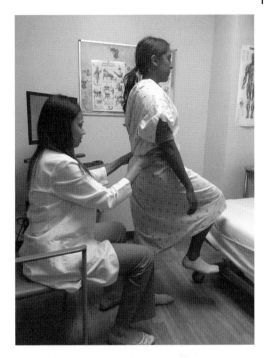

**Figure 15.1** Testing pelvic girdle for incoordination – Stork test/Trendelenberg test.

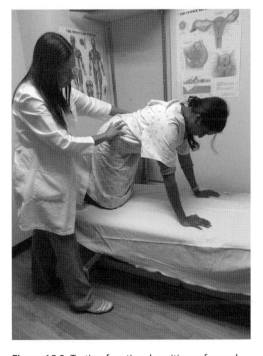

**Figure 15.2** Testing functional positions of sexual activity – quadriped with pelvic tilting.

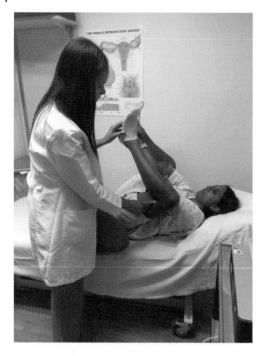

**Figure 15.3** Functional testing for sexual positions – "happy baby" pose.

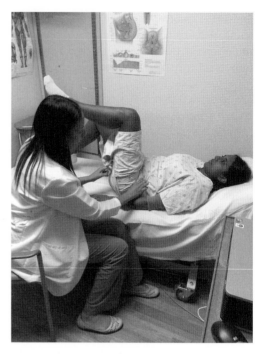

**Figure 15.5** Abdominal strength testing – Sarhmann progression.

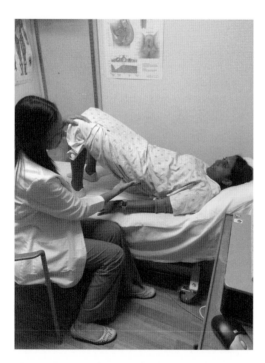

**Figure 15.4** Coordination of pelvic girdle for sexual function – bridge with breathing.

findings, such as lack of range of motion, strength, or impaired control, should be further assessed and special tests included to assign a musculoskeletal impairment diagnosis and determine if it has a relationship to the presenting complaint.

Once complete explanation of the anatomy and purpose of the examination is completed and consent for genital examination is obtained from the patient, the physical therapist continues to ensure patient control [15] and participation with the examination with ongoing but brief narrative of examination, "checking in" while observing nonverbal communication, and taking breaks at appropriate times to summarize the findings.

Initially the genitalia are observed as a screening before proceeding with an internal examination. The physical therapist notes the presence of discharge, swelling, rash, fissures or erythema. Labia majora are observed as well as separating them to look at the labia minora, vestibule, and clitoral hood. As the clinician describes what they are assessing, they can ask the patient to pull back the clitoral hood or indicate they will do so to evaluate the clitoral glans and mobility of the hood if there is underlying clitoral adhesions. It is important to visualize the corona of the glans; failure to visualize the corona may signal the presence of clitoral adhesions. Clitoral glans is observed for color and size; the size should be approximately the size of end of the cotton swab. If indicated, a vestibule Q-tip test can be performed, as well as a light touch sensation test for S2-S4 dermatomes. The purpose of this information is to identify any red flags regarding integrity of the tissue and the neural innervation. If all of these areas have been documented as screened recently by a physician, physician's assistant or nurse practitioner, then there is no need to subject the patient to in-depth testing, unless there has been a change in status or significant time since initial assessment. Those trained to use a vulvoscope (colposcope) are able to more clearly observe abnormalities in the vulvar, vestibular, and vaginal tissues; however, most physical therapy offices do not have this equipment and still have to refer the patient back to the physician, physician's assistant or nurse practitioner for care of conditions not of musculoskeletal origin.

Next, the clinician requests a pelvic floor volitional contraction, relaxation, and elongation and observes the correctness, timing, and excursion of the muscle unit. Involving the patient with use of a mirror can aid in execution of the request, as well as understanding the muscle function and feedback of effort. Verbal cues can be modified to achieve the desired demonstration. Following this, the clinician describes the superficial layer of pelvic floor muscles and bilaterally palpates the bulbospongiosus, superficial transverse perineal muscles, and perineal body for tenderness and identifies presence of any myofascial restriction [16].

The clinician then explains the next step of the examination, which is internal, and asks permission to start that component. One gloved lubricated finger is carefully introduced into the vaginal introitus to the hymenal ring, which is evaluated for extensibility. Next, the superficial layer of muscle can again be palpated between the index finger inserted and the thumb externally for tenderness and myofascial restriction and screening for Bartholin's gland tenderness. Internal assessment of the ischiocavernosus by the internal finger can be completed. Moving to deeper palpation the puborectalis, pubococcygeus, and iliococcygeus can be examined next for tenderness, tension, and stiffness. When a contraction and relaxation is requested, further quality and quantification of pelvic floor muscle strength (such as the modified Oxford grading scale), length, and coordination can be assigned. Palpation of obturator internus, ischiococcygeus, and piriformis muscles for the same functions can be completed and should be compared bilaterally. Any referred pain on palpation should be noted. As indicated, palpation of viscera including urethra, base of the bladder, cervix, base of the uterus, and rectum can rule out involvement of these structures if nontender and having normal mobility [17].

## Other Assessments of the Pelvic Floor

Electromyography of the pelvic floor is often used to establish pelvic floor recruitment patterns and identify hyperactivity or hypoactivity [18, 19]. Although there is limited reliability when measuring amplitude [20, 21], the information gained using surface electromyography to measure resting state (tonic), responsiveness for volitional contraction, endurance, and return back to baseline (phasic) can contribute to the totality of understanding the muscle function [22]. It should not be used as determinant of muscle force. Further information can be gathered regarding the force measurement using intravaginal dynamometry [23], while pelvic floor muscle resting tone and force can be measured with perineometry and manometry [24].

Use of 4D transperineal ultrasound can demonstrate both morphological differences from normal in resting states [25] by measuring the levator plate angle; it can also demonstrate dynamic displacement of the urethrovesicular junction and anorectal angle relating to the pelvic floor excursion capability [26]. These adjunctive tools of assessment are included to describe pelvic floor function more comprehensively, contributing to defining the "state of operation" of the muscle unit. Their use in concert with signs, symptoms, and standard physical examination may give a more comprehensive picture of their function *in vivo*.

## Categories of Myofascial and Musculoskeletal Dysfunction

After completing the examination, the clinician determines the relationships between symptoms and findings. It is important that the physical therapist clarifies if female orgasmic disorder diagnosis is multimodal and if musculoskeletal impairments may contribute a percentage to the dysfunction but may not explain the entire condition. While there are many definitions for muscle function and updates are perpetual, the current terminology in pelvic floor muscle function and dysfunction standardized by the International Continence Society will be used [27].

*Overactivity* of pelvic floor muscles is demonstrated with concurrent findings of tenderness on palpation, impaired volitional relaxation or elongation, possible elevated resting activity, muscle stiffness upon palpation, or shortened contraction excursion. It can exist in the superficial pelvic muscle layers or the deep levator ani group. Overactivity can lead to pain but can also exist without pain and demonstrate dysfunction with an inability to achieve orgasm that is hypothesized to be due to shortened muscle length not allowing local tissue perfusion and potential compression of clitoral, perineal or rectal branches of the pudendal nerve [28]. It

can also be a contributor to persistent sensations of genital arousal in the absence of sexual desire or stimulation, also known as persistent genital arousal disorder (PGAD), due to the inability to relieve venous outflow obstructed by pelvic muscle overactivity [29]. Persistent genital arousal disorder can exist with and without pain; its etiologies include peripheral and central factors (Chapter 11).

Patients can also present with *underactivity* of deep pelvic floor muscles, demonstrated by low tone on palpation, poor compression or elevation on dynamometry, perineo/manometry or small displacement on ultrasound. Although studies exist that have evaluated the association between pelvic floor muscle weakness and sexual dysfunction [30], specific improvement in orgasm is not defined and has not been directly studied. For the older studies that evaluated pelvic floor muscle and orgasm, controversy exists regarding pelvic muscle strengthening and reported orgasm function [31]. More evidence is emerging that shows a relationship between a strong pelvic floor and improved quality and intensity of orgasm [32], possibly due to increased stretch and pressure receptors, but no study has demonstrated change from anorgasmia to orgasmic by increasing muscle strength alone. Ultimately, the lack of homogeneity in the research as to the baseline of pelvic floor muscle function, the symptom report/patient desired goal, and the outcome pertaining to specifically female orgasmic disorder allows only for speculation as to the relationships between pelvic floor muscle underactivity and reduction of orgasm dysfunction and requires individualization of interventions.

A final area to classify is *noncontractile connective tissue restriction* – any restriction that is demonstrated as immobility of the labia, vestibule, clitoral hood [33], hymenal ring, vaginal introital mucosa or perineal body that limits adequate access and use of the perineal structures for sexual stimulus. This can occur as a result of hormonal deficiencies, dermatopathologies, vaginal delivery trauma, surgical procedures, perineal injuries, or part of genital cutting practices. Health of the tissues must factor in their ability to stretch and also produce an adequate amount of tensioning. This condition can pertain to superficial scars as well as deep scars, such as with urogynecological procedures.

# Overview of Treatment Options

In recent years, increasing attention has been paid to addressing the patient as a whole from a biopsychosocial perspective. The role as clinicians is to contribute to a whole person view of the condition and in our practice scopes address the component of dysfunction found with specific skill and training. The interventions in physical therapy are wholly provided to aid the body in restorative processes in areas where it has lost mobility, stability, and strength. These can be considered myofascial, musculoskeletal or neuromotor in their approach. Within each area, there is a common goal but different techniques are available. It is also important to treat patients individually and remember they can have comorbidities that require sequential organization of interventions.

## Myofascial Interventions

Soft tissue mobilization can be termed to be a manual therapy that affects the skin, fascia and muscle to increase extensibility. It can be applied directly or indirectly to achieve a reduction in previously tested painful palpation, range of motion or lack of flexibility. In patients with restrictions in their connective tissue that limits mobility of tissues of the perineum, the clinician can manually mobilize the tissue away from (direct) or towards (indirect) the restriction. They can determine what structures and depth they want to evaluate and treat. Noncontractile structures adjacent to the muscles, such as viscerofascial and neuro-fascial connections, can be targeted. Mechanical interventions

can also include use of perineal small soft tissue balls or internal vaginal dilators/accommodators to stretch larger areas of tissue in the absence of pain.

## Musculoskeletal Interventions

To the extent that the pelvic floor muscles are attached to the bony pelvis, there is always room for static or dynamic structural imbalances along the entire kinetic chain from the foot to the head. While the body adapts significantly to many alterations in length tension relationships, at times it may be assessed that the joint position or available arthrokinematics are not optimized for efficient function. After a fall onto one's hip or a macrosomic vaginal delivery, it is possible that a structural dysfunction is contributing to pelvic floor muscle dysfunction. If so, address the arthokinematic limitation with joint mobilization in any of the effective forms and then ensure that the new range is used and supported well with the muscular structures. It is also important to recognize that physical patterns occur through the whole body once an orgasm is triggered and musculoskeletal impairments can prohibit them, alter them or even make them painful.

## Neuromotor Interventions

All targeted exercise that involves volitional or responsive contraction requires neuromotor training. It includes contractions towards strength and coordination as well as reducing tone and relaxation. In addition, there is the potential for peripheral input to effect a central change. Pelvic muscle exercise can be practiced to increase correctness, speed, stamina, endurance of contraction or to release or elongate the muscle. All exercises should focus on functional positions and demands. Because sexual function has variety, multiple demands of the trunk, hips, and pelvic floor muscle require a variety of motor patterns. It should also include an awareness of training for actively relaxing the pelvic floor.

## Outcomes/Follow-Up

There are few studies on physical therapy interventions specific to improving sexual dysfunction with orgasm [34–36]. There are more that studied evaluating the benefits of physical therapy, specifically for overactive pelvic floor in sexual pain disorders that showed good efficacy [29, 37–39]. Nevertheless, it is important that an assessment of the pelvic floor muscle and the related musculoskeletal system be completed to properly direct care of the individual impairments in an effort to address the entire clinical picture. More research that includes musculoskeletal and myofascial impairments found in those classified with female orgasmic disorders would help clarify impairment based treatments that could then be studied with randomized, controlled trials.

## Screening/prevention

It is recommended that clinicians carry out screening and early intervention to address alterations in musculoskeletal structures after surgery or parity that cause change in sexual function related to arousal or orgasm. Giving patients counsel on possible changes to sexual function, whether transient, adaptable or permanent, is important to affirming that the patient's sexuality is an important part of their quality of life and that every effort is made to address what can be improved medically.

## Conclusion

Assessment of the structures involved in orgasm must include an evaluation of the connective tissue and muscular units of the pelvic floor to rule out musculoskeletal contributions to dysfunction. Further assessment of the trunk, pelvic girdle, and hips can demonstrate barriers to freedom of movement or adequate coordination of pelvic floor muscle for the purpose of participating in the orgasmic response. Specific interventions targeting restoration of mobility or strength can be valuable in patients who have female orgasmic dysfunction after local trauma, skeletal changes or connective tissue restrictions.

## References

1 Georgiadis JR. Doing it … wild? On the role of the cerebral cortex in human sexual activity. *Socioaffect Neurosci Psychol.* 2012;2:17337.

2 Komisaruk BR, Whipple B. Functional MRI of the brain during orgasm in women. *Annu Rev Sex Res.* 2005;16(1):62–86.

3 Stoleru S, Fonteille V, Cornelis C, *et al.* Functional neuroimaging studies of sexual arousal and orgasm in healthy men and women: a review and meta-analysis. *Neurosci Biobehav Rev.* 2012;36(6):1481–1509.

4 Maseroli E, Fanni E, Cipriani S, *et al.* Cardiometabolic risk and female sexuality: focus on clitoral vascular resistance. *J Sex Med.* 2016;13(11):1651–1661.

5 Meston CM, Hull E, Levin RJ, Sipski M. Disorders of orgasm in women. *J Sex Med.* 2004;1(1):66–68.

6 Reider B. Role of pelvic floor muscles in female orgasmic response. *J Womens Health Issues Care.* 2016;5(6). doi:10.4172//2325-9795.1000250.

7 Meston CM, Hull E, Levin RJ, Sipski M. Disorders of orgasm in women. *J Sex Med.* 2004;1(1):66–68.

8 Mould DE. Women's orgasm and the muscle spindle. In: Graber B (ed) *Circumvaginal Musculature and Vaginal Function.* Omaha, NE: Karger; 1982, pp. 93–100.

9 Bohlen JG, Held JP, Sanderson MO, Ahlgren A. The female orgasm: pelvic contractions. *Arch Sex Behav.* 1982;11(5):367–386.

10  Basson R, Leiblum S, Brotto L, *et al.* Revised definitions of women's sexual dysfunction. *J Sex Med.* 2004;1(1):40–48.

11  Pauls RN, Rogers RG, Parekh M, *et al.* Sexual function in women with anal incontinence using a new instrument: the PISQ-IR. *Int Urogynecol J.* 2015;26(5):657–663.

12  Rosen R, Brown C, Heiman J, *et al.* The Female Sexual Function Index (FSFI): a multidimensional self-report instrument for the assessment of female sexual function. *J Sex Marital Ther.* 2000;26(2):191–208.

13  Quirk F, Haughie S, Symonds T. The use of the sexual function questionnaire as a screening tool for women with sexual dysfunction. *J Sex Med.* 2005;2(4):469–477.

14  Keller A, McGarvey EL, Clayton AH. Reliability and construct validity of the Changes in Sexual Functioning Questionnaire short-form (CSFQ-14). *J Sex Marital Ther.* 2006;32(1):43–52.

15  Rosenbaum TY. Pelvic floor involvement in male and female sexual dysfunction and the role of pelvic floor rehabilitation in treatment: a literature review. *J Sex Med.* 2007;4(1):4–13.

16  Sarton J. Assessment of the pelvic floor muscles in women with sexual pain. *J Sex Med.* 2010;7(11):3526–3529.

17  Hartmann D, Sarton J. Chronic pelvic floor dysfunction. *Best Pract Res Clin Obstet Gynaecol.* 2014;28(7):977–990.

18  Podnar S, Mrkaic M, Vodusek DB. Standardization of anal sphincter electromyography: quantification of continuous activity during relaxation. *Neurourol Urodyn.* 2002;21(6):540–545.

19  Capson AC, Nashed J, McLean L. The role of lumbopelvic posture in pelvic floor muscle activation in continent women. *J Electromyogr Kinesiol.* 2011;21(1):166–177.

20  Auchincloss CC, McLean L. The reliability of surface EMG recorded from the pelvic floor muscles. *J Neurosci Methods.* 2009;182(1):85–96.

21  Peschers UM, Gingelmaier A, Jundt K, *et al.* Evaluation of pelvic floor muscle strength using four different techniques. *Int Urogynecol J Pelvic Floor Dysfunct.* 2001;12(1):27–30.

22  Pullman SL, Goodin DS, Marquinez AI, *et al.* Clinical utility of surface EMG: report of the therapeutics and technology assessment subcommittee of the American Academy of Neurology. *Neurology.* 2000;55(2):171–177.

23  Miller JM, Ashton-Miller JA, Perruchini D, DeLancey JO. Test-retest reliability of an instrumented speculum for measuring vaginal closure force. *Neurourol Urodyn.* 2007;26(6):858–863.

24  Naess I, Bo, K. Can a pelvic floor muscle contraction reduce vaginal resting presssure and resting EMG activity? *Neurourol Urodyn.* 2013;32(8).

25  Morin M, Bergeron S, Khalife S, *et al.* Morphometry of the pelvic floor muscles in women with and without provoked vestibulodynia using 4D ultrasound. *J Sex Med.* 2014;11(3):776–785.

26  Braekken IH, Majida M, Engh ME, Bo K. Test-retest reliability of pelvic floor muscle contraction measured by 4D ultrasound. *Neurourol Urodyn.* 2009;28(1):68–73.

27  Messelink B, Benson T, Berghmans B, *et al.* Standardization of terminology of pelvic floor muscle function and dysfunction: report from the pelvic floor clinical assessment group of the International Continence Society. *Neurourol Urodyn.* 2005;24(4):374–380.

28  Both S, van Lunsen R, Weijenborg P, Laan E. A new device for simultaneous measurement of pelvic floor muscle activity and vaginal blood flow: a test in a nonclinical sample. *J Sex Med.* 2012;9(11):2888–2902.

29  Laan E, van Lunsen RHW. Overactive pelvic floor: sexual functioning. In: Padoa A, Rosenbaum TY (eds) *The Overactive Pelvic Floor.* New York: Springer; 2016, pp. 17–29.

30  Lara LA, Montenegro ML, Franco MM, *et al.* Is the sexual satisfaction of postmenopausal women enhanced by physical exercise and pelvic floor muscle training? *J Sex Med.* 2012;9(1):218–223.

31 Roughan PA, Kunst L. Do pelvic floor exercises really improve orgasmic potential? *J Sex Marital Ther.* 1981;7(3):223–229.

32 Kanter G, Rogers RG, Pauls RN, *et al.* A strong pelvic floor is associated with higher rates of sexual activity in women with pelvic floor disorders. *Int Urogynecol J.* 2015;26(7):991–996.

33 Morrison P, Kellogg Spadt S, Golstein, A. The use of specific myofascial release techniques by a physical therapist to treat clitoral phimosis and dyspareunia. *J Womens Health Phys Therap.* 2015; 39(1):17–28.

34 Wurn LJ, Wurn BF, Roscow AS, *et al.* Increasing orgasm and decreasing dyspareunia by a manual physical therapy technique. *MedGenMed.* 2004;6(4):47.

35 Dorey DG. CASE REPORT: Pelvic floor muscle exercises for female orgasmic.

*J Womens Health Phys Therap.* 2006;30(2):40.

36 Beji NK, Yalcin O, Erkan HA. The effect of pelvic floor training on sexual function of treated patients. *Int Urogynecol J.* 2003; 14(4):234–238.

37 Rosenbaum TY, Owens A. The role of pelvic floor physical therapy in the treatment of pelvic and genital pain-related sexual dysfunction (CME). *J Sex Med.* 2008;5(3):513–523; quiz 524–525.

38 Rosenbaum TY, Padoa A. Managing pregnancy and delivery in women with sexual pain disorders. *J Sex Med.* 2012;9(7):1726–1735; quiz 1736.

39 Butrick CW. Pelvic floor hypertonic disorders: identification and management. *Obstet Gynecol Clin North Am.* 2009;36(3):707–722.

16

# Pathophysiology and Medical Management of Female Orgasm Disorder

*Irwin Goldstein and Barry R. Komisaruk*

### Abstract

Female orgasm disorder, the second most reported sexual problem among women, is characterized by a persistent or recurrent distressing compromise of orgasm frequency, intensity, timing, and/or pleasure. Multiple diagnostic procedures may be used to help resolve the various aspects of the underlying female orgasm disorder. Risk factors include psychosocial issues, psychiatric disorders, certain medications, central nervous system neurotransmitter imbalances associated with pelvic floor dysfunction, high- or low-tone pelvic floor dysfunction, male partner sexual dysfunctions, genital medical conditions, or endocrine, neurologic or vascular disorders or debilitating disease. There has been limited research on the physiology of orgasm in women and the pathophysiologies, diagnoses, and treatments of the multiple female orgasm disorders.

Therapeutic strategies include treatment considered disease modification aimed to cure the female orgasm disorder condition or symptomatic treatment aimed to reduce the female orgasm disorder symptoms so that the orgasm function is improved. More research is needed.

**Keywords:** *female orgasm disorder; orgasm; sympathetic efferent activity to pelvic organs; intense pleasure/well-being/contentment; brain neurotransmitter imbalance; anorgasmia; delayed orgasm; orgasm anhedonia; pleasure dissociative orgasm dysfunction; radiculopathy of the sacral spinal nerve root*

---

Female orgasm disorder is characterized by a persistent or recurrent distressing compromise of orgasm frequency, intensity, timing, and/or pleasure, associated with sexual activity for a minimum of six months.

Multiple diagnostic procedures may be used to help resolve the various underlying female orgasm disorder biopsychosocial pathophysiologies.

Therapies may be considered disease modification to either cure the female orgasm disorder condition or to reduce the female orgasm disorder symptoms.

---

## Introduction

Female orgasm disorder is the second most reported sexual problem for women [1, 2]. There has been limited research on the physiology of orgasm in women and the pathophysiologies, diagnoses, and treatments of the multiple female orgasm disorders.

## Genital Responses Prior to, During and Immediately after Orgasm in Women

The drive to experience orgasm occurs, in part, because orgasm achieves several objectives. Firstly, orgasm is associated with memorable events that are often expressed as

*Textbook of Female Sexual Function and Dysfunction: Diagnosis and Treatment*, First Edition. Edited by Irwin Goldstein, Anita H. Clayton, Andrew T. Goldstein, Noel N. Kim, and Sheryl A. Kingsberg.
© 2018 John Wiley & Sons Ltd. Published 2018 by John Wiley & Sons Ltd.

ecstasy, euphoria, and extreme pleasure and act to motivate the individual to want to experience orgasm again in the future and, thereby, encourage reproduction. Secondly, orgasm is associated with increased sympathetic efferent activity to the pelvic organs that acts to undo physiologic pelvic vasocongestion associated with the peak of sexual arousal in various genital and pelvic structures including the clitoris, labia, urethral glands, vagina, uterus, and pelvic ligaments [3–6].

An operational definition of orgasm in women may be considered as: "… a variable transient peak sensation of intense pleasure creating an altered state of consciousness, usually with an initiation accompanied by involuntary, rhythmic contractions of the pelvic striated circumvaginal musculature, often with concomitant vaginal, uterine and anal contractions, and myotonia that resolves the sexually induced vasocongestion (sometimes only partially) and myotonia, generally with an induction of well-being and contentment" [6]. In general, the most apparent physical sign of orgasm is the sense of vaginal and/or pelvic striated muscle rhythmic contractions [3–6].

There have been inadequate investigations characterizing physiologic changes that occur in women just prior to, during, and immediately after orgasm. At the peak of female sexual arousal just before orgasm, maximal heart rate, blood pressure, and respiration values are detected. Furthermore, progressive sexual arousal physiological changes of engorgement, tumescence and vasocongestion are observed in the genitalia [3, 4].

During orgasm, repeated pelvic muscle contractions of varying intensity and duration are noted. In some women, these are intense, repetitive and can last for several seconds, while in others, contractions are weaker, less intense, and contract only for a limited duration. Sensitivity to pain is also reduced at orgasm [3, 4].

Brain imaging by functional magnetic resonance imaging or positron emission tomography have characterized regions activated or inhibited or unchanged before, during, and after orgasm. There is no current consensus as to what regions of the brain are specifically activated or inactivated during orgasm in women [7, 8]. One group claims areas that are inactivated include the temporal and prefrontal areas. The brain region associated with increased orgasm-related activation included the left anterior vermis and deep cerebellar nuclei [9]. Another group [10] reported increased functional magnetic resonance imaging activity in the nucleus accumbens, the paraventricular nucleus of the hypothalamus, the hippocampus, amygdala, insula, anterior cingulate cortex, cerebellum, paracentral lobule of the sensory cortex, and prefrontal cortex. Unfortunately, comparisons of these studies are difficult because of various factors, including dissimilarity in the arousal stimulation used, difference in maneuvers used to limit head movement artifacts, the diverse basal levels used for subtraction from arousal images to obtain the specific levels associated with sexual arousal, and the lack of agreement for what comprises significant activation above basal levels.

Immediately after orgasm, there are rapid reductions in heart rate, blood pressure and respiration. There are changes in the genitalia, including detumescence or decongestion and return of basal labial hue. The heightened arousal-induced vaginal lubrication ends and the excess fluids are reabsorbed osmotically returning the vaginal eputhelium to basal or "just moist" conditions [3, 4].

Blood levels of hormones such as epinephrine, vasoactive intestinal peptide, oxytocin, vasopressin, and prolactin have been measured before, during, and after orgasm in women. Prolactin and oxytocin are increased during orgasm [3, 4].

## ISSWSH Consensus Conference Nomenclature – Female Orgasm Disorder

In the DSM IV, female orgasm disorder was considered: a female sexual disorder, associated with negative personal consequences, that was not better accounted for by a general medical or psychiatric condition and not due exclusively to the direct physiologic effects of a substance or medication, in which women had "persistent or recurrent delay in, or absence of orgasm after a normal sexual excitement phase" [11]. In the DSM-5, female orgasm disorder was considered: a female sexual disorder that persisted a minimum of six months and was not better explained by a nonsexual mental disorder or consequence of severe relationship distress or other significant stressors and not due to effects of substance/medication or other medical conditions, with the presence of the following "on all or almost all (75–100%) occasions of sexual activity: (i) marked delay in, marked infrequency of, or absence of orgasm and (ii) marked reduced intensity of orgasmic sensations" [12]. In summary, as it relates to specific patient complaints about female orgasm disorder, combining the two most recent DSM system classifications, female orgasm disorder has been defined by compromises in orgasm quality relating to: (i) absence of orgasm, (ii) delay in orgasm, (iii) infrequency of orgasm or (iv) reduced intensity of orgasm, after adequate sexual stimulation and arousal, causing personal distress.

Sexual medicine health-care providers, however, manage women who complain of far more broad, diverse, and differing orgasmic complaints than that represented in the DSM system. The past or current DSM definitions for women with orgasm disorders actually fail to characterize and include the various other kinds of bothersome and distressing female orgasmic disorders seen, observed, and managed by biopsychosocial sexual health-care providers of women with sexual dysfunction. A more inclusive, user-friendly, sexual medicine health-care provider-oriented classification of women with distressing orgasm is required. For example, biopsychosocial sexual medicine health-care providers manage women distressed with compromises in orgasm pleasure, such as reduced or absent pleasure (anhedonic orgasm, or pleasure dissociative orgasm disorder). Biopsychosocial sexual medicine

health-care providers also manage women distressed with compromises in orgasm timing, such as orgasms that occur spontaneously or too early (premature orgasm). Biopsychosocial sexual medicine health-care providers manage women distressed with aversive peripheral and/or central symptoms that occur prior to, during or following orgasm (female orgasmic illness syndrome). Additionally, biopsychosocial sexual medicine health-care providers manage women distressed with symptoms of persistent genital arousal not associated with concomitant sexual interest (persistent genital arousal disorder, genital dysesthesia), where orgasm may be aversive and/or compromised.

A broader, more diverse view of orgasm disorder in women would include female orgasmic disorders, where the primary orgasm complaint is a compromise of orgasm frequency, intensity, timing, and/or pleasure. Alternatively, the primary orgasm complaint may be aversive symptoms that occur prior to, during, or following the orgasm (female orgasm illness syndrome) and are not related, *per se*, to a compromise of orgasm quality.

The prevalence of the DSM-based female orgasmic disorder, which is characterized by orgasm concerns plus distress, is 4.7% [1]. There are no prevalence data on the current broader ISSWSH definition of orgasm disorders. There are no prevalence data on female orgasm illness syndrome

This chapter addresses female orgasm disorder. Separate chapters address female orgasm illness syndrome (Chapter 17) and persistent genital arousal disorder (Chapter 11).

# Female Orgasm Disorders (ISSWSH Consensus Conference Nomenclature)

Female orgasm disorder is characterized by a persistent or recurrent, distressing compromise of orgasm frequency, intensity, timing, and/or pleasure, associated with sexual activity for a minimum of six months [13].

- *Frequency*: orgasm occurs with reduced frequency (diminished frequency of orgasm) or is absent (anorgasmia).
- *Intensity*: orgasm occurs with reduced intensity (muted orgasm).
- *Timing*: orgasm occurs either too late (delayed orgasm) or too early (spontaneous or premature orgasm) than desired by the woman.
- *Pleasure*: orgasm occurs with absent or reduced pleasure (anhedonic orgasm, pleasure dissociative orgasm disorder).

Female orgasm disorder may be classified as "lifelong" if the condition is present throughout the person's life or "acquired" if the condition develops later in life. Female orgasm disorder may be classified as "generalized" if the condition is present at all times or "situational" if the condition is present only in certain situations.

## Risk Factors for Women with Female Orgasm Disorder

Multiple biopsychosocial pathophysiologies of female orgasm disorder can result in the symptoms typically associated with female orgasm disorder.

Female orgasm disorder may exist, in part, from psychosocial issues. Spectatoring (obsessive self-observation during sex), unresolved marital conflict, religious guilt, fear of pregnancy, ineffective sexual communication, traumatic relationship experiences, mood disorders, fatigue, emotional concerns, past trauma and abuse history, cultural and religious prohibitions, and feeling excess pressure to have a sexual experience, all represent examples in which psychosocial issues may result in insufficient central nervous system sexual excitatory processes or increased central nervous system sexual inhibitory processes. Female orgasm disorder may also exist, in part, associated with

psychiatric disorders including anxiety and/or depression [14–16].

Female orgasm disorder may also exist, in part, associated with use of certain medications, such as selective serotonin reuptake inhibitors typically used for treatment of depression. Serotonin, a central nervous system sexual response inhibitor, is elevated with the use of selective serotonin reuptake inhibitors, such that the medication inhibits orgasm capability. Other drug classes that negatively affect orgasm include antipsychotics, antihypertensives, benzodiazepines, histamine 2 receptor antagonists, and anticonvulsants [17–19].

Female orgasm disorder may exist, in part, from various factors.

- Brain central nervous system neurotransmitter imbalances in excitatory and inhibitory critical nuclei [20].
- Associated with pelvic floor dysfunction, both high-tone and low-tone pelvic floor dysfunction [21, 22].
- Male partner sexual dysfunctions, such as erectile dysfunction or premature ejaculation, or female partner sexual dysfunctions, such as low sexual interest or sexual pain disorder. The inadequate sexual arousal that may occur in these cases represent examples where partner issues may result in insufficient central nervous system sexual excitatory processes or increased central nervous system sexual inhibitory processes [23, 24].
- Endocrine disorders, such as low testosterone, low estradiol states including menopause and genitourinary syndrome of menopause, prolactinoma, or hypothyroidism [25–27].
- Genital medical conditions that are distracting, such as: genital dermatologic conditions such as lichen plannus, lichen sclerosus, or from vestibulodynia conditions such as hormonally-mediated vestibulodynia, neuro-proliferative vestibulodynia, vulvar granuloma fissuratum, and/or desquamative inflammatory vaginitis [28, 29].

- Neurologic disorders [30–32]: these may be subclassified as peripheral nervous system disorders (neuropathy of the dorsal nerve, perineal nerve, inferior hemorrhoidal nerve, pelvic or pudendal nerve) or central nervous system disorders (traumatic head injury, spinal cord injury, phantom orgasms, epilepsy, Parkinson's Disease, multiple sclerosis, radiculopathy of the sacral spinal nerve roots.

## Neurologic Disorders

### Traumatic Brain Injury

The variable and multiple regions of brain damage resulting from traumatic brain injury may induce female orgasm disorder, along with other sexual dysfunction symptoms such as decreased or increased libido, loss of genital sensation, and reduced lubrication. The sexual dysfunction produced by the traumatic brain injury may be direct, on physiologic control [e.g. orgasm), or indirect (e.g. emotional reactions to one's self-esteem, body image, or sexual identity) [33–35].

### Spinal Cord Injury

Depending on the location and "completeness" of the spinal cord injury and the specific genital response, the effects of spinal cord injury on sexual response vary because the afferent and efferent genital nerves connect to the spinal cord at different levels of the spinal cord. The pudendal nerves, which convey clitoral sensation, enter the spinal cord at sacral levels S2–S4, so "complete" spinal cord injury at that level or above, blocks the ability to perceive clitoral stimulation. The hypogastric nerves, which convey cervical and uterine sensation, enter the spinal cord much higher (i.e. at thoracic levels T10–T12, bypassing the lumbar and sacral levels). Consequently, pregnant women who have complete spinal cord injury below thoracic level T12 can feel their uterus contracting and their fetus moving, because the hypogastric nerve afferents enter above the level of the injury and their access to the brain remains intact [36]. Because the effer-

ents of the hypogastric nerve regulate blood flow and, thereby, control vaginal lubrication, women with complete spinal cord injury below thoracic T12 can experience psychogenic vaginal lubrication, but women with complete spinal cord injury above thoracic T10 cannot. However, women with complete spinal cord injury above thoracic T10 have intact pudendal nerve afferents and hypogastric nerve efferents, so they can experience reflexive, although not psychogenic, vaginal lubrication.

Genital afferent activity is conveyed within the spinal cord to the brain via the spinothalamic tract. If this pathway is interrupted, clitoral stimulation-induced orgasm is blocked. However, women with complete spinal cord injury above thoracic T10 may retain cervical and vaginal sensibility and experience orgasms from that stimulation via the vagus nerves [37]. Functional magnetic resonance imaging brain scanning provided evidence that the brain region to which the vagus nerves project (i.e. the nucleus of the solitary tract in the medulla oblongata of the brainstem) is activated by cervical or vaginal self-stimulation in women with complete spinal cord injury above thoracic T10. Furthermore, three of the five women with complete spinal cord injury experienced orgasm from the vaginal or cervical self-stimulation, which resulted in widespread activation throughout the brain. Thus, there is evidence of two separate genital-orgasmic neural pathways in women: the main, spinothalamic, pathway within the spinal cord and the "auxiliary" vagus nerve pathway, which bypasses the spinal cord and projects directly to the brain, capable of activating orgasm [37].

In cases of pregnant women with complete spinal cord injury who have intact hypogastric nerve input to the spinal cord because their complete spinal cord injury is below T12, those women can "feel their uterine contractions and fetal movements normally" [38]. There are assertions in the literature that vaginal and anal sensation is lost after complete spinal cord injury at S4 and above

[39], that there is "total loss of sensitivity of the internal organs in patients with complete transection of the spinal cord above T-10", and that genital sensations are lost and orgasm is not possible after complete spinal cord injury at T10 or above [40]. But contrary to these assertions, Cole stated, "However difficult it may be to understand, spinal injured women report orgasms in spite of complete denervation of all pelvic structures" [41]. Cole's assertion is supported by more recent reports of orgasm in "complete quadriplegic" women [42], women with complete spinal cord injury between C4 and T9. Women with spinal cord injury or complete spinal cord injury above T10 reported feeling spontaneous menstrual discomfort or cramps, further evidence of the existence of a spinal cord bypass pathway (i.e. the vagus nerves) [37].

### "Phantom" Orgasms

Patients with complete spinal cord injury and no genital sensation have reported "phantom" orgasms in their dreams, indicating the critical role of the brain in orgasm, independent of the genitals. Patients with an intact spinal cord and with an amputated foot reported that in response to genital stimulation (which, in the sensory cortex, is represented adjacent to the foot [43] they felt orgasms extending into their phantom foot.

Money presented the concept of "phantom orgasm" in characterizing patients with spinal cord injury and no genital sensation who experienced orgasm in their sleep [44]. In this case, at least in some patients, the "phantom" is the orgasm experienced as genital. Of 14 patients who had spinal cord injury between C5 and L1, all had experienced orgasm before injury. Eight of the patients reported experiencing sexual intercourse in their dreams and five of these patients reported orgasm imagery in dreams after their injuries. In Money's words, these patients with paraplegia, "had no genitopelvic gratification (none ejaculated after their injury]. It is therefore all the more remarkable a phenomenon that some of them had

orgasm imagery in dreams almost as vividly as though it were the real thing. ... [This finding] offers conclusive evidence that cognitional eroticism can be a variable of sex entirely independent of genitopelvic sensation and action. The brain, in other words, can work independently of the genitalia in the generation of erotic experience, just as the genitalia of paraplegics can work reflexly and independently of the brain. ... The occurrence of orgasm imagery in the sleep dreams of paraplegics may be regarded as a special example of phantom imagery. It is of interest that this phantom experience was restricted to sleep. Awake or asleep, there were no other reported examples, from any of the patients, of phantom sensation or imagery attributable to the genitalia" [44].

Money described the case of a woman, 32 years of age, who was injured in a fall three years earlier that produced a fracture dislocation at C6 and C7. The injury left her incontinent and completely paralyzed from the waist down, except for minimal toe movements that disappeared following rhizotomy. She described that when she had a "sexy dream" she always "reached a climax" [44].

### Epilepsy

Epilepsy is reported to exert potent and variable effects on sexuality; patients with epilepsy may experience states of hypo- or hypersexuality, and their seizures may feel as if they are genital orgasms or "nongenital orgasms". The seizure-related orgasms may be described as "unwelcome" or pleasurable [45]; in the latter case, a woman refused antiepileptic medication or brain surgery, claiming that she enjoyed her orgasmic auras and did not want to have them eliminated [46]. In the case of a 57-year-old woman with a tumor in the left anterior medial temporal lobe, she had a two-month history of daily seizures that she described as a sudden pleasure-provoking feeling "like an orgasm". Antitumor medication regressed the tumor and the seizures subsided. There are numerous reports of men and women experiencing orgasmic feelings just prior to the onset of an epileptic seizure, termed an "orgasmic aura" [45–48]. The most common brain region from which these orgasmic auras originate, based on electroencephalographic recordings, is the right temporal lobe of the forebrain, which contains the hippocampus and the amygdala. The aura may have a spontaneous onset or may be triggered by some specific stimulus, e.g. brushing the teeth. There are reports of epileptic seizures that originate in the genital-projection zone (paracentral lobule) of the sensory cortex. In those cases the individuals report that they experience genital sensation that develops into an orgasm, and the orgasm feels as if it were generated by genital stimulation [48]. However, some orgasmic auras are not necessarily experienced as originating in the genitals, and are described as "nongenital" orgasms [49]. In a study of 29 patients with temporal lobe epilepsy, 20 were characterized by "global hyposexuality", experiencing orgasms less than once per year or never. After these patients received temporal lobectomy, their seizures ceased, and they became "chronically hypersexual" [50].

## Parkinson's Disease

Although not universally observed [51], significant deleterious effects on sexuality and orgasm have been reported in patients with Parkinson's disease. In a study of patients with Parkinson's disease, 7/10 women reported that, since their diagnosis, they had reduced sexual interest and orgasm frequency, and 4/10 were unable to experience orgasm. The spouses noted a decrease in their affected partner's sexual interest in the majority of the cases [52]. On the basis of the extensive evidence of the role of dopamine in sexual response and orgasm [53], it is likely that the loss in sexual response and orgasm in Parkinson's disease – as well as the loss of motor function – is closely related to the deterioration of the dopaminergic neuron system, which is characteristic of this disease.

## Multiple Sclerosis

Multiple sclerosis in women is characterized by genital sensory dysfunction, loss of libido, decreased vaginal lubrication, increased spasticity during sexual activity, loss of orgasmic capacity [54], and bladder and bowel dysfunction [55, 56]. Orgasmic dysfunction in women with multiple sclerosis was reported to evolve independently of disease duration and physical disability. Abnormality of genital sensation in women with multiple sclerosis is likely related to absent or decreased cortical evoked responses to electrical stimulation of the pudendal nerve, which innervates the clitoris [57, 58]. Lesions of the pons [59] are involved in cases of anorgasmia [60]. Lesions of the left temporal periventricular and right visual association areas were also reported to be associated with decreased orgasmic function [61]. However, lesions of the frontotemporal cortex or midbrain were correlated with higher female sexual function index scores, indicating a disinhibiting effect of these brain regions on orgasmic function [62].

## Radiculopathy of the Sacral Spinal Nerve Roots

The pudendal and pelvic nerves involved in orgasm convey sensation from the clitoris, vagina, prostate, vulva, vestibule, perineum, and anal sphincter and enter the sacrum at levels Sacral 2-4. Upon entering the sacrum, these nerves pass superiorly as individual nerve root components of the cauda equina. The cauda equina also consists of sensory and motor nerve roots from the lower lumbar dermatomes, which convey sensation from the feet, legs, and buttocks. The sacral nerve roots first synapse in the sacral division of the spinal cord proper at the conus medullaris, typically located at vertebral level Thoracic 12 just below the lowest rib. Efferent sacral and lumbar nerve roots comprise part of the cauda equina, providing the parasympathetic (but not sympathetic) and somatic innervation of the genitalia and somatic motor innervation of the lower limbs [63].

As a result of this innervation pattern, when there is irritation of, or damage to, the cauda equina by physical herniation/compression by one or more intervertebral discs, most commonly at Lumbar 5-Sacral 1 or Lumbar 4-5, a constellation of one or more of the following symptoms may occur: altered (increased or decreased) genital sensation including paresthesias and persistent genital arousal disorder, less intense orgasm, anorgasmia, and lumbar root sensorimotor deficits, such as lower extremity weakness, sensory deficit below the knee, leg reflex change, low back pain, and/or sciatica [63].

Female orgasm disorder may also exist, in part, associated with vascular disorders including hypertension, metabolic syndrome, and diabetes. In a meta-analysis of 24 studies relating cardiovascular disease to sexuality in women, the authors concluded that cardiovascular disease detrimentally affected all the measured domains of sexual function (i.e. desire, arousal, vaginal lubrication, orgasm, sexual satisfaction, and pain). Hypertensive women were found to have more difficulty in experiencing lubrication and orgasm than the healthy comparison group [64]. A study of the effect of heart attack on sexuality compared one hundred women hospitalized for myocardial infarction with an age-matched sample of one hundred women hospitalized for other reasons. All of the women underwent a 57-item interview about their sex lives, including specifically whether they lacked sexual intercourse due to a partner's illness or erectile dysfunction, lacked enjoyment of sexual intercourse, or were emotionally distressed about being unable to experience orgasm during intercourse. The authors reported a significant correlation between positive responses on the above specific questions and the women's history of myocardial infarction [65].

Metabolic syndrome, which is associated with the risk of developing cardiovascular disease and type 2 (insulin-resistant) diabetes, consists of three or more of the following conditions: abdominal obesity, hypertension, elevated fasting plasma glucose, high serum triglycerides, and low levels of high-density lipoprotein [66]. Based on a study of 376 postmenopausal women (mean age 73) to whom the female sexual function index was administered, the women who fulfilled the criteria for a diagnosis of metabolic syndrome showed a significant correlation with low sexual activity and desire, arousal, orgasm, and satisfaction. Furthermore, low sexual activity was correlated with angina, heart attack, and coronary bypass surgery [65].

In an earlier study of women with diabetes, 35% of 125 had lost the ability to experience orgasm after the onset of their disorder, whereas only 6% of a comparison group of 100 nondiabetic women were anorgasmic (and had never experienced orgasm). There was no association between the diabetes-related anorgasmia and age, diabetes duration, or severity of neuropathy [67]. In a subsequent study, women with type 1 diabetes (insulin-dependent) showed an overall 40% incidence of sexual disorders (including decreased capacity to experience orgasms, decreased vaginal lubrication, and decreased sexual desire), whereas the age-matched comparison group showed only a 7% incidence of any kind of sexual disorder [68]. In the diabetic group compared with the comparison group, there were additional indicators of peripheral neuropathy, i.e. higher vibration perception thresholds measured at the clitoris and hands, incontinence, and reduced foot perspiration.

Female orgasmic disorder may also exist, in part, associated with debilitating diseases (e.g. cancer, degenerative diseases). A study assessed sexual well-being (using the sexual relationships and activities questionnaire) in 3708 women at least 50 years old who were either cancer survivors or cancer-free. Compared with the cancer-free women, the cancer survivors reported greater difficulty in experiencing orgasm (61 versus 28%), becoming aroused (55 versus 32%), and were more concerned about their orgasmic experience (18 versus 7%)

and their sexual desire (15 versus 7%). The authors did not propose a mechanism to account for these differences [69].

## Diagnosis of Women with Female Orgasm Disorder

Women with bothersome and distressing female orgasmic disorder should undergo a thorough biopsychosocial history and physical examination, and laboratory tests. Diagnostic efforts should be made to identify if there are any reversible causes of female orgasmic disorder. In this case, modification of any reversible causes would be recommended prior to focus on the initiation of symptomatic therapeutic interventions for female orgasmic disorder.

Multiple pathophysiologies of female orgasmic disorder have been proposed that can result in the symptoms typically associated with female orgasmic disorder.

- Psychological problems in part causing female orgasmic disorder: psychosocial assessment should be performed [14–16].
- Medication-related pathophysiologies, in part, causing female orgasmic disorder: a full history of medication use should be performed. Certain medications negatively affect orgasm, such as selective serotonin reuptake inhibitors, antipsychotics, antihypertensives, benzodiazepines, histamine 2 receptor antagonists, and anticonvulsants [17–19].
- Partner-related pathophysiologies, in part, causing female orgasmic disorder: partner sexual dysfunction assessment should be performed.
- Pelvic floor pathophysiologies, in part, causing female orgasmic disorder: pelvic floor physical therapy assessment should be performed. For women with female orgasmic disorder who may be considered to have high-tone pelvic floor dysfunction, a diagnostic local anesthesia nerve block to the specific suspected location

(trigger point injection) may result in reduction of the female orgasmic disorder symptoms. For women with female orgasmic disorder who may be considered to have low-tone pelvic floor dysfunction, strategies that would increase muscle tone may result in reduction of the female orgasmic disorder symptoms [21, 22].

- Distracting and bothersome genital medical conditions that may be associated with discomfort and cause female orgasm disorder: physical examination, including diagnostic procedures such as vulvoscopy, cotton swab (Q-tip) testing, and vaginal wet mount and smear testing, should be performed to assess for such pathologies as: lichen plannus, lichen sclerosus, vulvar granuloma fissuratum, and desquamative inflammatory vaginitis [28, 29].
- Endocrine disorders in part causing female orgasm disorder, such as low testosterone, low estradiol, low thyroid and elevated prolactin hormones: diagnostic blood testing can be performed to obtain baseline and then post-treatment values. These endocrinopathy states may be classically noted in the genitourinary syndrome of menopause or in reproductive age women on hormonal birth control. The diagnostic blood tests include: total testosterone, sex hormone binding globulin, dihydrotestosterone, luteinizing hormone, follicle stimulating hormone, prolactin, thyroid stimulating hormone, estradiol and progesterone. Calculated free testosterone can be performed using the law of mass action calculator and the values of total testosterone and sex hormone binding globulin [70–72].
- Neurologic pathophysiologies in part causing female orgasm disorder: diagnostic testing can be performed to help localize the sites of neurologic impairment. Diagnostic neuro-genital tests may be considered, such as quantitative sensory testing, sacral dermatome testing, bulbocavernosus reflex latency testing, and urodynamic testing [63]. Diagnostic

magnetic resonance imaging studies of the sacral and lumbar spine areas should further be considered. If a suspicious lesion is noted on magnetic resonance imaging, a diagnostic epidural local steroid injection to the specific lesion that resulted in marked reduction of the female orgasm disorder symptoms and enhanced genital sensitivity would provide evidence that the female orgasm disorder symptoms resulted from the spinal lesion.

- Vascular pathophysiologies in part causing female orgasm disorder, such as cardiovascular disease or metabolic syndrome: duplex Doppler ultrasonography or clitoral/vulvar thermography may be considered [73].

## Treatment of Women with Female Orgasm Disorder

There are two types of treatment for women with female orgasm disorder. Firstly, disease modification treatment strategies are designed to cure the female orgasm disorder and resolve the underlying pathophysiology(ies).

### Female Orgasm Disorder Disease Modification Treatment Strategies

For women with female orgasm disorder who have underlying psychological concerns: psychological treatment strategies, such as formal psychotherapy including sensate focus therapy, cognitive behavior therapy, and/or mindfulness therapy, typically focusing on modifying feelings, attitudes, actions, sentiments, and relationship communication/behaviors that may be causatively related to the female orgasm disorder condition. More conservative strategies to reduce anxiety may include yoga and acupuncture [74–76].

For women with female orgasm disorder who have underlying pelvic floor pathophysiologies, in part, causing persistent genital arousal disorder: pelvic floor physical therapy strategies should be performed. For women with high-tone pelvic floor dysfunction, traditional physical therapy strategies may be

considered to lower the high tone state. Adjunctive use of trigger point injections, vaginal or rectal diazepam or baclofen, and/or intramuscular onabotulinum toxin A may result in improvement of the female orgasm disorder symptoms. For women with low-tone pelvic floor dysfunction, traditional physical therapy strategies may be considered to raise the low tone state [77–81].

For women with female orgasm disorder who have underlying medication-related pathophysiologies, such as use of agents known to reduce orgasm function, including selective serotonin reuptake inhibitors, antipsychotics, antihypertensives, benzodiazepines, histamine 2 receptor antagonists, and anticonvulsants: identifying strategies to eliminate these agents, if possible, or to switch to agents with less orgasm interfering properties, should be considered [17–19].

For women with female orgasm disorder who have underlying endocrine pathophysiologies, such as low testosterone, low estradiol, low thyroid and elevated prolactin hormones: various treatment strategies may be considered. For women with female orgasm disorder and low testosterone, discussion should ensue as to the carefully monitored use of biologically-identical testosterone. There are no FDA-approved testosterone products for women, so the choices include off-label use of FDA-approved testosterone products for men dosed at approximately one-tenth of the intended male dose or off-label use of compounded testosterone products. An ideal goal of testosterone therapy is a calculated free testosterone values of 0.6–0.8 ng/dl. Follow-up blood tests for total testosterone, sex hormone binding globulin, and dihydrotestosterone should initially be made at three-month intervals and then as needed, such as every 6–12 months if stable. The three choices of testosterone therapy include: daily topical products typically applied to the back of the calf, weekly intramuscular injections of testosterone typically into the vastus lateralus, and 4–6-monthly testosterone pellets. A 75 mg testosterone pellet product is FDA-approved for men.

Side effects of testosterone treatment typically are cosmetic and include increased facial hair, thinning of scalp hair, acne, and oily facial skin. Usually the dose of testosterone is decreased if side effects occur. If testosterone treatment results in improvement of orgasm function, the patient should consider staying on testosterone treatment for 6–12 months and taking a drug holiday from the treatment to see if the treatment is still required. In most cases, testosterone therapy is needed to maintain the orgasm function improvement [71, 72].

For women with female orgasm disorder and low estradiol, typically women in menopause: discussion should ensue as to the carefully monitored use of biologically-identical estradiol. There are many FDA-approved estradiol products for women in menopause, including oral pills, patches, gels, vaginal rings, and intramuscular injections. For women with a uterus, those who have not had a hysterectomy, concomitant use of progesterone will act to protect the endometrial lining of unopposed stimulation. The ideal goal of estradiol therapy is a value of approximately 35–50 pg/ml, the usual upper value of normal for many reference laboratories in menopause and values consistent with 8–10% of peak estradiol values in the reproductive years. Follow-up blood tests for estradiol should initially be made at three-month intervals and then as needed, such as every 6–12 months if stable. Side effects of estradiol treatment include: breast cancer, thromboembolic disease, breast pain, nipple discharge, uterine bleeding. Usually the dose of estradiol is decreased if side effects occur. If estradiol treatment results in improvement of orgasm function, the patient should consider staying on estradiol therapy for 6–12 months and taking a drug holiday from the treatment to see if the treatment is still required. In most cases, estradiol therapy is needed to maintain the orgasm function improvement [71, 72].

For women with female orgasm disorder and low thyroid hormone: discussion should ensue as to the carefully monitored use of biologically-identical thyroid hormone. There are FDA-approved thyroid hormone products. The ideal goal of thyroid therapy is a thyroiod stimulating hormone value of 1–2 μU/ml. The typical starting daily dose of thyroid hormone is 25 μg/d. Follow-up blood tests for thyroid stimulating hormone, free triiodothyronine, total triiodothyronine, free thyroxine, and total thyroxine should initially be made at three-month intervals and then as needed, such as every 6–12 months if stable. Side effects of thyroid treatment typically are: headache, insomnia, nervousness, irritability, fever, hot flushes, sweating, pounding heartbeats or fluttering in the chest region. Usually the dose of thyroid hormone is decreased if side effects occur. If thyroid hormone treatment results in improvement of orgasm function, the patient should consider staying on thyroid hormone treatment for 6–12 months and taking a drug holiday from the treatment to see if the treatment is still required. In most cases, thyroid hormone therapy is needed to maintain the orgasm function improvement [25, 82, 83].

For women with female orgasm disorder and increased prolactin hormone levels: discussion should ensue as to obtaining magnetic resonance imaging of the pituitary with gadolinium. In most cases, a microadenoma will be identified and medical management with cabergoline will follow. In rare cases of local mass lesion symptom – producing macroadenomas, neurosurgical referral is indicated. In most cases, medical management will involve use of carefully-monitored FDA-approved cabergoline. The ideal goal of cabergoline therapy is a normal prolactin value of 4–23 ng/ml. The typical starting dose of cabergoline is 0.5 mg twice a week on Monday and Thursday. Follow-up blood tests for prolactin should initially be made at three-month intervals and then as needed, such as every 6–12 months if stable. Side effects of cabergoline treatment typically are: feeling short of breath on exertion, chest discomfort, dry cough, feeling weak or tired, loss of appetite, rapid weight loss, and lower back pain. Usually the dose of cabergoline is decreased if side effects occur. If treatment with cabergoline, which is a dopamine receptor stimulant (and prolactin secretion inhibitor), results in improvement of orgasm function, the patient should consider staying on cabergoline treatment for 6–12 months. A follow-up pituitary magnetic resonance imaging is indicated. Taking a drug holiday from the cabergoline may be attempted to see if the treatment is still required. In most cases, cabergoline therapy is needed to maintain the lowered prolactin levels and for orgasm function improvement [84, 85].

Concerning distracting and bothersome genital medical conditions that may be associated with discomfort and cause female orgasm disorder: management should be offered based on the underlying pathophysiology. Treatment of the genital dermatologic conditions, including lichen plannus and lichen sclerosus, typically involve initial use of daily ultra-potent steroids, such as clobetasol propionate 0.05% ointment. The condition of vulvar granuloma fissuratum is often cured by posterior vestibulectomy with vaginal advancement flap reconstruction. The condition of desquamative inflammatory vaginitis, a sterile form of vaginitis, can be caused by an irritant or allergic reaction to chemicals or be caused by a lack of estrogen. The characteristic sign of desquamative inflammatory vaginitis is a copious yellowish discharge that dries like glue. Sheets of white blood cells and parabasal cells are seen on smear. Typical treatment requires using 2 g each night for one month of a compound – hydrocortisone 10%; estradiol 0.02%; and clindamycin 2% in a vaginal cream base (VersaBase). Diflucan 150 mg once per week is also used [86, 87].

Concerning women with female orgasm disorder from suspected reduced sensory information (radiculopathy) passing from hypofunctioning sacral spinal nerve roots within the cauda equina from various sacral and lumbar pathologies: minimally invasive endoscopic and navigational spine surgery may be considered. Sacral spine nerve radiculopathy in general, and Tarlov cysts and/or herniated intervertebral disc or stenosis-induced chronic cauda equina syndrome in particular, may cause female orgasm disorder. It is hypothesized that female orgasm disorder may occur as a manifestation of mechanical irritation of the genital sensory (and possibly autonomic) nerve roots, which could result in hypofunction of sacral nerve roots. Our hypothesis is based in part on our recent findings that administration of epidural steroids at the site of the genital nerve roots, and subsequent surgical reduction of the intervertebral discs, or surgical treatment of Tarlov cysts, successfully alleviated the female orgasm disorder symptoms. This hypothesis supports the concept that the female orgasm disorder hypofunction is a form of genital radiculopathy due to hypofunction of the genital sensory nerve roots. It is suggested that female orgasm disorder be included as a subtype of the chronic form of cauda equina syndrome, on the basis that mechanical impingement of intervertebral discs on the cauda equina seems to be a clear etiological factor in certain cases of female orgasm disorder [63].

## Female Orgasm Disorder Symptomatic Treatment Strategies

Symptomatic therapeutic strategies for female orgasm disorder are based on pharmacologic agents used to rebalance brain central nervous system excitatory and inhibitory neurotransmitter imbalances. In female orgasm disorder management, it is hypothesized that increasing central nervous system sexual excitatory processes with agonists of dopamine, oxytocin, and/or norepinephrine, or decreasing central nervous system sexual inhibitory processes with antagonists of opioid and/or serotonin, would improve orgasm function. As there are no FDA-approved agents to safely or effectively treat female orgasm disorder, all such pharmaceutical therapies are off-label.

Off-label pharmaceutical agonist agents potentially for female orgasm disorder that may act on excitatory neurotransmitters, and the doses one of the authors recommends initially to women with female orgasm disorder, include: bupropion 75 mg/d in the AM; cabergoline 0.5 mg q Monday and q Thursday; ropinirole 0.25 mg qdaily – TID; oxytocin lozenges 250 U sublingually – one hour prior to sexual activity; and/or amphetamine, dextroamphetamine mixed salts, 2.5–10 mg taken 30 minutes prior to sexual activity, but if taken after 2:00 p.m. difficulty with sleep should be considered.

Off-label pharmaceutical antagonist agents potentially for female orgasm disorder that may act on inhibitory neurotransmitters, and the doses one of the authors recommends initially to women with female orgasm disorder, include: buspirone 10 mg twice a day, and/or naltexone 50 mg/d.

Off-label pharmaceutical agonist and antagonist agents potentially for female orgasm disorder that may act on both excitatory and inhibitory neurotransmitters include use of flibanserin at a dose of 100 mg/night. Flibanserin is a nonhormonal, centrally acting, postsynaptic serotonin 1A receptor agonist and a serotonin 2A receptor antagonist, and is classified as a multifunctional serotonin agonist and antagonist. Flibanserin use results in a decrease in serotonin activity and an increase in dopamine and norepinephrine activity, based on laboratory animal studies. While flibanserin is currently an FDA-approved treatment for generalized acquired hypoactive sexual desire disorder in premenopausal women, studies have reported that all domains in the female sexual function index, including orgasm function, are increased.

To prescribe flibanserin, the health-care provider needs to be certified in the risk evaluation and mitigation strategy program. Efficacy for libido improvement may not develop for up to 8–12 weeks, and it may be similar for the orgasm function improvement. The most common adverse events reported, in terms of placebo-corrected rates of occurrence, included mild-to-moderate severity dizziness (9.2%), somnolence (8.3%), nausea (6.5%), and fatigue (3.7%). These side effects are not uncommon with central nervous system active medications that influence serotonin [88–93].

## Conclusions

Female orgasm disorder is a relatively common sexual medicine condition. The ISSWSH Nomenclature for Female Sexual Dysfunctions has broadened the definition such that female orgasm disorder is characterized by a persistent or recurrent, distressing compromise of orgasm frequency, intensity, timing, and/or pleasure, associated with sexual activity for a minimum of six months. Multiple diagnostic procedures may be used to help resolve the various underlying female orgasm disorder biopsychosocial pathophysiologies. Therapies may be considered disease modification aimed to cure the female orgasm disorder condition. Therapies may be considered symptomatic, aimed to reduce the female orgasm disorder symptoms, so that the orgasm function is improved. More research is needed in female orgasm disorder.

## References

1 Shifren J, Monz BU, Russo PA, *et al.* Sexual problems and distress in United States women: prevalence and correlates. *Obstet Gynecol.* 2008;112:970–978.

2 Laumann E, Paik A, Rosen RC. Sexual dysfunction in the United States: Prevalence and predictors. *JAMA.* 1999;281.

3 Levin R. The pharmacology of the human female orgasm – its biological and physiological backgrounds. *Pharmacol Biochem Behav.* 2014;121:62–70.

4 Levin R. Female orgasm: correlation of objective physical recordings with subjective experience. *Arch Sex Behav.* 2008;37(6):855.

5 Meston C, Levin RJ, Sipski M, *et al.* Women's orgasm. *Annu Rev Sex Res.* 2004;15:173–257.

6 Meston C, Hull E, Levin RJ, Sipski M. Disorders of orgasm in women. *J Sex Med.* 2004;1(1):66–68.

7 Salonia A, Giraldi A, Chivers ML, *et al.* Physiology of women's sexual function: basic knowledge and new findings. *J Sex Med.* 2010;7(8):2637–2660.

8 Stoléru S, Fonteille V, Cornélis C, *et al.* Functional neuroimaging studies of sexual arousal and orgasm in healthy men and women: a review and meta-analysis. *Neurosci Biobehav Rev.* 2012;36(6):1481–1508.

9 Georgiadis J, Kringelbach ML. The human sexual response cycle: brain imaging evidence linking sex to other pleasures. *Prog Neurobiol.* 2012;98(1):49–81.

10 Komisaruk B, Whipple B. Functional MRI of the brain during orgasm in women. *Annu Rev Sex Res.* 2005;16:62–86.

11 American Psychiatric Association. *Diagnostic and Statistical Manual of Mental Disorders IV, Text Revision (DSM-IV-TR).* Washington, DC: American Psychiatric Association; 2003.

12 American Psychiatric Association. *Diagnostic and Statistical Manual of Mental Disorders,* 5th edn. Arlington, VA: American Psychological Association; 2013.

13 Parish SJ, Goldstein AT, Goldstein SW, *et al.* Toward a more evidence-based nosology and nomenclature for female sexual dysfunctions – Part II. *J Sex Med.* 2016;13(12):1888–906.

14 Leeners B, Hengartner MP, Rössler W, *et al.* The role of psychopathological and personality covariates in orgasmic difficulties: a prospective longitudinal evaluation in a cohort of women from age 30 to 50. *J Sex Med.* 2014;11(12):2928–2937.

15 Merwin K, O'Sullivan LF, Rosen NO. We need to talk: disclosure of sexual problems is associated with depression, sexual functioning, and relationship satisfaction in women. *J Sex Marit Ther.* 2017:43(8):786–800.

16 Rowland D, Kolba TN. Understanding orgasmic difficulty in women. *J Sex Med.* 2016;13(8):1246–54.

17 Baldwin D, Manson C, Nowak M. Impact of antidepressant drugs on sexual function and satisfaction. *CNS Drugs.* 2015;29(11):905–913.

18 Montejo A, Montejo L, Navarro-Cremades F. Sexual side-effects of antidepressant and antipsychotic drugs. *Curr Opin Psychiatry.* 2015;28(6):418–423.

19 Gelenberg A, Delgado P, Nurnberg HG. Sexual side effects of antidepressant drugs. *Curr Psychiatry Rep.* 2000;2(3):223–327.

20 Holstege G. How the emotional motor system controls the pelvic organs. *Sex Med Rev.* 2016;4(4):303–328.

21 Roos A, Thakar R, Sultan AH, *et al.* Pelvic floor dysfunction: women's sexual concerns unraveled. *J Sex Med.* 2014;11(3):743–752.

22 Knoepp L, Shippey SH, Chen CC, *et al.* Sexual complaints, pelvic floor symptoms, and sexual distress in women over forty. *J Sex Med.* 2010;7(11):3675–3682.

23 Maseroli E, Fanni E, Mannucci E, *et al.* Which are the male factors associated with female sexual dysfunction (FSD)? *Andrology.* 2016;4(5):911–920.

24 Rosen R, Heiman JR, Long JS, *et al.* Men with sexual problems and their partners: findings from the international survey of relationships. *Arch Sex Behav.* 2016;445(1):159–173.

25 Pasquali D, Maiorino MI, Renzullo A, *et al* Female sexual dysfunction in women with thyroid disorders. *J Endocrinol Invest.* 2013;36(6):729–733.

26 Atis G, Dalkilinc A, Altuntas Y, *et al.* Hyperthyroidism: a risk factor for female sexual dysfunction. *J Sex Med.* 2011;8:2327–2333.

27 Nappi R, Albani F, Santamaria V, *et al.* Menopause and sexual desire: the role of testosterone. *Menopause Int.* 2010;16(4):162–168.

28 Anderson A, Rosen NO, Price L, Bergeron S. Associations between penetration cognitions, genital pain, and sexual well-being in women with

provoked vestibulodynia. *J Sex Med.* 2016;13(3):444–542.

29  Bois K, Bergeron S, Rosen N, *et al.* Intimacy, sexual satisfaction, and sexual distress in vulvodynia couples: An observational study. *Health Psychol.* 2016;35(6):531–540.

30  Jones K, Kingsberg S, Whipple B (eds) *Women's Sexual Health in Midlife and Beyond.* ARHP Clinical Proceedings. Washington, DC: Association of Reproductive Health Professionals; 2005.

31  Phillips N. Female sexual dysfunction: evaluation and treatment. *Am Fam Physician.* 2000;62(1):127–136, 141–142.

32  Whipple B, Brash-Mcgreer K. Management of female sexual dysfunction. In: Sipski ML, Alexander CJ (eds) *Sexual Function in People with Disability and Chronic Illness: A Health Professional's Guide.* Gaithersburg, MD: Aspen; 1997, pp. 509–534.

33  Rees P, Fowler CJ, Maas CP. Sexual function in men and women with neurological disorders. *Lancet.* 2007;369:512–525.

34  Aloni R, Katz S. A review of the effect of traumatic brain injury on the human sexual response. *Brain Injury.* 1999;13:269–280.

35  Agha A, Rogers B, Sherlock M, *et al.* Anterior pituitary dysfunction in survivors of traumatic brain injury. *J Clin Endocrinol Metab.* 2004;89:4929–4936.

36  Komisaruk B, Gerdes CA, Whipple B. 'Complete' spinal cord injury does not block perceptual responses to genital self-stimulation in women. *Arch Neurol.* 1997;54:1513–1520.

37  Komisaruk B, Whipple B, Crawford A, *et al.* Brain activation during vaginocervical self-stimulation and orgasm in women with complete spinal cord injury: fMRI evidence of mediation by the vagus nerve. *Brain Res.* 2004;1024:77–88.

38  Berard E. The sexuality of spinal cord injured women: physiology and pathophysiology. *A review. Paraplegia.* 1989;27:99–112.

39  Perduta-Fulginiti P. Sexual functioning of women with complete spinal cord

injury: Nursing implications. *Sex Disabil.* 1992;10:103–118.

40  Szasz G. Sexual health care. In: Zejdlik C (ed) *Management of Spinal Cord Injury,* 2nd edn. Boston, MA: Jones and Bartlett; 1992, pp. 175–201.

41  Cole TM. Sexuality and physical disabilities. *Arch Sex Behav.* 1975;4(4):389–403.

42  Kettl P, Zarefoss S, Jacoby K, *et al.* Female sexuality after spinal cord injury. *Sex Disabil.* 1991;9:287–95.

43  Komisaruk BR, Wise N, Frangos E, *et al.* Women's clitoris, vagina, and cervix mapped on the sensory cortex: fMRI evidence. *J Sex Med.* 2011;8(10):2822–2830.

44  Money J. Phantom orgasm in the dreams of paraplegic men and women. *Arch Gen Psychiatry.* 1960;3:373–382.

45  Reading PWR. Unwelcome orgasms. *Lancet.* 1997;350:1746.

46  Janszky J, Ebner A, Szupera Z, *et al.* Orgasmic aura – a report of seven cases. *Seizure.* 2004;13:441–444.

47  Janszky J, Szucs A, Halasz P, *et al.* Orgasmic aura originates from the right hemisphere. *Neurology.* 2002;58:302–304.

48  Calleja J, Carpizo R, Berciano J. Orgasmic epileps. *Epilepsoa.* 1988;29:635–639.

49  Komisaruk BR, Whipple B. Non-genital orgasms. *Sex Relation Ther.* 2011;26:356–372.

50  Blumer D. Hypersexual episodes in temporal lobe epilepsy. *Am J Psychiatry.* 1970;126(8):1099–1106.

51  Ferrucci R, Panzeri M, Ronconi L, *et al.* Abnormal sexuality in Parkinson's disease: fact or fancy? *J Neurol Sci.* 2016;369:5–10.

52  Waters C, Smolowitz J. Impaired sexual function. In: Pfeiffer R (ed) *Parkinson's Disease and Nonmotor Dysfunction.* New York: Humana Press; 2005, pp. 127–138.

53  Komisaruk B, Beyer C, Whipple B. *The Science of Orgasm.* Baltimore, MD: Johns Hopkins University Press; 2006.

54  Rees PM, Fowler CJ, Maas CP. Sexual function in men and women with neurological disorders. *Lancet.* 2007;369(9560):512–525.

55 Ghezzi A. Sexuality and multiple sclerosis. *Scan J Sexology.* 1999;2:125–140.

56 Lundberg P, Hulter B. Sexual dysfunction in female patients with multiple sclerosis. *Int Rehab Med.* 1981;3:32–34.

57 Yang C, Bowen JR, Kraft GH, *et al.* Cortical evoked potentials of the dorsal nerve of the clitoris and female sexual dysfunction in multiple sclerosis. *J Urol.* 2000;164:2010–2013.

58 DasGupta R, Kanabar G, Fowler C. Pudendal somatosensory evoked potentials in women with female sexual dysfunction and multiple sclerosis. *Int J Impot Res.* 2002;14:S83.

59 Zivadinov R, Locatelli L, Stival B, *et al.* Normalized regional brain atrophy measurements in multiple sclerosis. *Neuroradiology.* 2003;45(11):793–798.

60 Barak Y, Achiron A, Elizur A, *et al.* Sexual dysfunction in relapsing-remitting multiple sclerosis: magnetic resonance imaging, clinical, and psychological correlates. *J Psychiatry Neurosci.* 1996;21(4):255–258.

61 Winder K, Linker RA, Seifert F, *et al.* Neuroanatomic Correlates of Female Sexual Dysfunction in Multiple Sclerosis. *Annals Neurology.* 2016;80:490–8.

62 Winder K, Linker RA, Seifert F, *et al.* Neuroanatomic correlates of female sexual dysfunction in multiple sclerosis. *Ann Neurol.* 2016;80(4):490–498.

63 Goldstein I, Komisaruk BR, Rubin RS, *et al.* A novel collaborative protocol for successful management of penile pain mediated by radiculitis of sacral spinal nerve roots from tarlov cysts. *Sex Med.* 2017;5(3):e203–e211

64 Duncan LE, Lewis C, Smith CE, *et al.* Sex, drugs, and hypertension: a methodological approach for studying a sensitive subject. *Int J Impot Res.* 2001;13(1):31–40.

65 Trompeter S, Bettencourt R, Barrett-Connor E. Metabolic syndrome and sexual function in postmenopausal women. *Am J Med.* 2016;129(12):1270–1277.

66 Kaur J. A comprehensive review on metabolic syndrome. *Cardiol Res Pract.* 2014;2014: 943162. doi: 10.1155/2014/943162.

67 Kolodny RC. Sexual dysfunction in diabetic females. *Diabetes.* 1971;20(8):557–559.

68 Hulter B, Berne C, Lundberg P. Sexual function in women with insulin dependent diabetes mellitus: correlation with neurological symptoms and signs. *Scan J Sexology.* 1998;1:43–50.

69 Jackson SE, Wardle J, Steptoe A, Fisher A. Sexuality after a cancer diagnosis: A population-based study. *Cancer.* 2016;122(24):3883–3891.

70 Portman D, Gass M, Kingsberg S, *et al.* Genitourinary syndrome of menopause: new terminology for vulvovaginal atrophy from the International Society for the Study of Women's Sexual Health and the North American Menopause Society. *Menopause.* 2014;21:1063–1068.

71 Goldstein I, Alexander JL. Practical aspects in the management of vaginal atrophy and sexual dysfunction in perimenopausal and postmenopausal women. *J Sex Med.* 2005;2(Suppl 3):154–165.

72 Goldstein I. Current management strategies of the postmenopausal patient with sexual health problems. *J Sex Med.* 2007;4(Suppl 3):235–253.

73 Goldstein I, Goldstein S, Millheiser L. The impact of Fiera, a women's personal care device, on genital engorgement as measured by thermography: a proof-of-principle study. *Menopause.* 2017; 24(11):1257–1263.

74 Dhikav V, Karmarkar G, Gupta R, *et al.* Yoga in female sexual function. *J Sex Med.* 2010;7:964–970.

75 Brotto L, Krychman M, Jacobson P. Eastern approaches for enhancing women's sexuality: Mindfulness, acupuncture and yoga. *J Sex Med.* 2008;5:2741–2748.

76 Khamba B, Aucoin, M, Lytle, M, *et al.* Efficacy of acupuncture treatment of sexual dysfunction secondary to antidepressants. *J Altern Complement Med.* 2013;19(11):862–869.

77 Halder G, Scott L, Wyman A, *et al.* Botox combined with myofascial release physical therapy as a treatment for

myofascial pelvic pain. *Investig Clin Urol.* 2017;58(2):134–139.

78 Adelowo A, Hacker MR, Shapiro A, *et al.* Botulinum toxin type A (BOTOX) for refractory myofascial pelvic pain. *Female Pelvic Med Reconstr Surg.* 2013;19(5):288–292.

79 Crisp C, Vaccaro CM, Estanol MV, *et al.* Intra-vaginal diazepam for high-tone pelvic floor dysfunction: a randomized placebo-controlled trial. *Int Urogynecol J.* 2013;24(11):1915–1923.

80 Carrico D, Peters KM. Vaginal diazepam use with urogenital pain/pelvic floor dysfunction: serum diazepam levels and efficacy data. *Urol Nurs.* 2011;31(5):279–284.

81 Rogalski M, Kellogg-Spadt S, Hoffmann AR, *et al.* Retrospective chart review of vaginal diazepam suppository use in high-tone pelvic floor dysfunction. *Int Urogynecol J.* 2010;21(7):895–899.

82 Oppo A, Franceschi E, Atzeni F, *et al.* Effects of hyperthyroidism, hypothyroidism, and thyroid autoimmunity on female sexual function. *J Endocrinol Invest.* 2011;34(6):449–453.

83 Atis G, Dalkilinc A, Altuntas Y, *et al.* Sexual dysfunction in women with clinical hypothyroidism and subclinical hypothyroidism. *J Sex Med.* 2010;7:2583–2590.

84 Worsley R, Santoro, N, Miller, KK, *et al.* Hormones and female sexual dysfunction: beyond estrogens and androgens – Findings from the Fourth International Consultation on Sexual Medicine. *J Sex Med.* 2016;13:283–290.

85 Rastrelli G, Corona G, Maggi M. The role of prolactin in andrology: what is new? *Rev Endocr Metab Disord.* 2015;16(3):233–248.

86 Mitchell L, King M, Brillhart H, Goldstein A. Cervical ectropion may be a cause of desquamative inflammatory vaginitis. *Sex Med.* 2017;5(3):e212–e214.

87 Burrows L, Shaw HA, Goldstein AT. The vulvar dermatoses. *J Sex Med.* 2008;5(2):276–283.

88 Goldstein I, Kim NN, Clayton AH, *et al.* Hypoactive sexual desire disorder: International Society for the Study of Women's Sexual Health (ISSWSH) Expert Consensus Panel Review. *Mayo Clin Proc.* 2017;92(1):114–128.

89 Portman D, Brown L, Yuan J, *et al.* Flibanserin in postmenopausal women with hypoactive sexual desire disorder: results of the PLUMERIA study. *J Sex Med.* 2017;14(6):834–942.

90 Gao Z, Yang D, Yu L, Cui Y. Efficacy and safety of flibanserin in women with hypoactive sexual desire disorder: a systematic review and meta-analysis. *J Sex Med.* 2015;12(11):2095–2104.

91 Katz M, DeRogatis LR, Ackerman R, *et al.* Efficacy of flibanserin in women with hypoactive sexual desire disorder: results from the BEGONIA trial. *J Sex Med.* 2013;10:1807–1815.

92 Jayne C, Simon JA, Taylor LV, *et al.* Open-label extension study of flibanserin in women with hypoactive sexual desire disorder. *J Sex Med.* 2012;9(12):3180–3188.

93 Parish S, Hahn SR. Hypoactive sexual desire disorder: a review of epidemiology, biopsychology, diagnosis, and treatment. *Sex Med Rev.* 2016;4(2):103–120.

17

# Pathophysiology and Medical Management of Female Orgasmic Illness Syndrome

*Irwin Goldstein and Barry R. Komisaruk*

### Abstract

Female orgasmic illness syndrome refers to those rare aversive symptoms that have been reported to occur prior to, during, or following orgasm, arbitrarily divided into central or peripheral aversive symptoms. Central aversive symptoms may include disorientation, confusion, impaired judgment, decreased verbal memory, anxiety/agitation/akathisia, insomnia, laughter, dysphoria/crying/depression, fatigue, seizures, muscle weakness/paralysis, and/or headache. Peripheral aversive symptoms may include diarrhea, constipation, muscle ache, sneezing, abdominal pain, diaphoresis, chills, hot flashes, pruritus, facial/ear/foot pain, and genital pain. Symptoms may last for minutes, hours, or days post-orgasm and varies widely within individuals. More research is needed.

**Keywords:** *orgasm illness syndrome (OIS); central aversive symptoms associated with orgasm; peripheral aversive symptoms associated with orgasm; confusion associated with orgasm; crying associated with orgasm; depression associated with orgasm; headache associated with orgasm; abdominal pain associated with orgasm; genital pain associated with orgasm; sneezing associated with orgasm*

---

Symptoms may last for minutes, hours, or days post-orgasm, and can vary widely in individuals.

Central aversive symptoms include disorientation, confusion, impaired judgment, decreased verbal memory, anxiety/agitation/akathisia, insomnia, laughter, dysphoria/crying/depression, fatigue, seizures, muscle weakness/paralysis, and/or headache.

Peripheral aversive symptoms include diarrhea, constipation, muscle ache, sneezing, abdominal pain, diaphoresis, chills, hot flashes, pruritus, facial/ear/foot pain, and genital pain.

---

## Introduction

Female orgasmic illness syndrome refers to those rare aversive symptoms that have been reported to occur prior to, during, or following orgasm [1]. Such symptoms may be arbitrarily divided into either central aversive symptoms or peripheral aversive symptoms.

## ISSWSH Consensus Nomenclature – Female Orgasmic Illness Syndrome

Female orgasmic illness syndrome is not mentioned in either the DSM IV [2] or the DSM-5 [3]. Sexual medicine health-care providers do manage women who complain of

*Textbook of Female Sexual Function and Dysfunction: Diagnosis and Treatment*, First Edition. Edited by
Irwin Goldstein, Anita H. Clayton, Andrew T. Goldstein, Noel N. Kim, and Sheryl A. Kingsberg.
© 2018 John Wiley & Sons Ltd. Published 2018 by John Wiley & Sons Ltd.

varying bothersome and distressing orgasmic complaints, and, although rare, it is not helpful to such patients who seek help and counsel that such orgasmic phenomena are not represented in a nomenclature system [1]. Thus, a more comprehensive, biopsychosocial sexual medicine health-care provider-oriented classification of women with distressing orgasm symptoms, such as those denoted as female orgasmic illness syndrome was required in women whose primary complaint is aversive symptoms that occur prior to, during, or following the orgasm.

The ISSWSH Nomenclature Consensus Conference considered female orgasmic illness syndrome to be consistent with peripheral and/or central aversive symptoms that occur prior to, during, or following orgasm [1]. Central aversive symptoms may include disorientation, confusion, impaired judgment, decreased verbal memory, anxiety/agitation/akathisia, insomnia, laughter, dysphoria (post-coital dysphoria)/crying/depression (post-coital tristesse), fatigue, seizures (orgasmic epilepsy), muscle weakness/paralysis (cataplexy), and/or headache (coital cephalalgia). Peripheral aversive symptoms may include diarrhea, constipation, muscle ache, sneezing, abdominal pain, diaphoresis, chills, hot flashes, pruritus, facial/ear/foot pain, and genital pain (dysorgasmia). Such orgasm-associated symptoms may last for minutes, hours, or days post-orgasm and vary widely in individuals

In this chapter, some of the many examples of female orgasmic illness syndrome are examined. It is clear that more research is need to safely and efficaciously manage these patients.

## Central Aversive Symptoms

### Seizures (Orgasmolepsy)

Concerning women with female orgasmic illness syndrome and the occurrence of seizures with orgasm, multiple cases have been reported occurring at the time of orgasm or even several hours after orgasm [4–10]. Use of anti-epileptics has been reported to reduce these orgasm-induced seizures. The orgasm-induced seizure focus has often been found within the temporal lobe [4, 5, 7, 10] but numerous other locations such as paracentral lobule [6], cerebral hemisphere [8], superior postcentral gyrus [10], or parietal parasagittal regions [3] have been identified. Various brain pathologies have been reported, such as post-traumatic brain injury [6], or even secondary to an astrocytoma [5].

### Headache (Coital Cephalalgia)

Concerning women with female orgasmic illness syndrome and sexual headaches – coital cephalalgia – there is more peer reviewed published literature on this symptom of female orgasmic illness syndrome than any other [11–13]. These sexual headaches are rare and mostly benign. They typically begin as a dull headache in the head and neck and are bilateral in two thirds of cases. They increase with sexual excitement and become intense at orgasm [11–13]. The pathophysiology is likely related to the adrenalin release associated with orgasm, intense sexual excitement, and contraction of facial and neck muscles. [14]. For some patients, the female orgasmic illness syndrome headaches may be related to the elevated blood pressure that occurs during orgasm. The pain has a variable duration and variable intensity, lasting from one minute up to 72 hours [11–13]. If the painful headache is, however, sudden and severe, this may warrant evaluation by magnetic resonance angiography to rule out intracranial pathology [15]. It is estimated that female orgasmic illness syndrome headaches occur in approximately 1% of the population [13]. Concerning women with female orgasmic illness syndrome and sexual headaches, conservative treatment may consist of beta-blockers and/or antimigraine medication [13, 16]. In patients who do not improve on these medications, indomethacin or a calcium channel antagonist such as verapamil can be tried [11, 13]. We have found that anticonvulsants such as topirimate can be successful in some cases that are otherwise resistant to treatment.

## Sneezing

The association between sneezing and sexual excitement or even sexual ideation has been know for more than 100 years [17]. Concerning the association of sneezing and/ or rhinorrhea with orgasm, reports have hypothesized that activation of one auto-nomic regulated function (orgasm) may activate a different autonomic-regulated function (sneezing) [18–20] and that sneez-ing is an orgasm of the respiratory system [21]. Concerning treatment of orgasm-induced sneezing, various strategies have been employed, some with minimal efficacy, such as antihistamines, nasal decongestants, and nasal anesthetics [18–20].

## Muscle Weakness/Paralysis (Cataplexy)

Concerning women with female orgasmic ill-ness syndrome and muscle weakness/paraly-sis (cataplexy), symptoms of post-orgasmic loss of total muscle control for less than a minute have been reported as far back as approximately 100 years [22–25]. It is unclear at this time how to best safely and effectively manage such patients but it may be that use of amphetamine, dextroamphetamine mixed salts, 2.5–10 mg taken 30 minutes prior to sexual activity may help these patients as the pharmacologically mediated heightened adr-energic activity may counteract the cataplexic symptoms [23–25]. More research is needed.

## Dysphoria (Postcoital Dysphoria)/ Crying/Depression (Postcoital Tristesse)

Concerning women with female orgasmic ill-ness syndrome and the post-coital negative aspects of dysphoria (postcoital dysphoria)/ crying/depression (post-coital tristesse), this has been described in secure relationships,

after consensual sexual activity, that can include tearfulness and sadness, and that can last up to an hour [26–28]. This has been reported to occur in approximately one-third of women [27]. It is unclear at this time how to best safely and effectively manage such patients.

## Peripheral Aversive Symptoms

### Genital Pain (Dysorgasmia)

Concerning women with female orgasmic ill-ness syndrome and bothersome distracting genital pain with orgasm (dysorgasmia), after ruling out other causes of dyspareunia, reports claim low dose tricyclic antidepres-sant amitriptyline (50 mg) can be helpful [29]. We have seen female orgasmic illness syndrome and dysorgasmia related to radicu-litis of the sacral spinal nerve roots from both sacral and lumbar spine pathology where the afferent sensory pelvic nerve is inflamed and is responsible for the dysorgasmia. For such patients, it is recommended to undergo neuro-genital testing with quantitative sen-sory testing, sacral dermatome testing, and bulbocavernosus reflex latency testing [30]. If abnormal, magnetic resonance imaging of the sacral and lumbar spine should be con-sidered. If pathology is noted, a focal epidural steroid and local anesthesia nerve block is likely to reveal diminution of distracting genital pain wth orgasm (dysorgasmia) symptoms, in which case minimally invasive endoscopic and navigational spine surgery could be considered [30].

### Facial/Ear/Foot Pain

Facial/ear/foot pain in women in relation to orgasm is reported in the literature [31–33]. For women with female orgasmic illness syn-drome and foot pain, this may be explained by the homuncular somatosensory cortical representation, in which the representation of the clitoris and genitals lies inferior to that of the feet and toes [34, 35]. Foot pain with orgasm may even occur after a below-the-knee amputation [36]. An epidural nerve block localized to sacral dorsal root ganglia can temporarily stop the foot pain with orgasm [32]. For women with female orgasmic illness syndrome and face or ear pain with orgasm, one report showed that symptoms can last up to 15 minutes and successful treatment involved a sympathomimetic agent to counteract the reduced post-orgasmic sympathetic nervous system activity [33].

## Conclusions

It is evident that women may report unusual central and/or peripheral symptoms associated with orgasm. In this chapter, some information and direction for the clinician encountering such a patient is provided. Most of the data are derived from case reports. More research is needed in female orgasmic illness syndrome, as it is clear that the central and peripheral (neuro)physiology of orgasm is complex.

## References

1 Parish SJ, Goldstein AT, Goldstein SW, *et al.* Toward a more evidence-based nosology and nomenclature for female sexual dysfunctions – Part II. *J Sex Med.* 2016;13(12):1888–1906.

2 American Psychiatric Association. *Diagnostic and Statistical Manual of Mental Disorders IV, Text Revision (DSM-IV-TR).* Washington, DC: American Psychiatric Association; 2003.

3 American Psychiatric Association. *Diagnostic and Statistical Manual of Mental Disorders*, Fifth Edition: DSM-5. Arlington, VA: American Psychological Association, 2013.

4 Hoenig J, Hamilton CM. Epilepsy and sexual orgasm. *Acta Psychiatr Scand.* 1960;35:448–456.

5 Bancaud J, Favel P, Bonis A, *et al.* Paroxysmal sexual manifestations and temporal epilepsy. *Electroencephalogr Clin Neurophysiol.* 1971;1(30):371.

6 Bertheir M, Starkstein S, Leiguarda R. Seizures induced by orgasm. *Ann Neurol.* 1987;22:394–395.

7 Ozkara C, Ozdemir S, Yilmaz A, *et al.* Orgasm-induced seizures: a study of six patients. *Epilepsia.* 2006;47:2193–2197.

8 Sengupta A, Mahmoud A, Tun SZ, Goulding P. Orgasm-induced seizures: male studied with ictal electroencephalography. *Seizure.* 2010;19:306–309.

9 Chaukimath S, Patil PS. Orgasm-induced seizures: a rare phenomenon. *Ann Med Health Sci Res.* 2015;5:483–484.

10 Toone B. Sex, sexual seizures and the female with epilepsy. In: MR Trimble M (ed) *Woman and Epilepsy.* Chichester: John Wiley & Sons; 1991, 201–206.

11 Evans R, Pascual J. Expert opinion: orgasmic headaches: clinical features, diagnosis, and management. *Headache.* 2000;40:491–494.

12 Headache Classification Committee of the International Headache Society (IHS). The international classification of headache disorders, 3rd edition (beta version). *Cephalgia.* 2013;33(9):629–808.

13 Cutrer F, DeLange J. Cough, exercise, and sex headaches. *Neurologic Clinics.* 2014;32(2):433–450.

14 Staunton HP, Moore J. Coital cephalgia and ischaemic muscular work of the lower limbs. *J Neurol Neurosurg Psychiatry.* 1978;41(10):930–933.

15 Valença M, Valença LP, Bordini CA, *et al.* Cerebral vasospasm and headache during sexual intercourse and masturbatory orgasms. *Headache.* 2004;44(3):244–248.

16 Anand K, Dhikav V. Primary headache associated with sexual activity. *Sing Med J.* 2009;50(5):e176–e177.

17 Reinert A, Simon JA. "Did you climax or are you just laughing at me?"

Rare phenomena associated with orgasm. *Sex Med Rev.* 2017;5:275–281.

18  Everett H, Shapiro SL. Paroxysmal sneezing following orgasm. *JAMA.* 1972;219:1350–1351.

19  Bhutta M, Maxwell H. Sneezing induced by sexual ideation or orgasm: an under-reported phenomenon. *J R Soc Med.* 2008;101:587–591.

20  Bhutta M, Maxwell H. Further cases of unusual triggers of sneezing. *J R Soc Med.* 2009;102:49.

21  Komisaruk BR, Whipple B. Non-genital orgasms. *Sex Relation Ther.* 2012;26(4):356–372.

22  Levin M. Narcolepsy (Gélinaus syndrome). *Arch Neurol.* 1929;22:1172–1200.

23  Poryazova R, Khatami R, Werth E, Bassetti CL. Weak with sex: sexual intercourse as a trigger for cataplexy. *J Sex Med.* 2009;6:2271–2277.

24  Anic-Labat S, Guilleminault C, Kraemer HC, *et al.* Validation of a cataplexy questionnaire in 983 sleep-disorder patients. *Sleep.* 1999;22:77–87.

25 Guileminalt C. Cataplexy. In: Guilleminault C, Dement W, Passouant P, Weitzman E. (eds) Narcolepsy. New York: Spectrum Publications; 1976, pp. 125–141.

26  Schweitzer R, O'Brien J, Burri A. Postcoital dysphoria: prevalence and psychological correlates. *Sex Med.* 2015;3:2245–2243.

27  Bird B, Schweitzer R, Strassberg D. The prevalence and correlates of postcoital dysphoria in women. *Int J Sex Health.* 2011;23:14–25.

28  Sayin H. Altered states of consciousness occurring during expanded sexual response in the human female: preliminary definitions. *Neuroquantology.* 2011;9:882–891.

29  Ajay B, Penny J, Kurian J. Dysorgasmia or pain at orgasm: a case series. *Int J Gynecol Obstet.* 2009;107:S558.

30  Goldstein I, Komisaruk BR, Rubin RS, *et al.* A novel collaborative protocol for successful management of penile pain mediated by radiculitis of sacral spinal nerve roots from Tarlov cysts. *Sex Med.* 2017;5(3):e203–e211.

31  Locke R. Pain in the foot during orgasm. A case report. *J Am Podiatry Assoc.* 1983;73:271.

32  Waldinger M, de Lint GJ, van Gils AP, *et al.* Foot orgasm syndrome: a case report in a woman. *J Sex Med.* 2013;10:1926–1934.

33  Check J, Katsoff B. Transient sixth cranial nerve palsy following orgasm abrogated by treatment with sympathomimetic amines. *Clin Exp Obstet Gynecol.* 2014;41:468–470.

34  Komisaruk BR, Wise N, Frangos E, *et al.* Women's clitoris, vagina and cervix mapped on the sensory cortex, using fMRI. *J Sex Med.* 2011;8:2822–2830.

35  Di Noto P, Newman L, Wall S, Einstein G. The hermunculus: what is known about the representation of the female body in the brain? *Cereb Cortex.* 2013;23:1005–1013.

36  Ramachandran V, Blakeslee S. Phantoms in the brain: Probing the mysteries of the human mind. New York: William Morrow; 1998.

**Part IV**

**Sexual Pain Disorders**

## 18

# Nosology and Epidemiology of Dyspareunia and Vulvodynia

*Tami Serene Rowen and Andrew T. Goldstein*

### Abstract

Sexual pain is common can involve a wide array of disorders of the vulva, vagina, cervix, uterus, adnexa, pelvic floor muscles, and nerves that innervate these structures. The three most frequently used terms to describe sexual pain in women are: vulvodynia, dyspareunia, and vaginismus. There has been an evolution in terminology of sexual pain that allows for a better understanding of the source of the pain. Vulvodynia specifically can be associated with inflammation, hormonal changes, neurological, musculoskeletal, embryologic, genetic as well as psychosocial factors. The outcomes can lead to severe impact on a woman's quality of life.

**Keywords:** *vulvodynia; vestibulodynia; vaginismus; dyspareunia; genito-pelvic pain disorder; sexual pain; inflammation; hormonal changes; quality of life*

---

Sexual pain can involve the vulva, vestibule, pelvis muscles as well as internal organs and has both a physiological and psychological basis.

Sexual pain has been described for centuries: the nosology has changed significantly. Contemporary terminology takes into account the many factors contributing to this condition.

Sexual pain is highly prevalent and carries a significant cost to society.

---

## Background

Sexual pain is common and can have severe negative effects on women and their partners. Sexual pain can involve a wide array of disorders of the vulva, vagina, cervix, uterus, adnexa, pelvic floor muscles, and the nerves that innervate these structures. In order to fully understand sexual pain and urogenital pain, a thorough examination of the historical and current terminology is very useful.

In addition, an understanding of the epidemiology of these disorders is essential in order to properly screen and counsel patients.

## Nosology

The three most frequently used terms to describe sexual pain in women are: vulvodynia, dyspareunia, and vaginismus. The term "vulvodynia" (chronic vulvar pain) is

*Textbook of Female Sexual Function and Dysfunction: Diagnosis and Treatment*, First Edition. Edited by Irwin Goldstein, Anita H. Clayton, Andrew T. Goldstein, Noel N. Kim, and Sheryl A. Kingsberg.
© 2018 John Wiley & Sons Ltd. Published 2018 by John Wiley & Sons Ltd.

derived from the combination of the words "vulva" (the external genitalia in females) and Odyne, the Greek goddess of pain. Descriptions of vulvodynia can be found in ancient texts such as the Ramesseum Papyrus and in the writings of Soranus of Ephesus [1]. The term "dyspareunia" (i.e. pain during intercourse) was first used by Robert Barnes in 1878 in his treatise "*A Clinical History of the Medical and Surgical Disease of Women*" [2]. Lastly, the term vaginismus (an involuntary contraction of the musculature of the vagina that interferes with intercourse) was coined by J Marion Sims in 1862 [3]. The first scientific examination of vulvodynia was began in the late nineteenth century by Thomas [4], who described this condition as an "excessive sensibility of the nerves supplying the mucous membrane of some portion of the vulva, sometimes confined to the vestibule... [and] other times to one labium minus." In addition, the Scottish gynecologist Alexander Skene, for whom the periurethral glands are named, reported "a supersensitiveness of the vulva. When, however, the examining finger comes in contact with the hyperaesthetic part, the patient complains of pain, which is sometimes so great as to cause her to cry out" [5].

By the mid-twentieth century, Dickinson documented that in a majority of women suffering from dyspareunia the source of pain could be localized to the hymen, urethra, and fourchette [6]. Additional research documented the role of inflammation in vulvodynia [7–10]. To reflect the importance of the role of inflammation on vulvar pain, various authors coined the terms "focal vulvitis", "vestibular adenitis", "focal vestibulitis vulvae", and later "vulva vestibulitis syndrome" [1].

In the 1980s, Freidrich and Woodruff published a detailed description of the vulvar vestibule, addressing anatomic features that are most associated with pain [11]. Friedrich also published an early account of 28 women with symptoms of vulvodynia, which he called vulvar vestibulitis syndrome (VVS). He defined the diagnosis as pain on touch, localized to the vestibule and with associated vestibular findings [12]. Friedrich went on to become a founding member of the International Society for the Study of Vulvovaginal Disease (ISSVD), which has since become the preeminent society in terms of research, advocacy, and nosology related to vulvodynia. The ISSVD was formed in 1970 and had its first Congress in 1971 [13]. In 1975, the ISSVD described generalized vulvodynia (GVD), also known as "essential" or "dysesthetic" vulvodynia, as "burning vulva syndrome" at its world congress [1]. Eight years later, the ISSVD adopted the first standard definition of GVD as chronic vulvar discomfort, characterized by the patient's complaint of burning and sometimes stinging, irritating, or raw sensations [1, 14].

As more providers showed an interest in vulvodynia, the focus narrowed onto the different subtypes of this condition, describing vestibular pain as distinct from generalized vulvar pain and pain that is not solely related to sexual activity [15, 16]. In 1992, a thorough review on vulvodynia incorporated the role of dermatoses, infection, inflammation, and neuralgia [17]. In 1999, the ISSVD replaced vestibulitis with "vestibulodynia", acknowledging that the condition is not solely related to inflammation [10]. Later, the ISSVD expanded on the term of vulvodynia to classify it based on whether or not there was a stimulus, calling it "provoked" or "unprovoked" as well as "localized or generalized". The term provoked vestibulodynia (PVD) refers to provoked pain that is localized to the vulvar vestibule, whereas generalized vuvoldynia refers to unprovoked, diffuse vulvar pain affecting the entire vulvar region.

The 2003, ISSVD terminology formed the foundation of vulvodynia research for the next decade. Many of these studies explored possible causative factors for vulvodynia, such as hormonal, inflammatory, neuroproliferative, musculoskeletal, and genetic. Other studies have focused on treatment options. Lastly, additional studies introduced new modifying descriptors, such as primary/secondary and intermittent/persistent.

---

**Box 18.1  2015 Consensus terminology and classification of persistent vulvar pain and vulvodynia.**

A)  Vulvar pain caused by a specific disorder*
  i)  Infectious (e.g. recurrent candidiasis, herpes)
  ii)  Inflammatory (e.g. lichen sclerosus, lichen planus, immunobullous disorders)
  iii)  Neoplastic (e.g. Paget disease, squamous cell carcinoma)
  iv)  Neurologic (e.g. postherpetic neuralgia, nerve compression, or injury, neuroma)
  v)  Trauma (e.g. female genital cutting, obstetrical)
  vi)  Iatrogenic (e.g. postoperative, chemotherapy, radiation)
  vii)  Hormonal deficiencies (e.g. genitourinary syndrome of menopause [vulvovaginal atrophy], lactational amenorrhea)

B)  Vulvodynia – vulvar pain of at least three months' duration, without clear identifiable cause, which may have potential associated factors.

The following are the descriptors:

- Localized (e.g. vestibulodynia, clitorodynia) or generalized or mixed (localized and generalized)
- Provoked (e.g. insertional, contact) or spontaneous or mixed (provoked and spontaneous)
- Onset (primary or secondary)
- Temporal pattern (intermittent, persistent, constant, immediate, delayed)

*Women may have both a specific disorder (e.g. lichen sclerosus) and vulvodynia

---

Because of the substantial advances in the understanding of vulvodynia made over the last dozen years, in 2015 the ISSVD, the International Society for the Study of Women's Sexual Health (ISSWSH), the International Pelvic Pain Society (IPPS), and representatives from the American Congress of Obstetricians and Gynecologists (ACOG) and the National Vulvodynia Association (NVA) convened a consensus congress to revise the vulvar pain and vulvodynia nomenclature. The final terminology was accepted by all three societies during July and August 2015 (Box 18.1) [18].

The terminology is divided into two sections. The first part is called "vulvar pain caused by a specific disorder". This part contains vulvar pain conditions for which a cause can be clearly identified (e.g. pain due to herpes genitalis, lichen sclerosus, genital cutting, etc.). The second section is the new definition of vulvodynia: vulvar pain of at least three months duration, without clear identifiable cause, which may have potential associated factors. A special section of part two defines the descriptors of vulvodynia. These descriptors help to describe the location of the pain as well as the temporal pattern of the pain. This section reflects the findings that pain characteristics typically used to define persistent pain conditions may be more useful for classifying vulvodynia subtypes than specifiers based on hypothesized etiology. Examples, therefore, might include "primary provoked vestibulodynia" or "secondary spontaneous intermittent clitorodynia".

However, the greatest difference between the 2015 terminology and the 2003 terminology is the addition of "potential associated factors" (Box 18.2). This addition represents a paradigm shift in the approach to vulvodynia, resulting from research that has shown that several factors may be associated with the development and maintenance of the condition, rendering vulvodynia likely the result of a multifactorial process. Given that these associated factors may be leading the direction of future basic science studies and treatment trials, it is worth examining them:

---

**Box 18.2 2015 Consensus terminology and classification of persistent vulvar pain and vulvodynia – potential associated factors.**

Appendix: potential factors associated with vulvodynia

- Comorbidities and other pain syndromes (e.g. painful bladder syndrome, fibromyalgia, irritable bowel syndrome, temporomandibular disorder; level of evidence 2)
- Genetics (level of evidence 2)
- Hormonal factors (e.g. pharmacologically induced; level of evidence 2)
- Inflammation (level of evidence 2)
- Musculoskeletal (e.g. pelvic muscle overactivity, myofascial, biomechanical; level of evidence 2)

- Neurologic mechanisms
- Central (spine, brain; level of evidence 2)
- Peripheral: neuroproliferation (level of evidence 2)
- Psychosocial factors (e.g. mood, interpersonal, coping, role, sexual function; level of evidence 2)
- Structural defects (e.g. perineal descent; level of evidence 3)

---

## Genetic Factors

Several studies suggest that some women have a genetic predisposition to developing this condition via at least three (potentially overlapping), mechanisms: genetic polymorphisms that increase the risk of candidiasis or other infections, genetic changes that allow prolonged or exaggerated inflammatory responses, and increased susceptibility to hormonal changes associated with oral contraceptive pills [19–22].

## Hormonal Factors

The tissues of the vulva and vagina are both responsive and dependent on sex steroids (hormones) for proper health and function. There are many causes of decreased sex steroids, both natural and iatrogenic, that can lead to dyspareunia. The most common cause of decreased sex steroids in women is menopause. Other natural causes include anovulation secondary to: lactation, anorexia, hypothalamic amenorrhea, excessive physical activity or physiological stress, and hyperprolactinemia. Iatrogenic causes of decreased circulating sex steroids include

oophorectomy and hysterectomy (without oophorectomy) and commonly prescribed medications, such as combined hormonal contraception, which include combined oral contraceptive pills [23]. Combined hormonal contraception use leads to a reduction in serum estradiol and free testosterone by decreasing ovarian production of estrogen and total testosterone and by inducing the liver to produce increased levels of sex hormone binding globulin. In addition, some combined hormonal contraceptives contain synthetic progestogins that act as testosterone antagonists at the androgen receptor. It has been shown that combined hormonal contraceptives cause histopathologic changes in the vestibular mucosa, thereby increasing vulnerability to mechanical strain and decreasing mechanical pain thresholds [24].

Given their effects on sex steroids, it is perhaps not surprising that studies have shown that combined hormonal contraceptives are associated with symptoms consistent with provoked vestibulodynia. Bazin and colleagues showed, in a case-controlled study, that women who used combined hormonal contraceptives prior to the age of 17 had a relative risk of 11 of developing vulvodynia

[25]. In addition, Burrows and Goldstein described a case series of 50 consecutive women who developed vestibulodynia while on oral contraceptive pills, and who were successfully treated with topical estradiol and testosterone [26].

## Inflammation

Although both women with vestibulodynia and healthy women have inflammatory cells in the vestibular mucosa, the relative abundance and organization of these cells may differ between women with and without vestibulodynia. A recent paper demonstrated that women with vestibulodynia have higher densities of B lymphocytes and mature mucosal IgA-plasma cells. In addition, both B and T lymphocytes were arranged into germinal centers in women with vestibulodynia, but not in controls [27]. Furthermore, other authors have found an increase in mast cell density in the mucosa of women with vestibulodynia [28]. Many studies also show increased pro-inflammatory cytokines, neurokines, and chemokines in biopsies of women with vulvodynia [29, 30]. In addition, heightened systemic inflammatory response has been demonstrated by researchers using a topical cutaneous challenge with yeast in vulvodynia cases compared to controls [31].

## Musculoskeletal

The discomfort of vulvodynia can also be associated with pelvic floor muscle overactivity. Prolonged holding patterns can result in decreased tissue oxygenation, muscle overactivity, shortening of sarcomeres, and the development of myofascial trigger points [32]. Hypertonicity (overactivity) of the muscles that insert at the posterior vestibule – the pubococcygeus, puborectalis, and superficial transverse perineum – can lead to allodynia (as seen in vestibulodynia) in the posterior vestibule. Hypertonicity of deeper muscles (e.g. ileococcygeus, obturator internus) can lead to vaginal or deep thrusting dyspareunia [33]. In addition, overactivity of the bulbocavernosus and ischiocavernosus is associated with clitorodynia [34].

## Neurologic Mechanisms – Central

Several controlled studies have demonstrated that women with vulvodynia have evidence of central sensitization. Pukall *et al.* were the first to examine women with vulvodynia using functional magnetic resonance imaging [35]. The results of this study indicated that women with vestibulodynia exhibited evidence of augmented neural activity in response to painful vestibular stimulation in areas involved in pain modulation, such as the somatosensory, insular, and anterior cingulate regions – areas that are commonly activated in patients with other pain conditions. In addition, nonpainful pressure led to significant activation levels in insular, frontal, and somatosensory regions in women with vestibulodynia. These results suggest that women with vulvodynia have an increased perception of nonpainful and painful stimulation to the vestibule.

## Peripheral – Neuro-Proliferation

Researchers have found that women with provoked vestibulodynia have up to 10 times the density of c-afferent nociceptors nerve endings in their vestibular mucosa than normal women [36, 37]. In addition, Bornstein *et al.* found increased numbers of mast cells in vestibular tissue of women with vulvodynia [28]. Persistently activated mast cells release nerve growth factor and heparinase that allow newly sprouted nerve endings to invade the superficial mucosa of vestibule [38].

## Psychosocial Factors

Population-based studies have shown that anxiety, depression, childhood victimization, and post-traumatic stress are risk factors for the development of vulvodynia [39]. Women with vulvodynia were four times more likely among women to have a history of a prior mood or anxiety disorder as compared to women without vulvodynia. Psychological factors associated with greater pain intensity or sexual dysfunction in women with vulvodynia include pain catastrophizing, fear of pain, hypervigilance to pain, lower pain self-efficacy, negative attributions about the pain, avoidance, anxiety, and depression [40].

## Embryological/Congenital Factors

The cooccurrence of vulvodynia with interstitial cystitis/painful bladder syndrome may be related to a congenital disorder of urogenital sinus-derived endothelium [41]. Additional evidence to support this hypothesis is that women with primary vestibulodynia exhibit umbilical hypersensitivity more often than women with secondary vestibulodynia and nonaffected women, suggesting that some cases of primary vestibulodynia may be associated with a congenital neuronal hyperplasia in tissue derived from the primitive urogenital sinus [42].

## Associated Factors – Conclusion

It is likely that one or more of these associated factors may be clinically prominent, and may help in choosing further evaluation methods and treatments. For example, in the patient with significant pelvic floor overactivity, treatment may consist of pelvic floor physical therapy, possibly in combination with muscle relaxants (such as diazepam suppositories) and or intralevator botulinum toxin injections. Conversely, a woman with a history of endometriosis who gradually develops severe vestibulodynia after using combined hormone contraceptives might be better treated by stopping the combined hormone contraceptives and using topical hormonal therapy to the vestibule. A more thorough discussion of specific treatments can be found in the next chapters of this textbook.

## Additional Nosology

It is important to note that other professional societies have also tried to address terminology related to dyspareunia. For example, The International Association for the Study of Pain includes a section on "Pain of Vaginismus or Dyspareunia" [43]. These classifications were updated in 2011 to included generalized and provoked vulvar pain syndrome [43], reflecting the growing understanding that vulvar pain presents in a variety of ways. Vulvodynia is included in the International Classification of Disease (ICD-10) and includes modifiers of "other" and unspecified" [44].

The American Psychological Association's (APA) previous edition of the Diagnostic and Statistical Manual, 4th edition (DSM-IV) has two separate "Sexual Pain Disorders" that were included in the section on sexual dysfunctions, which it labeled on sexual dysfunc"vaginismus" [45]. The most recent edition combined these two into a single category of Genito-Pelvic Pain/Penetration Disorder (GPPPD) [46]. This change occurred for several reasons [18, 47–49]. Firstly, the defining feature required for diagnosis of vaginismus in previous generations of the DSM was the presence of vaginal muscle spasm. Research, however, has failed to prove the presence of muscle spasm as a valid or reliable diagnostic criteria. Secondly, diagnosis based solely on vaginal spasm does not address the elements of fear of penetration, anxiety, and pain, which are integral components of this condition. Lastly, several studies have shown that clinicians have a very difficult time distinguishing between dyspareunia, vestibulodynia, and vaginismus, thus the similarities outweigh the differences.

## Prevalence

Prevalence studies of vulvodynia have indicated that it is prevalent, with lifetime estimates ranging from 8 to 28%, in reproductive-aged women in the general population [50–52]. In a study comparing two separate geographical regions with differing access to health care there was still similar prevalence of about 8% [52]. Further, these authors show that prevalence is different with regards to race, where nonwhite Hispanic women had an odds ratio of 1.4 for vulvodynia. Further research showed that daily pain is worse in black women compared to white women and that they describe their pain differently as well [53]. When looking at just dyspareunia, however, nationally representative data in the United States suggest the prevalence is closer to 30% [54].

## Impact

Research looking into the economic impact of vulvodynia has shown significant cost on an individual and population level. During a six-month period of treatment, the individual costs were US$ 8862.40 per patient. This includes hospital and insurance payments, leave from work, and transportation costs among others. In a nonprobability study using a conservative estimate of vulvodynia prevalence, the authors estimated the annual cost of vulvodynia to be US$ 31–72 billion [55]. This study also demonstrated the very real impact on quality of life experienced by women with vulvodynia, which has been well described in the literature [56–59]. Ponte went even further in demonstrating that women with vulvodynia have worse quality of life scores that similar women with other skin and vulvar conditions [57].

## Conclusion

The history of modern medicine's understanding of vulvodynia reflects the slow progress that is being made in addressing women's sexual health concerns. We now understand that there are many etiologies of sexual pain, and pain confined to the vulva encompasses multiple systems, including neurological, musculoskeletal, hormonal, dermatological, and inflammatory. The importance of a thorough and accurate nosology allows providers and patients to understand both the causes and manifestations of vulvar pain in addition to directing them towards treatment options. Vulvodynia is highly prevalent during a woman's lifetime and as we train more providers to recognize its multifaceted nature, we are better able to offer solutions to this common and distressing condition.

## References

1 Amalraj P, Kelly S, Bachmann GA. Historical perspective of vulvodynia, In: Goldstein A, Pukall CF, Goldstein I (eds) *Female Sexual Pain Disorders*. Oxford, UK: Wiley-Blackwell, 2009, pp. 1–3.

2 Barnes R. *Clinical History of the Medical and Surgical Diseases in Women*. J. and A. Churchill; 1874.

3 Sims JM. *On Vaginismus. Transactions of the Obstetrical Society*. London; 1862.

4 Thomas TG. *A Practical Treatise on the Diseases of Women*. Philadelphia, PA: Lea Brothers & Co; 1891.

5 Skene A. *Treatise on the Dieases of Women*. 2nd edn. New York, NY: D Appleton and Company; 1892.

6  Dickinson R. *Human Sex Anatomy*. 2nd edn. Baltimore, MD: Williams & Wilkins; 1949.

7  Lynch PJ. Vulvodynia: a syndrome of unexplained vulvar pain, psychologic disability and sexual dysfunction. *J Reprod Med*. 1986;31:773–780.

8  Bornstein J, *et al*. Vestibulodynia – a subset of vulvar vestibulitis or a novel syndrome? *Am J Obstet Gynecol*. 1997;177:1439–1443.

9  Kirby B, Yell J. Vulvodynia is important cause of vulval pain. *BMJ*. 1999;318:1559.

10  Moyal-Barracco M, Lynch PJ. 2003 ISSVD terminology and classification of vulvodynia: a historical perspective. *J Reprod Med*. 2004;49:772–777.

11  Woodruff JD, Friedrich EG, Jr. The vestibule. *Clin Obstet Gynecol*. 1985;28:134–141.

12  Friedrich EG, Jr. The vulvar vestibule. *J Reprod Med*. 1983;28:773–777.

13  ISSVD. History and past congresses. https://www.issvd.org/about-us/history-and-past-congress/; last accessed 30 December 2017.

14  Bachmann GA, *et al*. Vulvodynia: a state-of-the-art consensus on definitions, diagnosis and management. *J Reprod Med*. 2006;51(6):447–456.

15  McKay M. Subsets of vulvodynia. *J Reprod Med*. 1988;33(8): 695–698.

16  McKay M. Vulvodynia. A multifactorial clinical problem. *Arch Dermatol*. 1989;125(2):256–262.

17  McKay M. *vulvodynia. diagnostic patterns*. *Dermatol Clin*. 1992;10(2):423–433.

18  Bornstein J, *et al*. 2015 ISSVD, ISSWSH, and IPPS consensus terminology and classification of persistent vulvar pain and vulvodynia. *J Sex Med*. 2016;13(4):607–612.

19  Babula O, *et al*. Altered distribution of mannose-binding lectin alleles at exon I codon 54 in women with vulvar vestibulitis syndrome. *Am J Obstet Gynecol*. 2004;191(3):762–766.

20  Foster DC, Sazenski TM, Stodgell CJ. Impact of genetic variation in interleukin-1 receptor antagonist and melanocortin-1 receptor genes on vulvar vestibulitis syndrome. *J Reprod Med*. 2004;49(7):503–509.

21  Goldstein AT, *et al*. Polymorphisms of the androgen receptor gene and hormonal contraceptive induced provoked vestibulodynia. *J Sex Med*. 2014;11(11):2764–2771.

22  Lev-Sagie A, *et al*. Polymorphism in a gene coding for the inflammasome component NALP3 and recurrent vulvovaginal candidiasis in women with vulvar vestibulitis syndrome. *Am J Obstet Gynecol*. 2009;200(3):303.e1–e6.

23  Siddle N, Sarrel P, Whitehead M. The effect of hysterectomy on the age at ovarian failure: identification of a subgroup of women with premature loss of ovarian function and literature review. *Fertil Steril*. 1987;47(1):94–100.

24  Burrows LJ, Basha M, Goldstein AT. The effects of hormonal contraceptives on female sexuality: a review. *J Sex Med*. 2012;9(9):2213–2223.

25  Bazin S, *et al*. Vulvar vestibulitis syndrome: an exploratory case-control study. *Obstet Gynecol*. 1994;83(1):47–50.

26  Burrows LJ, Goldstein AT. The treatment of vestibulodynia with topical estradiol and testosterone. *Sex Med*. 2013;1(1):30–33.

27  Tommola P, *et al*. Activation of vestibule-associated lymphoid tissue in localized provoked vulvodynia. *Am J Obstet Gynecol*. 2015;212(4):476 e1–e8.

28  Bornstein J, Goldschmid N, Sabo E. Hyperinnervation and mast cell activation may be used as histopathologic diagnostic criteria for vulvar vestibulitis. *Gynecol Obstet Invest*. 2004;58(3):171–178.

29  Foster DC, Hasday JD. Elevated tissue levels of interleukin-1 beta and tumor necrosis factor-alpha in vulvar vestibulitis. *Obstet Gynecol*. 1997;89(2):291–296.

30  Bohm-Starke N, *et al*. Neurochemical characterization of the vestibular nerves in women with vulvar vestibulitis syndrome. *Gynecol Obstet Invest*. 1999;48(4):270–275.

31  Ramirez De Knott HM, *et al*. Cutaneous hypersensitivity to Candida albicans in

idiopathic vulvodynia. *Contact Dermatitis.* 2005;53(4):214–218.

32 Morin M, *et al.* Morphometry of the pelvic floor muscles in women with and without provoked vestibulodynia using 4D ultrasound. *J Sex Med.* 2014;11(3):776–785.

33 King M, *et al.* Current uses of surgery in the treatment of genital pain. *Curr Sex Health Rep.* 2014. doi: 0.1007/ s11930-014-0032-8.

34 Shafik A. The role of the levator ani muscle in evacuation, sexual performance and pelvic floor disorders. *Int Urogynecol J Pelvic Floor Dysfunct.* 2000;11(6):361–376.

35 Pukall CF, *et al.* Neural correlates of painful genital touch in women with vulvar vestibulitis syndrome. *Pain.* 2005;115(1–2):118–127.

36 Westrom LV, Willen R. Vestibular nerve fiber proliferation in vulvar vestibulitis syndrome. *Obstet Gynecol.* 1998;91(4):572–576.

37 Bohm-Starke N, *et al.* Increased intraepithelial innervation in women with vulvar vestibulitis syndrome. *Gynecol Obstet Invest.* 1998;46(4):256–260.

38 Bornstein J, *et al.* Involvement of heparanase in the pathogenesis of localized vulvodynia. *Int J Gynecol Pathol.* 2008;27(1):136–141.

39 Pukall CF, *et al.* Vulvodynia: definition, prevalence, impact, and pathophysiological factors. *J Sex Med.* 2016;13(3):291–304.

40 Khandker M, *et al.* The influence of depression and anxiety on risk of adult onset vulvodynia. *J Womens Health (Larchmt).* 2011;20(10):1445–1451.

41 Fariello JY, Moldwin RM. Similarities between interstitial cystitis/bladder pain syndrome and vulvodynia: implications for patient management. *Transl Androl Urol.* 2015;4(6):643–652.

42 Burrows LJ, *et al.* Umbilical hypersensitivity in women with primary vestibulodynia. *J Reprod Med.* 2008;53(6):413–416.

43 Mersky H, Bodguk N (eds) *Classification of Chronic Pain*, 2nd edn. Seattle, WA: IASP

(International Association for the Study of Pain); 1994.

44 WHO. *Manual of the International Statistical Classification of Diseases and Related Health Problems.* Geneva: World Health Organization, 2010.

45 American Psychological Association. *Diagnostic and Statistical Manual-IV.* Washington, DC American Psychological Association; 2002.

46 American Psychological Association. *Diagnostic and Statistical Manual-V.* Washington, DC American Psychological Association; 2013.

47 IsHak WW, Tobia G. DSM-5 Changes in diagnostic criteria of sexual dysfunctions. *Reprod Sys Sexual Disorders.* 2013;2(122). doi: 10.4172/2161-038X.1000122.

48 Sungur MZ, Gunduz A. A comparison of DSM-IV-TR and DSM-5 definitions for sexual dysfunctions: critiques and challenges. *J Sex Med.* 2014;11(2):364–373.

49 Vieira-Baptista P, Lima-Silva J. Is the DSM-V leading to the nondiagnosis of vulvodynia? *J Low Genit Tract Dis.* 2016;20(4):354–355.

50 Harlow BL, Stewart EG. A population-based assessment of chronic unexplained vulvar pain: have we underestimated the prevalence of vulvodynia? *J Am Med Womens Assoc.* 2003;58(2):82–88.

51 Reed BD, *et al.* Vulvodynia incidence and remission rates among adult women: a 2-year follow-up study. *Obstet Gynecol.* 2008;112(2 Pt 1):231–237.

52 Harlow BL, *et al.* Prevalence of symptoms consistent with a diagnosis of vulvodynia: population-based estimates from 2 geographic regions. *Am J Obstet Gynecol.* 2014;210(1):40 e1–e8.

53 Pukall CF, *et al.* Recommendations for self-report outcome measures in vulvodynia clinical trials. *Clin J Pain.* 2017;33(8):756–765.

54 Herbenick D, *et al.* Pain experienced during vaginal and anal intercourse with other-sex partners: findings from a

nationally representative probability study in the United States. *J Sex Med.* 2015;12(4):1040–1051.

55 Xie Y, *et al.* Economic burden and quality of life of vulvodynia in the United States. *Curr Med Res Opin.* 2012;28(4): 601–608.

56 Schmidt S, *et al.* Vulvar pain. Psychological profiles and treatment responses. *J Reprod Med.* 2001;46(4):377–384.

57 Ponte M, *et al.* Effects of vulvodynia on quality of life. *J Am Acad Dermatol.* 2009;60(1):70–76.

58 Danby CS, Margesson LJ. Approach to the diagnosis and treatment of vulvar pain. *Dermatol Ther.* 2010;23(5):485–504.

59 LePage K, Selk A. What do patients want? A needs assessment of vulvodynia patients attending a vulvar diseases clinic. *Sex Med.* 2016;4(4):e242–e248.

19

# Anatomy and Physiology of Sexual Pain

*Melissa A. Farmer*

## Abstract

Efficient clinical assessment, diagnosis, and treatment of women with sexual pain requires a comprehensive knowledge of the physiological systems underlying acute and chronic nociception. Whereas acute episodes of sexual pain are mediated by end-organ pathology, persistent sexual pain must be conceptualized in terms of ongoing peripheral, spinal, and brain mechanisms that can lead to dramatic functional changes in nociception and enhanced pain perception. This state-of-the-art review draws from rigorous rodent and human research to explore potential mechanisms underlying the symptom configurations associated with sexual pain. A strong understanding of these mechanisms is essential for the assessment and strategic treatment of women who present with unremitting sexual pain.

**Keywords:** *sexual pain; physiology; anatomy; pelvic; nociception; mechanisms; sensitization; referred pain; chronic*

---

The initiation and maintenance of chronic pain reflects a combination of peripheral, spinal, and brain mechanisms.

Pain assessments based on symptom configurations, rather than existing diagnostic categories, are useful in deciphering mechanisms of referred pain.

Visceral nociceptors are poised to hijack cutaneous nociceptive circuits through spinally-mediated cross-talk.

---

## Introduction

Pain and nociception are indispensable contributors to female sexual function. Nociception refers to the physiological processes that mediate detection of environmental threats and the relay of this information through the peripheral and central nervous systems. In contrast, pain is the cortically mediated subjective experience that can emerge when nociceptive signals are integrated into the neural networks underlying consciousness. Therefore, nociception may not lead to pain perception, and pain perception is not solely dependent on nociceptive input.

Just as a woman's subjective experience of desire and arousal are central to the study of female sexual function, pain perception also guides our understanding of pain physiology. This chapter reviews the mechanisms of the acute and chronic pain physiology of genito-pelvic pain. Acute genito-pelvic pain arises from trauma, inflammation, or infection and usually resolves as tissue heals. Given that chronic pain persists beyond the normal healing period, by definition the mechanisms underlying chronic pain maintenance are

*Textbook of Female Sexual Function and Dysfunction: Diagnosis and Treatment*, First Edition. Edited by Irwin Goldstein, Anita H. Clayton, Andrew T. Goldstein, Noel N. Kim, and Sheryl A. Kingsberg.
© 2018 John Wiley & Sons Ltd. Published 2018 by John Wiley & Sons Ltd.

independent of acute tissue pathology. Therefore, the assessment and treatment of genito-pelvic pain requires an understanding of the "rules" of nociception in the periphery, spine, and brain and how these rules are violated in chronic pain states across time.

## Nociceptor Structure and Function

Across species, the close correspondence between sensory neuron firing properties and magnitude of pain perception indicates that general properties of neuronal function can be deduced from subjective pain perception [1, 2]. Nociceptors are free nerve endings that detect noxious or potentially harmful mechanical, thermal, chemical, and electrical stimuli that are usually perceived as painful. Their cell bodies are located in the dorsal root ganglion, with one peripheral process extending to the target tissue and one process terminating in the ipsilateral dorsal horn of the spinal cord. All nociceptors release the excitatory neurotransmitter glutamate and can be distinguished according to five structural and functional criteria that facilitate encoding of a broad variety of sensory stimuli: (i) nerve diameter (which determines conduction velocity and response latency) and the presence of myelination, (ii) stimulus modality (i.e. mechanical, thermal, and/or chemical input), (iii) functional response characteristics (rate of neuronal firing, threshold of activation, adaptation profile), (iv) receptor expression modulating these response properties, and (v) functional properties unique to somatic or visceral nociceptors [3, 4]. These criteria are not absolute, as new subpopulations of nociceptors will inevitably be identified in the coming decades. Nociceptive signals are transmitted by Aδ and C nerve fibers that detect either a single sensory modality (unimodal) or two or more sensory modalities (polymodal) (Table 19.1). Large, myelinated Aδ fibers rapidly conduct mechanical, thermal, and/or cold nociceptive signals (at rates

of 5–30 m/s), terminate in superficial lamina I and deep lamina V of the dorsal horn, and lead to the immediate perception of sharp pain. In contrast, unmyelinated C fibers transmit mechanical, thermal, and/or chemical nociceptive information more slowly (at rates of 0.5–2 m/s) and terminate in laminae I and $II_{outer}$ of the dorsal horn, yielding a gradual pain perception of dull or burning pain. More fine-grained nociception is achieved with specialized receptor proteins and ion channels located on nerve endings. These receptors and channels mediate (i) the transduction, or conversion, of a sensory stimulus into an electrical signal and (ii) the encoding, or one-to-one correspondence, of electrical signals to stimulus attributes that the brain can interpret (e.g. modality, location, threshold, intensity, timing). For instance, increased stimulus intensity is encoded by an increased rate of neuronal firing, and the timing of neuronal firing encodes stimulus duration. Collectively, the interface between a sensory stimulus and these functional properties of nociceptors contribute to complex sensory perceptions, such as pain.

Detection of mechanical stimulation is central to sexual arousal because sexual activity involves skin-on-skin contact, including manual, oral, and/or genital stimulation of oneself and/or one's partner. Gentle mechanical pressure is encoded by Aβ mechanoreceptors (including Merkel cells, Pacinian, Ruffini, and Meissner's corpuscles) that terminate in laminae $II_{inner}$, III, and IV of the dorsal horn, and by a non-nociceptive population of C fibers that mediates pleasant touch, mild heat analgesia, and potentially erotic touch [5, 6]. Recently described Piezo receptors encode more nuanced gradations of mechanical pressure and stretch, including stretch in urothelial cells (*piezo1*) and intraluminal pressure and fullness (*piezo2*) [7]. In particular, piezo2 will play an important role in our future understanding of genito-pelvic pain thresholds. Piezo2 expression mediates reduced pain thresholds (*mechanical allodynia*), is required for Merkel cell mechanosensitivity, and leads to activation of

**Table 19.1** Structure and function of peripheral sensory afferent neurons mediating genito-pelvic sensation and pain.

| Neuron structure | Cutaneous nerve | Muscle nerve | Fiber diameter (μm) | Conduction velocity (ms) |
|---|---|---|---|---|
| *Myelinated* | | | | |
| Large diameter | Aα | I | 13–20 | 80–120 |
| Small diameter | Aβ | II | 6–12 | 35–75 |
| Smallest diameter | Aδ | III | 1–5 | 6–25 |
| | Unimodal | Mechanical nociceptors | | |
| | Unimodal | Thermal nociceptors | | |
| | Polymodal | Mechano-heat nociceptors | | |
| *Unmyelinated* | C | IV | 0.2–1.5 | 0.5–2 |
| *Also warm temperature and itch | Unimodal | Thermal nociceptors | | |
| | Unimodal | Mechano-heat nociceptors | | |
| | Polymodal | Mechano-heat/chemical/cold nociceptors | | |
| | | Quickly adapting → sensitive to heat and mechanical stimulus under basal conditions | | |
| | | Slowly adapting → exhibits temperature-dependent sensitization, reduced heat detection threshold, greater heat hyperalgesia | | |

Aβ nerve fibers, which can acquire nociceptor characteristics in certain pathological states discussed later in this chapter [8].

Most noxious stimuli also involve some degree of mechanical stimulation. The transition from nonpainful to painful mechanical pressure (i.e. pain threshold) is encoded by the $P2X_3$ subclass of purinoreceptors. $P2X_3$ activation provokes the rapid release and detection of adenosine triphosphate to generate a rapid and time-limited inflammatory response [9]. $P2X_3$ expression is inhibited by estrogen receptor-α binding on C-fiber nociceptors (mediated by signaling pathways dependent on cyclic adenosine monophosphate, protein kinase A, and extracellular signal-regulated protein kinases 1 and 2 interactions), which strongly suggests that estrogen–$P2X_3$ interactions modulate nociceptive signaling via immune mechanisms. Reduced mechanical pain thresholds may reflect inadequate estrogen receptor-α regulation of $P2X_3$, leading to $P2X_3$ overexpression [10, 11]. This hypothesis is indirectly supported by data in postmenopausal women and rodents showing that tissue depletion of estrogen is associated with mechanical allodynia [12, 13]. Similarly, vulvar punch biopsies from women with provoked vestibulodynia exhibit dramatic reductions in estrogen receptor-α expression [14]. $P2X_3$ participates in the amplification of persistent pain signals at the peripheral and spinal levels. For instance, increased bladder urothelial $P2X_3$ expression in women with interstitial cystitis/bladder pain syndrome may implicate the presence of altered lumbosacral $P2X_3$ response properties observed in rodent models of bladder inflammation [15, 16]. These data also raise the possibility that aversive feelings of fullness and mechanical allodynia reported by women with persistent genital arousal disorder could, in part, reflect a basal state of $P2X_3$ disinhibition [17].

$P2X_3$ frequently colocalizes with the capsaicin receptor (i.e. the transient receptor potential cation channel subfamily V member 1 receptor, previously the vanilloid 1 receptor), which is a cation channel receptor located on polymodal C fiber nociceptors in skin and, especially, visceral organs. Under normal physiological conditions, the capsaicin receptor activates with noxious thermal ($>43\,°C$), chemical, and acidic stimuli (pH < 5) and facilitates the perception of burning heat pain [18]. Women with provoked vestibulodynia exhibit increased capsaicin receptor expression in subepidermal vulvar nerves, which implicates a greater capacity to detect noxious vulvar stimulation [19]. Capsaicin receptor expression in keratinocytes may also contribute to nociceptive signaling [20]. Capsaicin receptors exhibit a range of unique functions that can contribute to symptom variability in genitopelvic pain. Under acidic conditions capsaicin receptors activate at room temperature ($20–25\,°C$), which would allow these receptors in acidic vulvar tissue (pH 3.8–4.5) to transmit burning heat sensations in the absence of high temperatures. Sustained activation of these receptors with topical capsaicin promotes a calcium-dependent decrease in channel activity that prevents nerve firing for an extended period [21]. This desensitization mechanism may explain the treatment of vulvar pain with topical capsaicin, and brief trials combining capsaicin and lidocaine (for comfort) can be used to assess the degree of peripheral nerve contributions to vulvar pain [22]. Capsaicin receptors can sensitize the activity of neighboring receptors, like $P2X_3$, and provide a feasible mechanism for mechanical pressure-induced sensations of burning pain. Note that this phenomenon does not require nerve injury – it represents a phenotypic shift in how sensory input is detected [21]. Collectively, these data suggest that nociceptors encoding both mechanical and heat pain are functionally poised to play major roles in genito-pelvic pain. Use of $P2X_3$ antagonists, capsaicin receptor antagonists or extended treatment with agonists (e.g. topical capsaicin) to induce depolarization blockade, and/or estrogen receptor-α agonists may prove fruitful in managing pain.

The actions of receptors may differ between basal, inflammatory, and neuropathic states. For instance, acute inflammation is characterized by thermal hyperalgesia that is dependent on capsaicin receptor expression and mechanical hyperalgesia that relies on expression of transient receptor potential ankyrin 1 [18]. Blockade of transient receptor potential ankyrin 1 normalizes mechanical sensitivity without affecting inflammation or capsaicin receptor expression. Receptors that express transient receptor potential cation channel subfamily V member 4 encode innocuous warmth in basal conditions and mediate inflammation-induced visceral mechanical sensitivity. Notably, these three receptors, in variable combinations, are expressed by most abomino-pelvic visceral afferents.

## Hormonal Regulation

Estrogen is implicated in sensation and nociception at the peripheral, spinal, and supraspinal levels. In the brain, estrogen promotes endogenous opioid analgesia and spinal inhibition of pain, yet it also facilitates hippocampal capsaicin receptor-mediated pain hypersensitivity. [23–25]. Spinal estrogenic regulation of μ- and/or κ-opioid heterodimer expression is critical for a female-specific neural pathway for opioid analgesia [26–28]. Estrogen receptors are present in lumbosacral dorsal root ganglia and on peripheral terminals of putative nociceptors, with estrogen receptor-α expressed in the vulva, vagina, uterus, bladder, and ovaries, and estrogen receptor-β intensely expressed in the ovaries [29, 30]. Both receptors are distributed throughout the vaginal epithelium, labia minora epidermis, and vaginal smooth muscle [31]. In the periphery, rapid 17β-estradiol signaling of membrane-bound estrogen receptors -α and -β plays a key role in regulating mechanical nociception [9]. For example, $P2X_3$-dependent painful bladder distension is inhibited by estrogen receptor-$\alpha$ binding, and ovariectomy increases bladder $P2X_3$ receptor expression by 300% [32, 33]. The respective roles of estrogen receptors -$\alpha$ and -$\beta$ remain poorly understood and their functions vary based on site(s) of action (peripheral or central), levels of bioavailable sex steroid hormones in local tissue and in free circulation, presence of inflammation or disease, states of hormone depletion (e.g. oophorectomy, menopause, lactational amenorrhea, etc.), and physiological adaptations resulting from long-term supplementation (e.g. oral contraceptive use).

It is feasible that nociceptor signaling could qualitatively differ across the cycle as hormones fluctuate. During pre-ovulatory periods of high circulating estrogen, enhanced structural integrity of tissue and estrogenic inhibition of $P2X_3$ may allow genital tissue to withstand the physically rigorous act of intercourse. In contrast, depletion of female gonadal hormones in rodents induces mechanical and thermal pain hypersensitivity that parallels a three-fold increase of $P2X_3$ receptor expression in the dorsal root ganglion [13, 34, 35]. Restoration of sexual function with combination oral/topical estrogen treatment in hormonally deficient women may, therefore, reflect improved physical integrity of the vaginal epithelium and normalized mechanical pain thresholds [36–39]. Given the pivotal role of estrogen in bladder and uterine visceral nociception, it likely plays an important role in referred and comorbid pelvic pain [40, 41].

The long-term consequences of oral contraceptive use on genito-pelvic pain remain poorly understood. On the one hand, estrogen-dependent conditions like endometriosis can benefit from oral contraceptive and aromatase inhibitor use [42]. In contrast, extended use of oral contraceptives, especially low-estrogen formulations, may confer greater risk for developing provoked vestibulodynia [43, 44]. Chronic use of oral contraceptives reduces sex steroid hormones and may lead to insufficient estrogen receptor-$\alpha$ binding of $P2X_3$ receptors, yielding lower pressure and/or distension pain thresholds.

Notably, vulvar vestibule expression of estrogen receptor-$\beta$, the receptor subtype associated with increased nociceptive action, is upregulated in women taking oral contraceptives, a population that exhibits lower mechanical pain thresholds than naturally cycling women [45–47]. Pain hypersensitivity could develop with long-term alterations in estrogen and/or progesterone levels by promoting *de novo* nerve sprouting and hyperinnervation [48–50]. However, oral contraceptive use alone may not be sufficient to enhance the risk of developing chronic vulvar pain. A subgroup of women with low basal androgen receptor transcriptional function and low free testosterone levels may have a greater risk for developing provoked vestibulodynia [51, 52]. These data reinforce that acute and adaptive effects of sex steroid hormones on nociception are mechanistically distinct and clinically relevant.

## Somatic and Visceral Pain

Nociceptors exhibit unique functional properties based on the tissue type in which they are embedded (Figure 19.1). "Somatic" nociceptors innervate skin, muscle, and bone and contribute to pain perception that closely correlates with stimulus intensity, duration, and location, and it has distinctive qualities ("sharp", "pinching", etc.). Tissue depth can impact the spatial perception of somatic pain: for instance, deep muscle pain may be perceived across the length of the muscle. In contrast, "visceral" pain caused by hollow organ distension and traction is perceived along the midline of the body as diffuse discomfort that may lag seconds or minutes behind noxious stimulation. Visceral sensations include nausea, bladder and stomach filling, distension (vaginal, rectal, intestinal, esophageal), menstrual cramps, and bloating, but many visceral experiences lack an

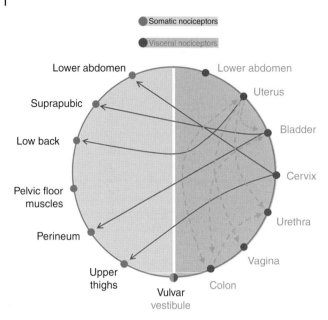

**Figure 19.1** A circle graph depicts pain referral patterns between 14 anatomically-distinct body locations that exhibit spinal "cross-talk." Depicted body regions are innervated by either somatic nociceptors (left, in blue) or visceral nociceptors (right, in red). The lines connecting body locations represent either (a) viscero–visceral (organ to organ) interactions, indicated in with grey dashed lines, or (b) viscero–somatic (organ to muscle/skin) interactions, indicated with solid red lines. Methods of data collection include electrophysiology, animal behavior with symptom comodulation, and quantitative sensory testing techniques in women. Note that additional pain referral patterns between structures on this circle graph almost certainly exist, but are not supported by current research.

adequate vocabulary (e.g. the sensations associated with catheter insertion, venous cannulation, or having food lodged in one's throat). The body must be able to tolerate some physiological discomfort associated with normal functions (e.g. with bowel or bladder distension). The viscera are, therefore, exclusively innervated with both high threshold nociceptors that transmit innocuous and noxious input and with intensity-encoding nociceptors, which allows visceral pain to emerge only with prolonged and/or intense noxious stimulation [53]. Moreover, high threshold nociceptors can create a time delay between visceral stimulation and its subjective perception (refer to Table 19.2).

The lower third of the female genital tract, including the vulva, urethra, and proximal vagina, receives a combination of both somatic and visceral innervation [54]. As a result, conditions like provoked vestibulodynia may be characterized by complex nociceptive signaling. Dynamic modeling has revealed that vulvar pain perception closely corresponds with the quality and time course of vulvar punctate pressure, whereas the delayed onset of distension-induced vulvovaginal pain is consistent with visceral transduction [55]. These findings imply that

genital quantitative sensory testing research that uses somatic tissue (e.g. volar forearm) as a "control" for lower genital tract sensitivity may be comparing fundamentally different types of pain [56]. The significant anatomical variability in vulvovaginal shape and size may also facilitate visceral pain through simple mechanical traction. Genital sensitivity testing should always be validated against clinical pain reports because different tissues may exhibit variable degrees of hypersensitivity [57].

## Referred Pain

Referred pain is one of the least appreciated mechanisms underlying genito-pelvic pain and other comorbid pain syndromes. Referred pain is a regular feature of visceral pain and can also account for many seemingly enigmatic pain symptoms [58]. Three major hypotheses should be considered when a woman reports pain in a specific location: (i) her pain is caused by tissue pathology in target tissue, (ii) pain is referred from another site exhibiting tissue pathology, and/or (iii) pain is cortically mediated as a sensory memory. In practice, genito-pelvic

**Table 19.2** Symptom patterns and mechanisms underlying different types of pain.

| Types of Pain / Adaptive function(s) | | Mechanisms | | |
| --- | --- | --- | --- | --- |
| | | Acute triggers | Pain maintenance | Symptoms |
| **Nociceptive**<br>Signals potential for tissue injury | **Somatic** | Detection of noxious stimuli at skin, muscle and bone | Requires continued presence of noxious stimulus | Transient pain (seconds to minutes) |
| | **Visceral** | Intense or prolonged organ distension or pressure | Requires continued presence of noxious stimulus | Transient pain (seconds to hours) |
| **Inflammatory**<br>Eliminates cause of injury and repairs tissue | | Pro-inflammatory cascades in response to tissue injury, detection of pathogens, radiation | Peripheral nerve sensitization, repeated inflammatory insults (e.g. infections); occult inflammation (e.g. mast cell proliferation) | Tissue hypersensitivity (days – weeks), edema, redness, itch |
| **Functional**<br>Limits physical activity and promotes fear learning of illness-related pain cues | | Sexual activity, dietary triggers, severe or recurrent infections, nervous system priming by early adverse events | Increased excitability of nociceptors and/or dorsal horn interneurons, referred pain and/or organ cross-sensitization | Pain with intercourse, bladder filling or voiding, digestion, defecation, secondary pelvic floor muscle dysfunction |
| **Neuropathic**<br>No adaptive function | | Presumed nerve injury or nerve compression | May include increased excitability of nociceptors and/or dorsal horn neurons | Gain of function (spontaneous burning or electric shock-like pain, dysesthesia) and/or loss of function (numbness, tingling, "pins and needles") |

pain rarely fits neatly into existing diagnostic categories, which is not surprising given that vulvodynia, bladder pain syndrome/interstitial cystitis, dysmenorrhea, pelvic girdle pain, and debatably (painful) endometriosis are diagnoses of exclusion. Therefore, pain assessments based on symptom configurations, rather than existing diagnostic categories, are useful in deciphering mechanisms of referred pain.

Somatic afferent fibers account for 90% of nerves that terminate in the spinal cord, while the remaining 7–10% are visceral afferent fibers that may synapse at, above, or below their originating dermatome (or even on the contralateral side of the spinal cord) [54, 59]. Visceral nociceptors synapse onto dorsal horn interneurons in laminae I, II, and V that also receive somatic terminations, and the resulting nociceptive signals – regardless of their tissues of origin – are then transmitted along specialized ventro-lateral funiculus projections to the brain. With intense noxious stimulation, the visceral–somatic convergence of nociceptors onto common interneurons allows neural discharges from one afferent to influence the electrical activity of another and to sensitize their shared interneuron [54]. Visceral nociceptors are, therefore, poised to hijack cutaneous nociceptive circuits.

This neuronal "cross-talk" establishes three types of functional interactions between the participating afferent fibers, including viscero–visceral (organ to organ), viscero–somatic (organ to muscle/skin), or somato–visceral (muscle/skin to organ) interactions (Figure 19.2). Rodent data have confirmed the functional convergence of abdominal and pelvic visceral organs in 13–60% of lumbosacral dorsal horn neurons, with variation observed between spinal segments [60]. Importantly, referred pain can manifest in neighboring dermatomes due to the broad arborization of visceral afferents onto multiple spinal cord segments [61, 62]. Classic accounts of visceral pain focused on referral between body sites with common embryological origins (e.g. tissue derived from the

urogenital sinus, including vulvar vestibule, bladder, urethra, umbilicus, and prostate); however, pain referral regularly deviates from such patterns. Clinical signs of pain referral from viscera to somatic tissue include cutaneous and deep muscle hyperalgesia (but not altered detection thresholds), which emerges over minutes to hours and may outlast the original visceral pain [63]. Referred visceral pain can generate one or more regions of referral to somatic tissue (e.g. referred uterine pain that is experienced in the lower back), or it can manifest as a radiating, burning, aching, prickling, and/or electrical shock-like pain that moves throughout the pelvic cradle, which is reminiscent of neuropathic pain features [64, 65]. Therefore, referred pain is an umbrella term that can indicate: (i) pain referred from a visceral structure to muscle, with no muscle hyperalgesia; (ii) pain referred from a visceral structure to muscle, resulting in muscle hyperalgesia; and (iii) expansion of referred hyperalgesia following intense and/or persistent nociceptive input and/or presence of co-occurring visceral pain conditions. Accordingly, more frequent visceral pain episodes are associated with greater pain threshold reductions at sites of pain referral [64]. Similarly, presence of comorbid chronic visceral pain conditions may promote increased intensity and greater spatial spread of referred hyperalgesia [66].

Referred deep muscle hyperalgesia in the pelvic floor musculature may contribute to diffuse pain sensations, given that muscle pain can be perceived along the length of the muscle. [67]. It is hypothesized that this hyperalgesia results from a viscero–muscular reflex that induces painful muscle contractions that can ultimately become maintained independent of the original visceral input. Muscle hyperalgesia referred from the viscera can, in turn, cause secondary referred pain across multiple dermatomes and promote a broad spectrum of extra-pelvic pain symptoms that are not due to sensitization, *per se*. It is plausible that localized muscle pain, or "trigger points" are the product of visceral

(a) Visceral pain referred to somatic and visceral tissue

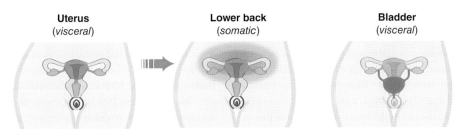

(b) Somatic/visceral pain referred to visceral tissue

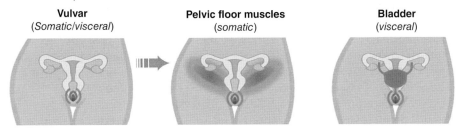

**Figure 19.2** Hypothetical referred pelvic pain patterns supported by the clinical literature that are suggestive of spinal cross-talk between visceral and somatic nociceptors. (a) Based on the clinical co-occurrence of uterine cramps and low back pain, this schematic depicts visceral pain originating in the uterus (far left) as a potential cause of somatic pain referred to muscles in the lower back (viscero–somatic referred pain, middle). Alternatively, uterine pain could also refer to a visceral structure like the bladder (viscero–visceral referred pain, far right) to create more diffuse pelvic pain. (b) Given the co-occurrence of pelvic floor muscle dysfunction/pain and chronic vulvar pain, this schematic depicts somatic–visceral pain originating at the vulvar vestibule (far left, due to dual innervation of the lower one-third of the female reproductive tract) as a potential cause of somatic pain referred to pelvic floor muscles (somato-/viscero–somatic referred pain, middle). In contrast, vulvar pain referral to the bladder has been described and is supported by high clinical comorbidity between chronic vulvar and bladder pain (somato-/viscero–visceral referred pain, far right). Both clinical presentations (a) and (b) would likely include both localized and diffuse pelvic pain. Note that referred pain is a normal feature of visceral pain and the interactions shown here are not "pathological" if the referred pain resolves in a timely manner.

pain referral, rather than primary dysfunctions. Care should be taken to parse referred muscle pain from reactive muscle tension, which is a natural defensive response to pain, and from the muscle tension and pain that emerge as the body attempts to compensate for functional deficits caused by genito-pelvic pain. Pelvic floor physical therapists have the ideal education and training to help disentangle the causes and consequences of referred genito-pelvic pain within a larger biopsychosocial framework [68].

Spinally mediated cross-talk can intensify or strategically alleviate pain symptoms. Viscero–visceral hyperalgesia caused by cross-organ sensitization in animals and humans confirms that referral can mutually

influence pain generated at either site [69]. Accordingly, the successful treatment of pain originating in one visceral organ can partially alleviate pain symptoms associated with other organs sharing overlapping innervation [69]. Pain referral is ultimately dependent on continued nociceptive input and its spinal mediation; as a result, anesthetic blocks at the site of pain referral provide only partial relief [70, 71].

## Vascular Pain

The discrepancy between pain perception and degree of arterio-venous pathology is a classic feature of visceral pain [54]. In general, vascular pain arises either from inadequate or excessive blood flow to a body region. Circulation is impaired when tissue, muscles, and tendons are deprived of oxygen or constricted by edema leading to elevated internal venous pressure. Visceral vasculature can also be compressed by surrounding muscle and fascia, depending on regional differences in pelvic floor muscle architecture. For example, shorter coccygeus muscle fibers can generate greater force than longer pubovisceral muscle fibers [67]. The generated biomechanical forces result in stretch, compression, shear, or injury of vasculature that contribute to pelvic pain through local inflammation and/or direct nerve compression. The resilience of vasculature is compromised by estrogen-mediated signaling cascades that promote vasodilation, compromise vascular smooth muscle contraction, alter vascular remodeling, and weaken venous walls.

Acute venous dilation is rarely painful, yet chronic venous reflux is considered a diagnostic indicator of pelvic congestion syndrome, a symptom complex characterized by aching, burning pain with muscle exertion (e.g. claudication) that radiates from the buttocks to feet, as well as neuropathic symptoms like numbness, paresthesia. Pelvic congestion syndrome is characterized by venous insufficiency, as corroborated by evidence of pelvic, abdominal, and thigh varicose veins. However, pelvic venous dilation and compromised venous integrity are also present in many healthy women who do not have these symptoms [72]. Again, this is not surprising given that superficial and deep venous reflux are not correlated with pain perception.

## Inflammation

As a normal feature of female reproductive physiology, inflammation is not an inherently pathological process. Menstruation is thought to be initiated by progesterone withdrawal-induced pro-inflammatory responses [73].

The lower genital tract (vagina and vulva) exhibits ongoing low-grade inflammation, presumably as a defense against pathogens introduced with invasive sexual contact or migrated from nearby body sites (e.g. anorectal bacteria) [74–76]. The degree of inflammation can vary based on a woman's vaginal and bladder flora (which changes across the menstrual cycle), presence of injury (e.g. vaginal fissures), tissue-specific inflammatory profiles (e.g. upper versus lower genital tract), exposure to new immune threats (e.g. sexually transmitted infections), priming by past immune threats, host resilience to new immune threats, genetic polymorphisms that bias the inflammatory response, and interactions between these factors [56, 77–79]. Therefore, inflammation results from, mediates, and fine-tunes nociception to enhance the sensitivity and specificity of nociceptive signaling. The presence of inflammation may reflect immune responses to current as well as past immune threats. As a result, inflammation *per se* may be a poor indicator of underlying pain pathology. Given the complexity of this process, the dynamics of inflammation are discussed in relation to the pathogen–host interactions that may facilitate emergence of the most common cause of dyspareunia, provoked vestibulodynia.

The standard clinical assumption is that vestibulodynia pain arises from vulvar vestibular inflammation that is secondary to repeated exposure to biological or synthetic inflammagens (e.g. recurrent yeast infections), neuroproliferation, and hormonal antagonists (not mutually exclusive). Regarding the first hypothesis, nonautoimmune inflammation reflects an interaction between stimulus severity (e.g. a pathogen's virulence, pathogen load, frequency of repeated exposures, etc.) and host resilience (e.g. genetic and developmental influences, microbial abundance/richness, immune suppression, etc.). Although the detection of pathogenic viruses, yeast, and bacteria by epithelial toll-like receptors immediately triggers a nonspecific "innate" immune cascade [80], each of these pathogens in isolation may contribute to clinically relevant pain: repeated yeast exposures cause persistent vulvar pain, postviral neuropathic pain can last years beyond primary infections, and bacteria may modulate nociception [81–83]. Some of these microorganisms have even evolved unique adaptations to evade dominant immune responses in human hosts [84]. Therefore, inflammation *per se* may account for a limited degree of pain pathophysiology observed in women with genito-pelvic pain.

Recent evidence has revealed one innate immune pathway that may play a major role in the initiation and maintenance of provoked vestibulodynia in women with histories of recurrent vulvovaginal candidiasis. An experimental mouse model of chronic vulvar pain following recurrent Candida albicans infections provided causal evidence that prolonged yeast exposure can initiate persistent pain and vulvar hyperinnervation [82]. The role of yeast exposure in the maintenance of provoked vestibulodynia is supported by the differential cytokine expression induced by yeast-exposed fibroblasts isolated from vestibule versus nonvestibule punch biopsies in women with and without the condition [75]. In both groups, vestibule fibroblasts expressed more interleukin-6 and prostaglandin than nonvestibule fibroblasts. This cytokine expression is mitigated by blocking Dectin-1 gene expression and is almost abolished with inhibition of nuclear factor-$\kappa$B phosphorylation [85]. Estrogen receptor-$\alpha$ binding directly inhibits nuclear factor-$\kappa$B pathways, which suggests a critical role of estrogen in regulating nociception and related immune reactivity [86]. Note that yeast-induced nociception can sensitize nociceptive pathways that are ultimately independent of the presence or absence of yeast, and such mechanisms are difficult to study *in vitro*.

These studies highlight the importance of anatomical and genetic factors in provoked vestibulodynia, a pain condition that is frequently comorbid with pelvic, abdominal, and temporomandibular pain. The unique immune profile of the vulvar vestibule, a urogenital sinus-derived tissue, may be shared by tissues of common embryological origin (urethra, bladder, umbilicus) [87, 88]. These shared immunological abnormalities may, therefore, predispose women with vulvar pain to develop comorbid bladder and/or urethral pain, a diagnostic overlap that is consistently observed in the literature [89]. Moreover, women with provoked vestibulodynia are 2.5 times as likely to exhibit loss-of-function melanocortin-1 receptor polymorphisms that may interfere with the downregulation of pro-inflammatory cytokines and adhesion molecules generated by the nuclear factor-$\kappa$B pathway [90, 91]. This polymorphism may impact a broad range of pain mechanisms because the melanocortin-1 receptor mediates $\kappa$-opioid analgesia in women, modulates $\mu$-opioid analgesia, and pain thresholds in women [92–95]. Indeed, most of the genetic polymorphisms identified in genito-pelvic pain populations appear to impact inflammatory cascades, host–pathogen interactions, and pain sensitivity [88].

The body cannot afford to sustain a biologically expensive response like inflammation indefinitely because these resources must be available to defend against new threats. Inflammation promotes physiological adaptations that maintain efficient nociceptive signaling as chronic pain persists, and these adaptive solutions will change over time. Sensory neurons are the only afferents that can regenerate in mammals, and *de novo* nerve sprouting is a well-documented consequence of chronic pain pathology observed with frank tissue injury, skin scratching, infection, and even radiation in rodent models [82, 96, 97]. Indeed, women with provoked vestibulodynia exhibit increased density of vulvar calcitonin gene-related peptide expressing C fiber nociceptors and area vulvar vestibular nerve fibers, compared to healthy controls [98, 99]. Therefore, vulvar neuroproliferation may in some cases evolve as a long-term consequence of inflammation. A pervasive bias continues to influence the field's understanding of inflammation and is based on the expectation that chronic inflammation will resemble the acute inflammatory state. Instead, one of the most common findings across pelvic pain populations is evidence of increased mast cell count and/or mast cell degranulation [100–103].

## Peripheral and Central Sensitization

The term "sensitization" is not in itself mechanistically useful because amplified nociceptive signaling can be sustained by the nociceptor that detects noxious input, and/or the spinal cord interneurons that relay these signals, and/or the brain that interprets and learns from these signals. However, this concept can be used to better interpret configurations of pain symptoms (Figure 19.3).

Repeated noxious stimulation can enhance the firing properties of C fiber nociceptors in a process called peripheral sensitization [65, 104]. Peripheral sensitization is defined by the following five functional changes in nociceptors: (i) reduced activation thresholds due to changes in membrane potentials, (ii) enhanced magnitude of signaling, (iii) generation of spontaneous signaling with no stimulus (i.e. ectopic discharges), (iv) enhanced magnitude of signaling with repeated stimulation (wind-up), and (v) recruitment of "silent nociceptors", which are previously non-nociceptive Aβ afferents that switch phenotypes to become nociceptors [105]. Inflammation is the most common cause of peripheral sensitization and it is a normal physiological process from which our

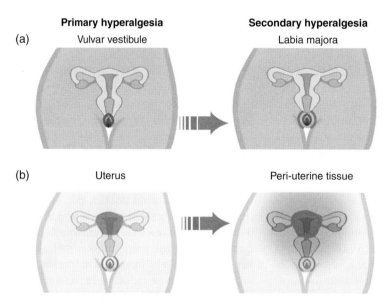

**Figure 19.3** Spatial characteristics of primary and secondary hyperalgesia (enhanced pain sensitivity) that would be expected with injury/inflammation at the (a) vulvar vestibule or (b) uterus. Primary hyperalgesia occurs at the site of injury as a natural consequence of peripheral nociceptor sensitization. These nociceptors may trigger spinal cord central sensitization of dorsal horn interneurons, which generates a region of secondary hyperalgesia that surrounds the region of primary hyperalgesia (injury/inflammatory site) that is only hypersensitive to noxious mechanical stimulation. This phenomenon can account for mechanical hyperalgesia in vulvar tissue surrounding the vulvar vestibule in women with provoked vestibulodynia (a). A parallel (and hypothetical) example is provided for primary hyperalgesia originating with uterine injury/inflammation (b). In this example, secondary hyperalgesia in surrounding uterine tissue may not be perceived as a distinct pain because both sites of visceral hyperalgesia produce similar diffuse sensations of pain. Note that central sensitization is a normal (albeit time-limited) consequence of strong inflammatory pain and the interactions shown here are not "pathological" if the secondary hyperalgesia resolves in a timely manner and the primary hyperalgesia dissipates soon thereafter.

bodies usually recover. It can generate clinical symptoms like mechanical and heat allodynia and hyperalgesia at the site of injury, without the independent participation of spinal cord interneurons.

Central sensitization is a powerful idea, as it provides a physiological mechanism for sustained pain in the absence of the precipitating stimulus. Prolonged activation of peripheral nociceptors can trigger enhanced activity of spinal cord cephalad projecting neurons in proportion to intensity, repetition, and duration of the nociceptive input [106]. Symptoms consistent with central sensitization include touch but not thermal hypersensitivity around the perimeter of the primary injury. This may include increased punctate pain sensitivity (*hyperalgesia*) mediated by A δ fibers, pain with moving tactile pressure (*dynamic tactile allodynia*) mediated by "silent nociceptors" (Aβ fibers), and pain sensations that persist long after vulvar or bladder stimulation has ceased [65]. Thermal hyperalgesia is rarely observed. When central sensitization and referred pain co-occur, secondary hyperalgesia may take a different form: silent nociceptors can mediate new regions of cutaneous or deep muscle hypersensitivity [64]. However, the most distinctive signature feature of central sensitization is the temporal dissociation between removal of the noxious stimulus and continued spinal interneuron firing that underlies pain after-sensations. This can be contrasted with the period of quiescence that separates the removal of a visceral stimulus and prolonged visceral pain. Mechanisms underlying central sensitization of visceral nociceptive signals remain poorly understood and may not follow the same "rules" as sensitization of somatic nociceptive signals.

Note that central sensitization may coexist with, but is not the same as, the following: (i) peripheral sensitization, (ii) "wind-up", which refers to the summation of excitatory input by a subset of hyperexcitable dorsal horn interneurons (without stimulus-response temporal dissociation), (iii) referred pain, (iv) neuropathic pain, which is caused by an identifiable lesion or disease of the somatosensory system, and (v) the hypothetical diagnoses of "central sensitivity" or "central sensitivity syndrome" [64, 65]. Similarly, symptoms like allodynia and hyperalgesia present with peripheral as well as central sensitization, and their relationship to other pain symptoms must be considered to decipher their underlying mechanisms [107].

Central sensitization shares key features with but is not synonymous with neuropathic pain. Although central sensitization is considered a key pathological process used to define the initiation of neuropathic pain, neuropathy encompasses a broader range of symptoms including spontaneous (unprovoked) fluctuations of burning or electrical shock-like pain. Neuropathic pain may include regional numbness or "pins and needles" sensations that indicate a loss of function; central sensitization exclusively reflects gain of function. Importantly, the maintenance of central sensitization, but not neuropathic pain, is dependent on continued provocation of peripheral nociceptors. However, it is possible for these processes to coexist in a woman with chronic genito-pelvic pain. To date, the presence of central sensitization in many types of genito-pelvic pain has not been supported by evidence due to confusion regarding its definition, variability between diagnoses, and methodological limitations [63, 108].

It is tempting to invoke central sensitization as a catch-all mechanism for unexplained clinical pelvic and nonpelvic pain. However, the mere presence of pain hypersensitivity is not evidence of this phenomenon [107]. It is a functional change unique to spinal cord interneurons that requires very specific conditions (moderate, repetitive noxious stimulation) to be maintained and rekindled; otherwise it will extinguish [109]. To date, no study has demonstrated a parallel phenomenon in cortical neurons, and therefore no empirical data supports the claims that maladaptive pain behaviors, catastrophization, or other psychological "amplifications" of pain are symptomatic of central sensitization. Similarly, the extrapolation of central sensitization to explain complex symptom patterns found in comorbid pain conditions is purely hypothetical at this point [65]. Worst case, the misuse of the term will promote the haphazard mixing and matching of heterogeneous chronic pain conditions in the absence of empirical or clinical data.

The spinal relay of nociceptive information to the brain is influenced by cortically-controlled descending pain modulation, which can be experimentally evaluated using conditioned pain modulation paradigms. Conditioned pain modulation is stable in healthy and chronic pain populations and may provide prognostic value; however, it has not been assessed in relation to clinical symptom change [110–112]. Two of three studies failed to identify abnormal spinal inhibition in vestibulodynia, as evidenced by intact diffuse noxious inhibitory control via conditioned pain modulation [113–115]. Indeed, symptoms like temporal summation suggests that spinally mediated facilitation (or gain) plays a more dominant role than descending inhibition. Conditioned pain modulation studies in other populations await replication.

## The Brain

Ultimately, pain perception is a cortically-mediated phenomenon. Therefore, all content discussed to this point – from the initial detection of sensory stimuli to the dynamic spinal relay of this information – culminates in a nociceptive signal that can be attended to, ignored, or even distorted by brain circuits. Although a thorough treatment of this topic cannot be achieved here, a brief review of the current state of pain neuroimaging is presented.

It was previously believed that the brain regions that mediate pain perception must represent a specialized neural network. This assumption was supported by many studies demonstrating that acute pain perception correlates with functional activation of the insula, anterior cingulate cortex, somatosen-sory cortices, prefrontal cortex, thalamus, brainstem, and other regions, and individual regions mediated distinct aspects of pain location, sensation, affect, intensity, and higher cognitive processing [116–119]. More recently, this interpretation has been questioned because the activation of brain regions originally associated with acute nociceptive processing are not specific to noxious stimulation and show limited overlap with neural "signatures" of chronic pain. Recent meta-analyses and large-scale studies have found that acute pain sensitivity has minimal prognostic value across chronic pain populations [120, 121]. Instead, more recent evidence suggests that mesocorticolimbic, rather than sensory encoding regions, mediate the transition to and maintenance of pain chronicity [122]. For instance, a longitudinal brain imaging study determined that the neural representation of spontaneous fluctuations of subacute low back pain shift from nociceptive to limbic regions as patients transitioned to chronicity [123]. These findings highlight the distinction between pain sensation and the long-term suffering it causes, given that both should ideally be targeted in pain management efforts.

Realistically, the transition from acute to chronic pain reflects three broad classes of mechanisms, including peripheral, spinal, and brain processes. The initiation and maintenance of chronic pain reflects a combination of these components that must evolve over time: spinal central sensitization will eventually extinguish without additional peripheral input, and it is not known whether additional insults (e.g. recurrent infections, pain flares) are sufficient to indefinitely sustain central sensitization [109, 124]. Likewise, initial formation of a strong emotional memory related to pain is naturally reinforced with continued exposure to the detrimental impact of chronic pain on mood, daily function, sexual relationships, and identity.

One of the most intriguing findings from the field of pain neuroimaging is that the degree of brain functional and structural reorganization can reflect clinically meaningful pain properties, such as subjective pain intensity, duration, and even emotional dimensions of pain. Whereas moment-to-moment changes in perception are reflected in brain functional properties, the longer-term consequences associated with chronic pain, such as symptom severity, correlate with neocortical gray matter (neuronal) density/volume and white matter (axonal) microstructure. This suggests that networks can manifest short- and long-term neuroplasticity by (i) adapting to brain state changes in order to optimize the representation of information, as well as (ii) evolving over time based on reinforced functional connections, which may in turn promote structural changes [125].

A final comment on the physiological substrates of pain perception: despite the clinical reliance on numerical rating scales, pain perception does not operate on an absolute scale. Pain is evaluated relative to the state that immediately preceded its onset and relative to predicted outcomes based on past experience [126]. A critical principle revealed by investigations of neural encoding of nociceptive input is that the experience of pain begins with pain anticipation. The dynamic nature of pain perception – including peripheral and central sensitization – is adaptive because it facilitates the accurate prediction and detection of future threats. Like somatic pain, fear is tightly coupled with a distinct threat that has a discrete beginning and end. Like visceral pain, anxiety is diffusely focused, without an identifiable threat to defend against (or with all threats being equally salient) and persists long after a significant threat has passed. The difference is that anxiety further distorts sensory and affective dimensions of potential threats (degree of threat, salience, context cues, and avoidance).

## Novel Future Directions

The temporal patterns of genito-pelvic pain may provide insight into the respective contributions of peripheral versus central nervous systems. Theoretically, more variability in pain perception – especially in response to environmental perturbation – may be indicative of a peripheral-dominant pain. In contrast, unprovoked pain with low variability is more consistent with centrally-mediated pain, potentially with intermittent peripheral nerve contributions. Importantly, genito-pelvic pain symptoms may reflect a combination of peripheral and central factors, thereby implying that concurrent treatment approaches targeting peripheral *and* central abnormalities may yield the greatest gains. The hypothesis that early and chronic genito-pelvic are maintained by distinct factors suggests the existence of (at least) two subtypes: the sub-clinical/early onset phenotype and the chronic phenotype. To date, the majority of genito-pelvic pain research has been conducted on the chronic phenotype based on etiological assumptions that preferentially reflect the early phenotype.

Visceral pain deserves special consideration here because it is not purely sensory in nature: it reflects (i) the diffuse sensations by which visceral nociception is currently defined; (ii) negative emotion; and (iii) increased sympathetic nervous system arousal [53, 54]. Targeting any combination of these dimensions can, in theory, diminish the subjective experience of visceral pain (Table 19.3). The co-occurrence of visceral discomfort with negative affect and sympathetic activation creates ideal physiological conditions for the consolidation and maintenance of robust emotional memories related to visceral pain [127–130].

## Summary

Genito-pelvic pain emerges from a series of dynamic interactions between molecular, cellular, systems, behavioral, and psychological factors. Nociceptive signals are functionally amplified by sensory afferent neurons that detect noxious stimuli, spatially generalized by spinal cross-talk, and temporally prolonged by spinal cord central sensitization.

**Table 19.3** Therapeutic mechanisms of action targeting nociception in genito-pelvic pain.

| Medications | Mechanism(s) of action | Pain indications |
|---|---|---|
| **Target: primary afferent excitability** | | |
| Capsaicin | • Hyperpolarization of capsaicin receptors with sustained use<br>• Possible inhibition of neighboring P2X$_3$ receptors | ○ Mechanical and thermal allodynia/hyperalgesia |
| Local anesthetics<br>*(lidocaine, lidocaine plaster, prilocaine, bupivacaine, mepivacaine)* | • Prevents neuronal firing by blocking voltage-gated sodium channels<br>• Possible desensitization of transient receptor potential ankyrin 1<br>• Reduced efficacy in inflamed tissue<br>• Reduced efficacy in nerve lesion pain, which alters functional properties of sodium channels Nav1.7 and Nav1.8 | ○ Cutaneous mechanical and heat hyperalgesia, including pain due to neuroproliferation<br>○ Can be used to assess contributions of cutaneous pain mechanisms<br>○ Nerve blocks may not alleviate referred pain |
| Corticosteroids<br>*(hydrocortisone, cortisone, prednisone, triamcinolone, betamethasone, dexamethasone)* | • Prevents formation of arachidonic acid by inhibiting phospholipase<br>• Limits degree of inflammation by curtailing lymphocyte migration and cytokine expression<br>• Inhibits delayed hypersensitivity reactions | ○ Inflammatory pain (may be limited to increased mast cells)<br>○ Pain associated with allergic reactions<br>○ Stop use if pain does not dissipate, as side effects with prolonged use can contribute to genito-pelvic pain |
| Topical estrogen<br>*(17β-estradiol, conjugated estrogens)* | • Increases epithelial thickness, elasticity and tissue integrity<br>• Improves vaginal lubrication<br>• Inhibits P2X$_3$ excitability through estrogen receptor-α binding on C-fiber nociceptors | ○ Pain onset associated with natural or pharmacologically-induced changes in estrogen levels<br>○ Lubrication reduces pain with traction |
| P2X$_3$ antagonists<br>*(AF-219)* | • Inhibits rapid inflammatory response induced by adenosine triphosphate | ○ Mechanical allodynia and hyperalgesia<br>○ Potentially "burning" pain induced by mechanical pressure |
| **Target: peripheral sensitization** | | |
| Nonsteroidal anti-inflammatories<br>*(ibuprofen, naproxen, aspirin)* | • Inhibits cyclooxygenase-1 and -2 activity<br>• Short-term reduction in inflammatory mediators, such prostaglandins | ○ Pain related to wounds (e.g. vulvar fissures)<br>○ Inflammatory pain |
| Reservatrol and salicylic acid | • Activates 5′ adenosine monophosphate-activated protein kinase<br>• Inhibits extracellular signal regulated kinase and mammalian target of rapamycin signaling pathways<br>• Reservatrol has poor bioavailability unless combined with salicylic acid | ○ Mechanical allodynia associated with interleukin-6 expression and primed hyper-responsivity to prostaglandin E2 |

**Target: spinal cord central sensitization**

| Medication | Mechanism | Indications/Notes |
|---|---|---|
| Gabapentinoids (*gabapentin, pregabalin*) | • Inhibits reuptake of γ-aminobutyric acid by modulating α-2-δ subunit voltage-dependent calcium channel activity in spine and brain<br>• Modulates spinal descending inhibition<br>• Inhibits primary afferent hyperactivity and ectopic activity in peripheral and wide dynamic range neurons<br>• Independent of endogenous opioid system | ○ Neuropathic pain<br>○ Mechanical allodynia, thermal hyperalgesia, cold hyperalgesia<br>○ Preoperative use to limit nociceptive sensitization in central nervous system |
| Other antiepileptic medications (*carbamazepine, benzodiazepines, topiramate*) | • Blocks potassium and voltage-gated sodium channels, yielding reduced glutamate and/or increased γ-aminobutyric acid activity<br>• Inhibits glutamate signaling<br>• Targets γ-aminobutyric acid receptors, transporters and/or enzymatic degradation | ○ Neuropathic pain |
| Tricyclic antidepressants (*amitriptyline, imipramine, nortriptyline, desipramine*) | • Blockade of voltage-gated sodium channels in periphery<br>• Blocks reuptake of serotonin and norepinephrine; dopamine to lesser extent<br>• Modulates endogenous opioid system<br>• Long-term: δ-opioid receptor modulation | ○ Neuropathic pain, including thermal and mechanical hyperalgesia<br>○ Potentially useful in pain due to central sensitization, through inhibition of N-methyl-D-aspartate-induced spinal hyperalgesia |
| Opioids (*codeine, hydrocodone, oxycodone, hydromorphone, oxymorphone, fentanyl, morphine*) | • Binds primarily to spinal μ-opioid receptors, with some δ- & κ-opioid receptor binding<br>• Duration of analgesia corresponds with duration of stable blood levels of medication<br>• Estrogen attenuates opioid receptor activity<br>• Sustained use suppresses hypothalamic-pituitary-gonadal axis<br>• Chronic use (>10years) increases nociception (poorly understood mechanisms) | ○ Alters subjective perception of pain severity and unpleasantness<br>○ Very effective for acute pain (e.g. postsurgical pain)<br>○ Preferred use after failed trials of other centrally-acting medications<br>○ Short-acting opioids used for intermittent "breakthrough" or "flare-like" pain<br>○ Physiological tolerance is expected and should not be confused with addiction |

**Target: emotional learning**

| Medication | Mechanism | Indications/Notes |
|---|---|---|
| d-Cycloserine | • Partial agonist at the glycine recognition site of the glutamatergic N-methyl-D-aspartate receptor that yields antagonist-like effects (50–300 mg) | ○ Thought to target fear memories at low doses when delivered 1 h prior to memory reactivation<br>○ With extended use (6–8 weeks), reduces neuropathic mechanical allodynia |
| Propranolol | • Blocks epinephrine and norepinephrine at β1- and β2-adrenergic receptors | ○ Reduces norepinephrine-induced strengthening of emotional (fear) memories when they are formed (consolidation) and revised (reconsolidation) |

Understanding the rules by which these nerves function – and especially how these rules are violated in the chronic pain state – is key in uncovering the mechanisms driving persistent genito-pelvic pain. Therefore, distinct sensory abnormalities can point to unique alterations in peripheral, spinal, and/or brain physiology that bias sensory perception.

Pain pathophysiology – caused by injury, infection, hormonal deficiency, pelvic floor dysfunction, or other insults – reflects the body's adaptations to a threat, not the original threat itself. Etiological factors are distinct from the physiological alterations that eventually become part of the disease of chronic pain over years and decades. The noble goal of identifying and treating suspected etiology (i.e. the acute phenotype) may ultimately detract from opportunities to target mechanisms of the chronic phenotypes of genito-pelvic pain.

## References

1 Gybels J, Handwerker HO, Van Hees J. A comparison between the discharges of human nociceptive nerve fibres and the subject's ratings of his sensations. *J Physiol.* 1979;292:193–206.

2 LaMotte RH, Thalhammer JG, Robinson CJ. Peripheral neural correlates of magnitude of cutaneous pain and hyperalgesia: a comparison of neural events in monkey with sensory judgments in human. *J Neurophysiol.* 1983;50(1):1–26.

3 Ringkamp M, Raja SN, Campbell JN, Meyer RA. Peripheral mechanisms of cutaneous nociception. In: McMahon SB, Koltzenberg M, Tracey I, Turk DC (eds) *Wall and Melzack's Textbook of Pain.* Philadelphia, PA: Elsevier Saunders; 2013, pp. 1–30.

4 Dubin AE, Patapoutian A. Nociceptors: the sensors of the pain pathway. *J Clin Invest.* 2010;120(11):3760–3772.

5 Jonsson EH, Backlund Wasling H, Wagnbeck V, *et al.* Unmyelinated tactile cutaneous nerves signal erotic sensations. *J Sex Med.* 2015; 12(6):1338–1345.

6 Liljencrantz J, Olausson H. Tactile C fibers and their contributions to pleasant sensations and to tactile allodynia. *Front Behav Neurosci.* 2014;8:37.

7 Woo SH, Ranade S, Weyer AD, *et al.* Piezo2 is required for Merkel-cell mechanotransduction. *Nature.* 2014;509(7502):622–626.

8 Woo SH, Lumpkin EA, Patapoutian A. Merkel cells and neurons keep in touch. *Trends Cell Biol.* 2015;25(2):74–81.

9 Chaban V. Estrogen and Visceral nociception at the level of primary sensory neurons. Pain research and treatment. *Pain Res Treat.* 2012;pii: 960780.

10 Bodin P, Burnstock G. Purinergic signalling: ATP release. *Neurochem Res.* 2001;26(8–9):959–969

11 Ford AP. P2X3 antagonists: novel therapeutics for afferent sensitization and chronic pain. *Pain Manag.* 2012;2(3):267–277.

12 De Icco R, Cucinella L, De Paoli I, *et al.* Modulation of nociceptive threshold by combined hormonal contraceptives in women with oestrogen-withdrawal migraine attacks: a pilot study. *J Headache Pain.* 2016;17(1):70.

13 Sanoja R, Cervero F. Estrogen modulation of ovariectomy-induced hyperalgesia in adult mice. *Eur J Pain.* 2008;12(5):573–581.

14 Eva LJ, MacLean AB, Reid WM, *et al.* Estrogen receptor expression in vulvar vestibulitis syndrome. *Am J Obstet Gynecol.* 2003;189(2):458–461.

15 Chen X, Gebhart GF. Differential purinergic signaling in bladder sensory neurons of naive and bladder-inflamed mice. *Pain.* 2010;148(3):462–472.

16 Fabbretti E. ATP P2X3 receptors and neuronal sensitization. *Front Cell Neurosci.* 2013;7:236.

17 Jackowich RA, Pink L, Gordon A, Pukall CF. Persistent genital arousal disorder: a review of its conceptualizations, potential origins, impact, and treatment. *Sex Med Rev.* 2016;4(4):329–342.

18 Julius D. TRP channels and pain. *Annu Rev Cell Dev Biol.* 2013;29:355–834.

19 Tympanidis P, Casula MA, Yiangou Y, *et al.* Increased vanilloid receptor VR1 innervation in vulvodynia. *Eur J Pain.* 2004;8(2):129–133.

20 Pang Z, Sakamoto T, Tiwari V, *et al.* Selective keratinocyte stimulation is sufficient to evoke nociception in mice. *Pain.* 2015;156(4):656–565.

21 Caterina MJ, Pang Z. TRP Channels in skin biology and pathophysiology. *Pharmaceuticals (Basel).* 2016;9(4):77.

22 Steinberg AC, Oyama IA, Rejba AE, *et al.* Capsaicin for the treatment of vulvar vestibulitis. *Am J Obstet Gynecol.* 2005;192(5):1549–1553.

23 Amandusson A, Blomqvist A. Estrogenic influences in pain processing. *Front Neuroendocrinol.* 2013;34(4):329–349.

24 Smith YR, Stohler CS, Nichols TE, *et al.* Pronociceptive and antinociceptive effects of estradiol through endogenous opioid neurotransmission in women. *J Neurosci.* 2006;26(21):5777–5785.

25 Wu YW, Bi YP, Kou XX, *et al.* 17-Beta-estradiol enhanced allodynia of inflammatory temporomandibular joint through upregulation of hippocampal TRPV1 in ovariectomized rats. *J Neurosci.* 2010;30(26):8710–8719.

26 Chakrabarti S, Liu NJ, Gintzler AR. Formation of mu-/kappa-opioid receptor heterodimer is sex-dependent and mediates female-specific opioid analgesia. *Proc Natl Acad Sci USA.* 2010;107(46):20115–20119.

27 Liu NJ, Chakrabarti S, Schnell S, *et al.* Spinal synthesis of estrogen and concomitant signaling by membrane estrogen receptors regulate spinal kappa- and mu-opioid receptor heterodimerization and female-specific spinal morphine antinociception. *J Neurosci.* 2011;31(33):11836–11845.

28 Niesters M, Dahan A, Kest B, *et al.* Do sex differences exist in opioid analgesia? A systematic review and meta-analysis of human experimental and clinical studies. *Pain.* 2010;151(1):61–68.

29 Fan X, Kim HJ, Warner M, Gustafsson JA. Estrogen receptor beta is essential for sprouting of nociceptive primary afferents and for morphogenesis and maintenance of the dorsal horn interneurons. *Proc Natl Acad Sci USA.* 2007;104(34):13696–13701.

30 Taleghany N, Sarajari S, DonCarlos LL, *et al.* Differential expression of estrogen receptor alpha and beta in rat dorsal root ganglion neurons. *J Neurosci Res.* 1999;57(5):603–615.

31 Hodgins MB, Spike RC, Mackie RM, MacLean AB. An immunohistochemical study of androgen, oestrogen and progesterone receptors in the vulva and vagina. *Br J Obstet Gynaecol.* 1998;105(2):216–222.

32 Carley ME, Cliby WA, Spelsberg TC. P2X(3) receptor subunit messenger RNA expression in the female mouse bladder after oophorectomy with or without estrogen replacement. *Am J Obstet Gynecol.* 2002;187(1):103–106.

33 Lu Y, Jiang Q, Yu L, *et al.* 17beta-estradiol rapidly attenuates P2X3 receptor-mediated peripheral pain signal transduction via ERalpha and GPR30. *Endocrinology.* 2013;154(7):2421–3243.

34 Pajot J, Ressot C, Ngom I, Woda A. Gonadectomy induces site-specific differences in nociception in rats. *Pain.* 2003;104(1–2):367–373.

35 Kao A, Binik YM, Amsel R, *et al.* Challenging atrophied perspectives on postmenopausal dyspareunia: a systematic description and synthesis of clinical pain characteristics. *J Sex Marital Ther.* 2012;38(2):128–150.

36 Burrows LJ, Goldstein AT. The treatment of vestibulodynia with topical estradiol and testosterone. *Sex Med.* 2013;1(1):30–33.

37 Cayan F, Dilek U, Pata O, Dilek S. Comparison of the effects of hormone therapy regimens, oral and vaginal estradiol, estradiol + drospirenone and tibolone, on sexual function in healthy postmenopausal women. *J Sex Med.* 2008;5(1):132–138.

38 Gast MJ, Freedman MA, Vieweg AJ, *et al.* A randomized study of low-dose conjugated estrogens on sexual function and quality of life in postmenopausal women. *Menopause.* 2009;16(2):247–256.

39 Sarrel PM. Effects of hormone replacement therapy on sexual psychophysiology and behavior in postmenopause. *J Womens Health Gend Based Med.* 2000;9(Suppl 1): S25–S32.

40 Chaban V. Estrogen modulation of visceral nociceptors. *Curr Trends Neurol.* 2013;7:51–55.

41 Papka RE, Hafemeister J, Storey-Workley M. P2X receptors in the rat uterine cervix, lumbosacral dorsal root ganglia, and spinal cord during pregnancy. *Cell Tissue Res.* 2005;321(1):35–44.

42 Stratton P, Berkley KJ. Chronic pelvic pain and endometriosis: translational evidence of the relationship and implications. *Hum Reprod Update.* 2011;17(3):327–346

43 Bouchard C, Brisson J, Fortier M, *et al.* Use of oral contraceptive pills and vulvar vestibulitis: a case-control study. *Am J Epidemiol.* 2002;156(3):254–261.

44 Greenstein A, Ben-Aroya Z, Fass O, *et al.* Vulvar vestibulitis syndrome and estrogen dose of oral contraceptive pills. *J Sex Med.* 2007;4(6):1679–1683.

45 Bohm-Starke N, Johannesson U, Hilliges M, *et al.* Decreased mechanical pain threshold in the vestibular mucosa of women using oral contraceptives: a contributing factor in vulvar vestibulitis? *J Reprod Med.* 2004; 49(11):888–892.

46 Coulombe MA, Spooner MF, Gaumond I, *et al.* Estrogen receptors beta and alpha have specific pro- and anti-nociceptive actions. *Neuroscience.* 2011;184:172–182.

47 Johannesson U, Sahlin L, Masironi B, *et al.* Steroid receptor expression in the vulvar vestibular mucosa-—effects of oral contraceptives and menstrual cycle. *Contraception.* 2007;76(4):319–325.

48 Bjorling DE, Beckman M, Clayton MK, Wang ZY. Modulation of nerve growth factor in peripheral organs by estrogen and progesterone. *Neuroscience.* 2002;110(1):155–167.

49 Liao Z, Smith PG. Persistent genital hyperinnervation following progesterone administration to adolescent female rats. *Biol Reprod.* 2014;91(6):144.

50 Teng J, Wang ZY, Bjorling DE. Estrogen-induced proliferation of urothelial cells is modulated by nerve growth factor. *Am J Physiol Renal Physiol.* 2002;282(6):F1075–1083.

51 Burrows LJ, Basha M, Goldstein AT. The effects of hormonal contraceptives on female sexuality: a review. *J Sex Med.* 2012;9(9):2213–2223.

52 Goldstein AT, Belkin ZR, Krapf JM, *et al.* Polymorphisms of the androgen receptor gene and hormonal contraceptive induced provoked vestibulodynia. *J Sex Med.* 2014;11(11):2764–2771.

53 Cervero F, Laird JM. Understanding the signaling and transmission of visceral nociceptive events. *J Neurobiol.* 2004;61(1):45–54.

54 Cervero F. Sensory innervation of the viscera: peripheral basis of visceral pain. *Physiol Rev.* 1994;74(1):95–138.

55 Farmer MA, Maykut CA, Huberman JS, *et al.* Psychophysical properties of female genital sensation. *Pain.* 2013;154(11): 2277–2286.

56 Bohm-Starke N. Medical and physical predictors of localized provoked vulvodynia. *Acta Obstet Gynecol Scand.* 2010;89(12):1504–1510.

57 Witzeman K, Nguyen RH, Eanes A, *et al.* Mucosal versus muscle pain sensitivity in provoked vestibulodynia. *J Pain Res.* 2015;8:549–555.

58 Vecchiet L, Vecchiet J, Giamberardino MA. Referred muscle pain: clinical and pathophysiologic aspects. *Curr Rev Pain.* 1999;3(6):489–498.

59 Sugiura Y, Terui N, Hosoya Y. Difference in distribution of central terminals between visceral and somatic unmyelinated (C) primary afferent fibers. *J Neurophysiol.* 1989;62(4):834–840.

60 Malykhina AP. Neural mechanisms of pelvic organ cross-sensitization. *Neuroscience.* 2007;149(3):660–672.

61 Hoheisel U, Mense S, Simons DG, Yu XM. Appearance of new receptive fields in rat dorsal horn neurons following noxious stimulation of skeletal muscle: a model for referral of muscle pain? *Neurosci Lett.* 1993;153(1):9–12.

62 Ustinova EE, Fraser MO, Pezzone MA. Cross-talk and sensitization of bladder afferent nerves. *Neurourol Urodyn.* 2010;29(1):77–81.

63 Giamberardino MA, Tana C, Costantini R. Pain thresholds in women with chronic pelvic pain. *Curr Opin Obstet Gynecol.* 2014;26(4):253–259.

64 Giamberardino MA. Referred muscle pain/hyperalgesia and central sensitisation. *J Rehabil Med.* 2003 (41 Suppl):85–58.

65 Woolf CJ. Central sensitization: implications for the diagnosis and treatment of pain. *Pain.* 2011;152(3 Suppl):S2–S15.

66 Giamberardino MA, De Laurentis S, Affaitati G, et al. Modulation of pain and hyperalgesia from the urinary tract by algogenic conditions of the reproductive organs in women. *Neurosci Lett.* 2001;304(1–2):61–64.

67 Tuttle LJ, Nguyen OT, Cook MS, et al. Architectural design of the pelvic floor is consistent with muscle functional subspecialization. *Int Urogynecol J.* 2014;25(2):205–212.

68 Vandyken C, Hilton S. Physical therapy in the treatment of central pain mechanisms for female sexual pain. *Sex Med Rev.* 2017;5(1):20–30.

69 Giamberardino MA, Costantini R, Affaitati G, et al. Viscero-visceral hyperalgesia: characterization in different clinical models. *Pain.* 2010;151(2):307–322.

70 Laursen RJ, Graven-Nielsen T, Jensen TS, Arendt-Nielsen L. Referred pain is dependent on sensory input from the periphery: a psychophysical study. *Eur J Pain.* 1997;1(4):261–269.

71 Laursen RJ, Graven-Nielsen T, Jensen TS, Arendt-Nielsen L. The effect of compression and regional anaesthetic block on referred pain intensity in humans. *Pain.* 1999;80(1–2):257–263.

72 Ball E, Khan KS, Meads C. Does pelvic venous congestion syndrome exist and can it be treated? *Acta Obstet Gynecol Scand.* 2012;91(5):525–528.

73 Maybin JA, Critchley HO. Menstrual physiology: implications for endometrial pathology and beyond. *Hum Reprod Update.* 2015;21(6):748–761.

74 Foster DC, Hasday JD. Elevated tissue levels of interleukin-1 beta and tumor necrosis factor-alpha in vulvar vestibulitis. *Obstet Gynecol.* 1997;89(2):291–296.

75 Foster DC, Falsetta ML, Woeller CF, et al. Site-specific mesenchymal control of inflammatory pain to yeast challenge in vulvodynia-afflicted and pain-free women. *Pain.* 2015;156(3):386–396.

76 Wira CR, Grant-Tschudy KS, Crane-Godreau MA. Epithelial cells in the female reproductive tract: a central role as sentinels of immune protection. *Am J Reprod Immunol.* 2005;53(2):65–76.

77 Ferrari LF, Araldi D, Levine JD. Regulation of expression of hyperalgesic priming by estrogen receptor alpha in the rat. *J Pain.* 2017;18(5):574–582.

78 Hilt EE, McKinley K, Pearce MM, et al. Urine is not sterile: use of enhanced urine culture techniques to detect resident bacterial flora in the adult female bladder. *J Clin Microbiol.* 2014;52(3):871–876.

79 Witkin SS, Linhares IM, Giraldo P. Bacterial flora of the female genital tract: function and immune regulation. *Best Pract Res Clin Obstet Gynaecol.* 2007;21(3):347–354.

80 Liston A, Masters SL. Homeostasis-altering molecular processes as mechanisms of

inflammasome activation. *Nat Rev Immunol.* 2017;17(3):208–214.

81 Chiu IM, Heesters BA, Ghasemlou N, *et al.* Bacteria activate sensory neurons that modulate pain and inflammation. *Nature.* 2013;501(7465):52–57.

82 Farmer MA, Taylor AM, Bailey AL, *et al.* Repeated vulvovaginal fungal infections cause persistent pain in a mouse model of vulvodynia. *Sci Transl Med.* 2011;3(101):101ra91.

83 Gabutti G, Bonanni P, Conversano M, *et al.* Prevention of Herpes Zoster and its complications: From clinical evidence to real life experience. *Hum Vaccin Immunother.* 2017;13(2):391–398.

84 Chai LY, Netea MG, Vonk AG, Kullberg BJ. Fungal strategies for overcoming host innate immune response. *Med Mycol.* 2009;47(3):227–236.

85 Falsetta ML, Foster DC, Woeller CF, *et al.* Identification of novel mechanisms involved in generating localized vulvodynia pain. *Am J Obstet Gynecol.* 2015;213(1):38 e1–e12.

86 Kalaitzidis D, Gilmore TD. Transcription factor cross-talk: the estrogen receptor and NF-kappaB. *Trends Endocrinol Metab.* 2005;16(2):46–52.

87 Fitzpatrick CC, DeLancey JO, Elkins TE, McGuire EJ. Vulvar vestibulitis and interstitial cystitis: a disorder of urogenital sinus-derived epithelium? *Obstet Gynecol.* 1993;81(5 (Pt 2)): 860–822.

88 Lev-Sagie A, Witkin SS. Recent advances in understanding provoked vestibulodynia. *F1000Res.* 2016;5:2581.

89 Bogart LM, Berry SH, Clemens JQ. Symptoms of interstitial cystitis, painful bladder syndrome and similar diseases in women: a systematic review. *J Urol.* 2007;177(2):450–456.

90 Foster DC, Sazenski TM, Stodgell CJ. Impact of genetic variation in interleukin-1 receptor antagonist and melanocortin-1 receptor genes on vulvar vestibulitis syndrome. *J Reprod Med.* 2004;49(7):503–509.

91 Starowicz K, Przewlocka B. The role of melanocortins and their receptors in inflammatory processes, nerve regeneration and nociception. *Life Sci.* 2003;73(7):823–847.

92 Chhajlani V. Distribution of cDNA for melanocortin receptor subtypes in human tissues. *Biochem Mol Biol Int.* 1996;38(1):73–80.

93 Liem EB, Joiner TV, Tsueda K, Sessler DI. Increased sensitivity to thermal pain and reduced subcutaneous lidocaine efficacy in redheads. *Anesthesiology.* 2005;102(3):509–514.

94 Mogil JS. Sex differences in pain and pain inhibition: multiple explanations of a controversial phenomenon. *Nat Rev Neurosci.* 2012;13(12):859–866.

95 Wikberg JE. Melanocortin receptors: perspectives for novel drugs. *Eur J Pharmacol.* 1999;375(1–3):295–310.

96 Niizeki H, Streilein JW. Hapten-specific tolerance induced by acute, low-dose ultraviolet B radiation of skin is mediated via interleukin-10. *J Invest Dermatol.* 1997;109(1):25–30.

97 Yamaoka J, Di ZH, Sun W, Kawana S. Changes in cutaneous sensory nerve fibers induced by skin-scratching in mice. *J Dermatol Sci.* 2007;46(1):41–51.

98 Bohm-Starke N, Hilliges M, Falconer C, Rylander E. Increased intraepithelial innervation in women with vulvar vestibulitis syndrome. *Gynecol Obstet Invest.* 1998;46(4):256–260.

99 Bohm-Starke N, Hilliges M, Falconer C, Rylander E. Neurochemical characterization of the vestibular nerves in women with vulvar vestibulitis syndrome. *Gynecol Obstet Invest.* 1999;48(4):270–275.

100 Anaf V, Chapron C, El Nakadi I, *et al.* Pain, mast cells, and nerves in peritoneal, ovarian, and deep infiltrating endometriosis. *Fertil Steril.* 2006;86(5):1336–1343.

101 Bornstein J, Goldschmid N, Sabo E. Hyperinnervation and mast cell activation may be used as histopathologic diagnostic criteria for vulvar vestibulitis. *Gynecol Obstet Invest.* 2004;58(3):171–178.

102 Bornstein J, Cohen Y, Zarfati D, *et al.* Involvement of heparanase in the pathogenesis of localized vulvodynia. *Int J Gynecol Pathol.* 2008;27(1):136–141.

103 Patnaik SS, Lagana AS, Vitale SG, *et al.* Etiology, pathophysiology and biomarkers of interstitial cystitis/painful bladder syndrome. *Arch Gynecol Obstet.* 2017;295(6):1341–1359.

104 Amir R, Kocsis JD, Devor M. Multiple interacting sites of ectopic spike electrogenesis in primary sensory neurons. *J Neurosci.* 2005;25(10):2576–2585.

105 Basbaum AI, Bautista DM, Scherrer G, Julius D. Cellular and molecular mechanisms of pain. *Cell.* 2009;139(2):267–284.

106 Fields HL, Basbaum AI. Central nervous system mechanisms of pain modulation. In: Wall PD, Melzack R (eds) *Textbook of Pain.* London: Churchill Livingstone; 1999, pp. 309–329.

107 Woolf CJ. What to call the amplification of nociceptive signals in the central nervous system that contribute to widespread pain? *Pain.* 2014;155(10):1911–1912.

108 Kaya S, Hermans L, Willems T, *et al.* Central sensitization in urogynecological chronic pelvic pain: a systematic literature review. *Pain Physician.* 2013;16(4):291–308.

109 Cavallone LF, Frey K, Montana MC, *et al.* Reproducibility of the heat/capsaicin skin sensitization model in healthy volunteers. *J Pain Res.* 2013;6:771–784.

110 Biurrun Manresa JA, Fritsche R, Vuilleumier PH, *et al.* Is the conditioned pain modulation paradigm reliable? A test-retest assessment using the nociceptive withdrawal reflex. *PloS One.* 2014;9(6):e100241.

111 Edwards RR, Dolman AJ, Martel MO, *et al.* Variability in conditioned pain modulation predicts response to NSAID treatment in patients with knee osteoarthritis. *BMC Musculoskelet Disord.* 2016;17:284.

112 Martel MO, Wasan AD, Edwards RR. Sex differences in the stability of conditioned pain modulation (CPM) among patients with chronic pain. *Pain Med.* 2013;14(11):1757–1768.

113 Grinberg K, Granot M, Lowenstein L, *et al.* A common pronociceptive pain modulation profile typifying subgroups of chronic pelvic pain syndromes is interrelated with enhanced clinical pain. *Pain.* 2017;158(6):1021–1029.

114 Johannesson U, de Boussard CN, Brodda Jansen G, Bohm-Starke N. Evidence of diffuse noxious inhibitory controls (DNIC) elicited by cold noxious stimulation in patients with provoked vestibulodynia. *Pain.* 2007;130(1–2):31–39.

115 Sutton KS, Pukall CF, Chamberlain S. Diffuse noxious inhibitory control function in women with provoked vestibulodynia. *Clin J Pain.* 2012;28(8):667–674.

116 Ingvar M. Pain and functional imaging. *Philos Trans R Soc Lond B Biol Sci.* 1999;354(1387):1347–1358.

117 Lee MC, Tracey I. Unravelling the mystery of pain, suffering, and relief with brain imaging. *Curr Pain Headache Rep.* 2010;14(2):124–131.

118 Porro CA, Cavazzuti M, Lui F, *et al.* Independent time courses of supraspinal nociceptive activity and spinally mediated behavior during tonic pain. *Pain.* 2003;104(1–2):291–301.

119 Rainville P. Brain mechanisms of pain affect and pain modulation. *Curr Opin Neurobiol.* 2002;12(2):195–204.

120 Grosen K, Fischer IW, Olesen AE, Drewes AM. Can quantitative sensory testing predict responses to analgesic treatment? *Eur J Pain.* 2013;17(9):1267–1280.

121 Samuelsen PJ, Nielsen CS, Wilsgaard T, *et al.* Pain sensitivity and analgesic use among 10,486 adults: the Tromso study. *BMC Pharmacol Toxicol.* 2017;18(1):45.

122 Mouraux A, Diukova A, Lee MC, *et al.* A multisensory investigation of the functional significance of the "pain matrix". *Neuroimage.* 2011;54(3):2237–2249.

123  Hashmi JA, Baliki MN, Huang L, *et al.* Shape shifting pain: chronification of back pain shifts brain representation from nociceptive to emotional circuits. *Brain.* 2013;136(Pt 9):2751–2768.

124  Goswami R, Anastakis DJ, Katz J, Davis KD. A longitudinal study of pain, personality, and brain plasticity following peripheral nerve injury. *Pain.* 2016;157(3):729–739.

125  Farmer MA, Baliki MN, Apkarian AV. A dynamic network perspective of chronic pain. *Neurosci Lett.* 2012;520(2):197–203.

126  Leknes S, Berna C, Lee MC, *et al.* The importance of context: when relative relief renders pain pleasant. *Pain.* 2013;154(3):402–410.

127  Cahill L, Haier RJ, Fallon J, *et al.* Amygdala activity at encoding correlated with long-term, free recall of emotional information. *Proc Natl Acad Sci USA.* 1996;93(15):8016–8021.

128  Logothetis NK. What we can do and what we cannot do with fMRI. *Nature.* 2008;453(7197):869–878.

129  McGaugh JL. Memory – a century of consolidation. *Science.* 2000;287(5451):248–251.

130  Rodrigues SM, LeDoux JE, Sapolsky RM. The influence of stress hormones on fear circuitry. *Annu Rev Neurosci.* 2009;32:289–313.

20

# Psychological Management of Provoked Vestibulodynia

*Caroline F. Pukall and Sophie Bergeron*

### Abstract

Vulvodynia represents a unique challenge for health-care professionals, as it intersects two poorly understood conditions: pain and sexual health problems. This chapter focuses on the psychosocial aspects of provoked vestibulodynia – the most common subtype of vulvodynia – highlighting its diagnosis and assessment, and emphasizing that measuring pain and sexuality outcomes are useful in terms of validating the patient's experience as well as tracking treatment progression. Psychosocial factors – including sexuality, sexual partners, relationship dynamics, mood, and cognitive/emotional responses to the pain – are discussed in light of the importance of these factors in the expression of vulvodynia. Psychological interventions and their efficacy are reviewed, and the conclusion that individual and group psychological treatments represent empirically validated and safe options for provoked vestibulodynia is made.

**Keywords:**  *vulvodynia; provoked vestibulodynia; psychosocial factors; mood; sexuality; pain; assessment; relationships; psychological interventions; cognitive behavioral therapy*

---

Take a multidimensional approach to the assessment of the woman's pain and sexuality, validate her pain experience, discuss contributing factors, and include the partner in the assessment when possible.

Address anxiety, mood, and post traumatic stress disease comorbidities, especially if they reach clinical levels.

Throughout treatment, target pain and sexuality concurrently; obtain pain ratings and re-assess sexual function periodically to facilitate the identification of factors that affect the pain experience and associated sexual difficulties, provide psychoeducation to help patients espouse a multifactorial view of their pain and its impact on sexuality; create specific short-term goals addressing pain reduction and improved sexual function and satisfaction to structure the treatment, and to instill hope in women and their partners

---

## Provoked Vestibulodynia

### Pain Characteristics

Vulvodynia, or unexplained chronic vulvovaginal pain, represents a unique challenge for health-care professionals in terms of the intersection of two poorly understood conditions: pain and sexual health problems.

Ideally, a comprehensive treatment program for women with vulvodynia will target these two components, as women complain as much about the pain as they do about the sexual difficulties associated with it, and these two symptom domains are relatively independent of one another [1]. Mental health-care professionals who treat women with vulvodynia, therefore, should be

*Textbook of Female Sexual Function and Dysfunction: Diagnosis and Treatment*, First Edition. Edited by Irwin Goldstein, Anita H. Clayton, Andrew T. Goldstein, Noel N. Kim, and Sheryl A. Kingsberg.
© 2018 John Wiley & Sons Ltd. Published 2018 by John Wiley & Sons Ltd.

comfortable in the domains of both pain management and sex therapy; an empirically validated treatment protocol combining these two complimentary approaches has been developed for groups [2], couples [3], and individuals [4, 5]; and can be obtained by contacting the authors of this chapter.

The pain of provoked vestibulodynia is typically characterized as severe, located at the vaginal entrance, and experienced in response to pressure [6]. Activities that elicit the pain can be sexual (e.g. those involving vaginal pressure/penetration) or nonsexual (e.g. tampon insertion, bicycle riding); usually, women with provoked vestibulodynia will present to health-care professionals with complaints of pain during sexual activities involving vaginal pressure/penetration. Although many adjectives are used to describe the pain of provoked vestibulodynia, some of the most common descriptors are burning, cutting, sharp, and searing [7]. Despite the fact that medical professionals often will cite "no observable cause" when diagnosing a patient with provoked vestibulodynia (a diagnosis of exclusion), many factors that are not routinely assessed in a typical examination room and/or via medical tests – from vestibular hyperinnervation resulting in hypersensitivity, to heightened pelvic floor muscle tension, to neural responses – are associated with the experience of this pain [6]. As such, the pain experience should be validated even in the face of a lack of observable findings, and the correlates should be explained to the person with provoked vestibulodynia.

## Diagnosis

The diagnosis and treatment of provoked vestibulodynia are discussed in depth in Chapter 22. Briefly, the diagnosis is typically made by a medical professional, who rules in/out known causes of vulvar pain such as an infection (e.g. candidiasis) or dermatologic disease of the vulva (e.g. lichen sclerosus). If a diagnosis of a known cause of vulvar pain is made, then the patient does not have vulvodynia. If the health-care provider is unable to make a diagnosis of a known cause of vulvar pain, then the patient is diagnosed with vulvodynia [8]. In the majority of cases, the patient has pain localized to the vulvar vestibule and, therefore, her diagnosis is provoked vestibulodynia. It is possible that the health-care provider believes that there is an associated biomedical factor that may be playing a role in the pain experience, such as inflammation or hormonal changes. In these cases, the provider may initiate treatment for this possible associated factor [9]. A referral to a pelvic floor physical therapist is also typically made if one is available because many women with provoked vestibulodynia have overactive pelvic floor muscles that may be contributing to the vestibulodynia. In addition, a referral to a mental health-care professional with knowledge of vulvodynia could then be made, so that the patient can focus on various biopsychosocial elements involved in the expression of the pain and associated psychological, relationship, and sexual difficulties.

## Assessment

A mental health-care professional should complete a comprehensive evaluation of the following: medical, psychological, and general health history; vulvar pain history, including pain characteristics, and treatment attempts and outcomes; sexuality, including current function, satisfaction, and distress, and any past childhood trauma and maltreatment; and individual and couple relationship factors (Table 20.1). This information would then be used to confirm or refine the initial diagnosis, and would lead to areas of focus in terms of psychotherapeutic intervention.

Ideally, the initial assessment as well as treatment progress should involve some validated measures and/or scales, especially for the core symptomatology of provoked vestibulodynia: pain and sexual dysfunction (see the referenced recommendations for vulvodynia clinical trials [10].) Scales and/or questionnaires assessing the following

**Table 20.1** General and specific domains for a comprehensive pain and psychosocial assessment.

| General domain | Specific domains |
| --- | --- |
| Medical history | Surgical history<br>Medical conditions and treatments (past and current)<br>Previous and current vulvodynia-related diagnoses<br>Bowel and bladder function<br>Past and current prescription medication use<br>Past and current use of nonprescriptives (e.g. vitamins, supplements) |
| Psychological history | Mental health conditions and treatments (past and present)<br>Past abuse (sexual, physical, verbal) or neglect, current abuse |
| General health history | History of injuries or falls affecting the genito-pelvic and lower back areas |
| Vulvar pain history | Time since onset<br>Temporal pattern<br>Duration<br>Location<br>Quality<br>Factors that elicit the pain<br>Intensity<br>Primary or secondary presentation<br>Treatment attempts and outcomes |
| Sexuality | Desire<br>Arousal<br>Orgasm<br>Pleasure<br>Frequency of sexual activity<br>Satisfaction with sexual activity<br>Sexual repertoire<br>Pain with sexual activity<br>Sexual distress<br>Sexual trauma/negative experiences/ongoing sexual victimization |
| Individual factors | Thoughts, emotions, and behaviors associated with the pain<br>(e.g. avoidance, fear of pain, pain coping) |
| Couple relationship factors, if relevant | Couple interactions that accompany the pain<br>Current relationship dynamic (e.g. strengths, areas of conflict, couple's pain coping style, sexual and nonsexual intimacy) |

aspects of the pain experience can be useful: vulvovaginal pain intensity, quality, and affect, as well as sexual function, the effects of the vulvovaginal pain on quality of life, interference of the pain with sexual activity, and depressive and anxiety symptoms. Using validated measures is useful for making comparisons with clinical norms and for tracking treatment progress. However, obtaining a large amount of information in this manner is not always feasible in a clinical setting.

A simple zero-to-ten numerical rating scale can be used to measure pain intensity at the beginning of treatment and to follow the progression of the patient throughout the treatment process. On this scale, zero would indicate "no pain at all" and ten would indicate "pain as bad as you can imagine" [10]. This basic information – especially when pain ratings decrease over the course of treatment – can contribute to instilling hope, further motivating the patient to be an active participant in her recovery. In the case where pain ratings change (increase or decrease), specific factors (e.g. levels of anxiety, relationship dynamics with partner, sexual arousal) related to those experiences can be discussed in order to delineate what factors affect the pain experience. To this end, a pain diary can also be useful in keeping track of such factors. In addition, a numerical rating scale can be used to track progress in the experience of sexual desire and arousal, and serve the same purpose of reinforcing treatment gains. Measuring pain and sexuality outcomes can validate the patient's experience and communicate the mental health professional's interest in seeing improvement in these domains. In addition, it is important to communicate to the patient that her progress is not expected to be linear, and that ups and downs are typical – and, in fact, useful in understanding the complexity of her experience. Indeed, many factors can impact the experience of vulvovaginal pain.

## Psychosocial Factors

### Sexuality and Sexual Partners

Numerous studies indicate that women with provoked vestibulodynia report significantly lower levels of sexual desire, arousal and satisfaction, more difficulty reaching orgasm, lower frequencies of intercourse, more negative attitudes toward sexuality, and more sexual distress than pain-free controls [6]. Studies have also shown that women with vulvodynia report more distress about their body image, more anxiety and self-awareness with exposure of their bodies during sexual activity, and a more negative genital self-image than control women [6]. With all of these negative sexual consequences, one might question why over 80% of women with provoked vestibulodynia continue to engage in sexual activities involving vaginal pressure/penetration [11]. Reasons can include the following: to feel closer to their partner, to avoid losing their partner, to protect their partner, and to fulfill their duties as a sexual partner [12–14]. At the same time, some studies have indicated that partners of women with provoked vestibulodynia also tend to report more sexual difficulties [15]. For example, they report more erectile problems and lower sexual satisfaction as compared to men who are partnered with women who do not have provoked vestibulodynia. But do these sexual issues affect the overall relationship in any way?

### Relationship Dynamics

A recent line of investigation has examined whether couples with provoked vestibulodynia report lower relationship adjustment than nonaffected couples. Although a systematic review concluded that affected couples do not experience lower relationship satisfaction in comparison to control groups or norms on validated measures [16], some studies have demonstrated evidence of significantly lower relationship adjustment in couples affected by vulvodynia [17]. This discrepancy has led some researchers to suggest that "relationship satisfaction" or "relationship adjustment" may be too global a construct; perhaps examining more specific aspects of relationship dynamics may yield differences between provoked vestibulodynia and nonprovoked vestibulodynia affected couples, and partly explain the development and maintenance of associated sexual difficulties.

Recently, specific relationship variables have been shown to be associated with sexuality and pain outcomes in women with provoked vestibulodynia, such as partner responses to the pain, degree of relationship and sexual intimacy, levels of empathy, and amount of self-disclosure and ambivalence over emotional expression. Partner responses to pain can be solicitous (providing attention and sympathy), negative (demonstrations of hostility), and facilitative (encouraging adaptive coping). For example, in provoked vestibulodynia, a solicitous response would be a partner suggesting to stop engaging in all sexual activity, a negative response would be a partner expressing anger, and a facilitative response would be a partner expressing positive feelings about the woman engaging in any sexual activity. In a series of studies conducted with couples coping with provoked vestibulodynia, Rosen, Bergeron, and colleagues found that both solicitous and negative responses were detrimental to women's pain and couples' sexual well-being, whereas facilitative responses were beneficial to both members of the couple [18–20]. In addition, a study examining women's intimacy found that higher levels of self-reported sexual intimacy were associated with higher sexual satisfaction, sexual function, and pain self-efficacy (i.e. the degree to which one believes that they can manage the pain effectively) [21]. Empathic responses and self-disclosure – two components of intimacy – have also been found to improve sexuality in couples: in an observational study involving 50 provoked vestibulodynia affected couples, both partners' observed and reported greater empathic responses were associated with their better sexual satisfaction and lower sexual distress. Furthermore, both partners' greater perceived self-disclosure was associated with their better sexual satisfaction [22]. In another study involving the same sample, greater observed empathic response and perceived self-disclosure in women were associated with their higher quality of life. Women and partners' greater empathic response were associated with both partners' higher relationship adjustment [23].

Ambivalence over emotional expression (AEE) has also been examined in couples with provoked vestibulodynia. Ambivalence over emotional expression is defined as the extent to which one is comfortable with the way they express emotions. Being high in ambivalence over emotional expression indicates that the way in which one expresses emotions (or does not) is personally problematic and carries with it negative personal consequences, such as feeling inadequate or fearing to hurt someone else, whereas being low in ambivalence over emotional expression involves managing emotions in a less internally conflicted way and, overall, is suggestive of better emotion regulation. In a sample of over 250 couples with provoked vestibulodynia, those in which both members were found to be low in ambivalence over emotional expression reported significantly better sexual function and satisfaction, less depressive symptoms, and better dyadic adjustment than couples in which both were high in ambivalence over emotional expression or in which one member was high and the other was low [24]. This recent pattern of findings suggests that couples who can be intimate, communicate more openly about sexuality, and coregulate emotions effectively together may experience less pain-related negative impacts on their sexuality, relationship, and mood.

## Other Relationships: Peers and the Health-Care Community

Provoked vestibulodynia can be considered by some people to be a "private" pain given its location and negative effects on sexuality. Although approximately two-thirds of women reported discussing their pain with their sexual partner, only 40% reported feeling comfortable talking about it with a family member. This number dropped to just over one quarter when asking about comfort talking about the pain with female acquaintances [25]. Coupled with the findings that many affected women believe that people think their condition is an excuse to avoid intercourse, and that approximately half of them who sought medical care reported feeling stigmatized by their physicians [26], these results highlight affected women's sense of feeling alone in dealing with their pain and may explain some of their hesitancy and difficulties in finding appropriate health care. Indeed, many women with chronic vulvar pain are silent sufferers; one study reported that less than 50% of women who met criteria for vulvodynia sought treatment and, of these, only 1.4% received an appropriate diagnosis [11]. Anecdotal evidence suggests that women with vulvodynia receive little validation for their symptoms in health-care settings, with many being told their pain is "all in their heads" due to the absence of visible pathology. It has been well established that women with vulvodynia are apprehensive to speak about their pain with others, and that feelings of isolation and invalidation of their pain are common [27].

## Cognitive and Emotional Responses to the Pain

Many women with provoked vestibulodynia report feelings of shame, inadequacy, and low self-esteem; these feelings should be examined in treatmen,t as they may play a role in the pain experience. Psychological factors that have been associated with higher pain intensity and sexual impairment include: pain catastrophizing, fear of pain, pain hypervigilance, lower vulvar pain self-efficacy (the degree to which one believes that one can manage the pain effectively), negative attributions about the pain, avoidance, anxiety, and depression [6]. Although prospective studies examining the role of psychological factors in provoked vestibulodynia are rare, one such study that followed 222 women with provoked vestibulodynia over two years found that increases in pain self-efficacy were associated with reductions in pain intensity [28]. This relationship was partially mediated by lower avoidance of painful activities (i.e. engaging in more intercourse attempts). The same pattern of results was found for changes in sexual satisfaction as the outcome.

## Mood

Several studies indicate that women with vulvar pain report higher levels of depressive symptoms than nonaffected women [6], although these results have not been consistently replicated. It is noteworthy that in many of the studies that do report higher levels of depressive symptoms, the levels are not necessarily within the clinical range. A similar pattern emerges with anxiety symptoms: many studies report that women with provoked vestibulodynia exhibit higher levels of anxiety symptoms compared to women without provoked vestibulodynia [6]. Indeed, it has been well established that depressive

and anxiety symptoms tend to be comorbid in the general population as well as in chronic pain populations, and this association appears to play a role in provoked vestibulodynia as well. Results of an epidemiological study suggest that anxiety and depression may both precede and follow the development of vulvodynia. This study reported that the odds of chronic vulvar pain were four times more likely among women with a history of depression or anxiety as compared to nonaffected women. Furthermore, vulvodynia was associated with a new or recurrent onset of mood or anxiety disorder, suggesting a reciprocal relationship among anxiety, depression, and vulvodynia [29]. In another multiethnic population-based study, Iglesias-Rios *et al.* found that women who screened positive for posttraumatic stress disorder were twice as likely to report vulvodynia [30]. Posttraumatic stress disorder is a debilitating psychiatric disorder that may develop after unresolved trauma, such as childhood victimization. It is characterized by intrusive re-experiencing of the traumatic event, avoidance behaviors, hypervigilance, and emotional numbing, as well as by activation of the physiological and neuroendocrine systems. In sum, psychological factors, including psychiatric disorders, may be associated with both the onset and maintenance of vulvodynia and, thus, warrant clinical attention by mental health professionals.

## The Role of Childhood Victimization

Childhood sexual and physical abuse may play a role in the development of chronic vulvar pain. In two population-based studies, women with vulvodynia were more likely to have reported sexual abuse and severe physical abuse, as well as living in fear of abuse, when compared to nonaffected women [31, 32]. This pattern was also shown in a large-scale cross-sectional study of sexually active female adolescents with dyspareunia. Those with dyspareunia were more likely to report a history of sexual abuse and fear of physical abuse compared to sexually active adolescents without dyspareunia [33]. It appears as though childhood victimization can increase one's risk for developing chronic vulvar pain, and there is some suggestion that it might also affect sexual function and mood. In a study of women with dyspareunia, victims of childhood sexual abuse reported significantly lower levels of sexual functioning and psychological well-being compared to women reporting no sexual abuse [33]. However, less is known about the impact of broader forms of childhood interpersonal trauma on provoked vestibulodynia affected couples' adaptation to current symptomatology. In a recent study involving 50 such couples, women's greater occurrence of childhood maltreatment was associated with their lower sexual function and higher anxiety, whereas partners' maltreatment was associated with their lower sexual function, lower couple satisfaction, and higher anxiety, as well as women's lower couple satisfaction and higher anxiety. Both women's and partners' greater occurrence of childhood maltreatment were associated with higher affective pain intensity ratings for women [34]. Overall, findings suggest that childhood interpersonal trauma is not only a risk factor for the onset of provoked vestibulodynia but also complicates couples' adjustment to the sexual, psychological, and relationship repercussions of vulvodynia and, as such, should be given careful attention in the treatment plan.

## Treatment

The typical treatment plan for a woman with provoked vestibulodynia starts with treatments that are considered noninvasive (e.g. psychological interventions, pelvic floor physical therapy) and, depending on her response to treatment, may progress to medical treatments (e.g. gabapentin, topical hormones). If these treatments fail, surgical intervention (if the pain is limited to the vestibule) may be recommended. Treatment progression is usually consecutive and based on 'trial-and-error'; however, recently, King and colleagues have suggested a more algorithmic approach based on physical examination findings and laboratory tests when deciding on specific treatments [35]. Lastly, some have argued that starting with more invasive treatments, such as surgical intervention, should be considered given its high effectiveness and low side-effect profile [36]. Still others have stated that concurrent or integrative (i.e. multidisciplinary) treatments, if possible, might be more efficacious in terms of outcome [37, 38], although, at present, there is no empirical evidence to support any particular combination and/or sequence of treatments [9].

### Psychological Interventions: What do they Target?

Psychological interventions focus on reducing pain and distress, improving sexual function and satisfaction, and strengthening the romantic relationship by targeting the thoughts, emotions, behaviors, and couple interactions associated with the experience of pain and sexual difficulties. Such interventions can be delivered in individual, couple, or group formats [36, 39, 40]. Cognitive behavioral therapy is the most commonly used and most studied psychological treatment for provoked vestibulodynia to date [9]. In the first phase of cognitive behavioral therapy, psycho-education is provided about a multidimensional view of pain and its negative impact on sexuality, as well as on the role of psychological and relationship factors in the maintenance of provoked vestibulodynia. Self-exploration of the genitals and localization of the pain are generally introduced at this stage, as is the regular use of a pain and sexuality diary to raise awareness about which psychological and relationship factors influence pain, arousal, and desire, and to track progress. The second step involves targeting individual coping strategies that may lead to increased pain and sexual difficulties, such as pain catastrophizing, hypervigilance to pain, avoidance of sexual activity, fear of pain, and excessive anxiety. If in a couple therapy format, securing the attachment bond is another relationship factor that can be addressed, as well as partner solicitous and negative responses, emotion coregulation between partners, and sexual and relationship intimacy within the couple. One helpful multitarget strategy is to increase each partner's capacity for empathic response and self-disclosure. The aim of this second step is to enable women and their partners to make better use of approach behaviors, i.e. engaging in sexual activity to achieve a positive outcome, optimal emotion regulation, communication, and self-assertiveness, while reconnecting with each other through nonsexual physical and emotional intimacy, expanding their sexual repertoire to steer the focus away from intercourse, and sharing mutual experiences of desire and arousal in a nonthreatening, nonpainful context. Exercises associated with this step may include breathing and meditation; discussing views about the impact of the pain on their romantic and sexual relationship; identifying distressing thoughts, emotions and couple interactions; familiarizing themselves with what facilitates arousal and desire; communicating sexual preferences and needs; and using cognitive defusion to decatastrophize pain-related thoughts and emotions.

Although traditionally prescribed in sex therapy, Kegel exercises and vaginal dilation exercises are best done with a pelvic floor physical therapist. Toward the end of treatment, the mental health professional will help in skill consolidation and maintenance of gains, helping the woman or couple attribute these gains to the efforts they deployed in and outside of therapy. Follow-up sessions are recommended when possible. Finally, in terms of a timeline, cognitive behavioral therapy can be delivered in 10–12 sessions, but mental health professionals are encouraged to adapt their pace and sequence of interventions to the specific clinical presentation of the woman or couple.

## Significant Psychological Distress: How to Deal with it

In some cases, psychological distress will reach clinical levels and this aspect of the woman's presentation will become more central. At this point, mental health professionals may need to move beyond pain and sexuality-focused cognitive behavioral therapy. Reasons for elevated psychological distress can range from a history of childhood maltreatment to significant relationship conflict, including intimate partner physical, sexual and/or psychological violence. Childhood maltreatment can become the focus of treatment if briefer cognitive behavioral therapy interventions are ineffective in reducing pain and improving sexual function, and the woman is ready to attend to this aspect of her past more directly. In such instances, the mental health professional should have sufficient experience and training in trauma-informed psychotherapy, and childhood maltreatment should not be presented as the sole cause of provoked vestibulodynia given that chronic pain is a complex, multifactorial phenomenon. Namely, focusing on childhood maltreatment to the exclusion of other potential exacerbating factors could prolong treatment unnecessarily and be less helpful. Focusing on childhood maltreatment should not eclipse the need to work on reducing pain and improving sexuality.

Significant relationship conflict, disengagement, or trauma should be addressed in couple therapy, especially since these factors may interfere with other ongoing treatments for provoked vestibulodynia. Women with pre-existing psychiatric disorders could be in need of more intensive psychotherapy to cope with the added burden of provoked vestibulodynia. In addition, women with primary provoked vestibulodynia onset (i.e. the pain has been present since the first occasion of vaginal pressure/penetration) may benefit less from treatment than those who have secondary provoked vestibulodynia (i.e. the pain developed after a period of time during which pain-free vaginal pressure/penetration activities were possible) [41]. For example, a nonrandomized treatment study assessing outcome of women with provoked vestibulodynia who received various multimodal interventions (ranging from topical lidocaine gel to surgery) demonstrated that women with primary provoked vestibulodynia had lower success rates than women with secondary provoked vestibulodynia [42]. Taking pain onset into consideration may help guide treatment planning and allow for more reasonable goals to be set. Finally, women who have tried multiple treatments with no success, or women who have experienced many negative side effects or complications from past treatments – leading them to lose faith in ever improving their condition and quality of life – may prove more challenging to treat. They may require additional psychological support and/or psychotherapy targeting their lack of trust in the mental health professional or their difficulty engaging in treatment for fear of being disappointed yet again.

## Efficacy of Psychological Interventions

Bergeron and colleagues investigated the efficacy of a combination of group cognitive behavioral therapy in two randomized trials of women diagnosed with provoked vestibulodynia. In the first study, which compared vestibulectomy, electromyographic biofeedback, and cognitive behavioral therapy, intent-to-treat analyses indicated that participants who took part in cognitive behavioral therapy reported significant improvements in pain at a six-month follow-up, although significantly less than vestibulectomy participants [43]. At a 2.5-year follow-up, their ratings of pain during intercourse – the most relevant functional outcome – were equivalent to those of women having undergone vestibulectomy [44]. In another study, women with provoked vestibulodynia were randomly assigned to either a corticosteroid cream or to group cognitive behavioral therapy for a

13-week treatment period [2]. Intent-to-treat multilevel analyses showed that participants of both groups reported statistically significant reductions on pain from baseline to post-treatment and six-month follow-up, although the cognitive behavioral therapy group reported significantly more pain reduction at the six-month follow-up. At post-treatment, women randomized to the cognitive behavioral therapy condition were significantly more satisfied with their treatment, displayed significantly less pain catastrophizing, and reported significantly better global improvements in the domain of sexuality than women assigned to the topical application. Findings suggest that cognitive behavioral therapy may yield positive outcomes on more dimensions of provoked vestibulodynia than does a topical treatment.

In a randomized trial involving a mixed group of 50 women with vulvodynia, Masheb *et al.* also found that cognitivebehavioral therapy, delivered in an individual format, yielded significantly greater pain reduction and improved sexual function than supportive psychotherapy [5]. In a pilot study, Corsini-Munt *et al.* prospectively examined the preliminary efficacy of a 12-session manualized cognitive behavioral therapy couple intervention in nine couples in which the woman was diagnosed with provoked vestibulodynia [3]. Findings showed significant improvements in women's pain, as well as in sexuality outcomes, pain-related thoughts, anxiety, and depressive symptoms for both members of the couple, in addition to high treatment satisfaction. In an effort to apply third generation cognitive behavioral therapy interventions to provoked vestibulodynia, Brotto and colleagues prospectively evaluated a four-session mindfulness-based, group psychoeducational intervention in an uncontrolled study of 85 women with provoked vestibulodynia [45]. Participants reported significant improvements from pre- to post-treatment in pain self-efficacy, catastrophizing, hypervigilance, as well as sexual distress and pain during gynecological examination. Overall, these studies demonstrate that individual and group psychological treatments represent empirically validated, noninvasive, and safe therapeutic options for provoked vestibulodynia, whereas couple interventions remain to be rigorously assessed using randomized controlled trial designs.

## Predictors of Psychological Treatment Outcome

Very few studies to date have focused on identifying predictors of treatment outcome for psychological approaches to provoked vestibulodynia. One randomized controlled trial comparing cognitive behavioral therapy to a medical management option showed that for the cognitive behavioral therapy condition higher levels of pretreatment fear of pain and catastrophizing predicted higher pain intensity at six-month follow-up, whereas higher levels of pretreatment pain self-efficacy were associated with less pain at follow-up. Psychological factors did not predict sexual functioning outcomes for cognitive-behavioral therapy in this study [46]. This pattern of results suggests that such intra-individual factors may not be the most relevant for understanding women's response to psychological interventions. Given that relationship factors have been found to play an important role in the experience of sexual difficulties associated with provoked vestibulodynia, they may be more meaningful predictors of sexuality outcomes following treatment. It may also be fruitful to examine in future research whether they play a role in mediating change during couple cognitive-behavioral therapy.

## Alternative Treatments

When traditional treatment options fail, some women turn to alternative treatments in an effort to relieve their pain. Two uncontrolled prospective pilot studies showed that participants reported improvements in pain and sexuality after taking part in acupuncture and hypnosis [47, 48]. One randomized wait-list controlled pilot study examined the use of acupuncture in a mixed group of women with vulvodynia [49]. Thirty-six participants were randomly assigned to the acupuncture or to the wait-list control condition. Women who took part in acupuncture received 10 sessions, at a pace of twice weekly for five weeks. At post-treatment, relative to those in the control condition, participants in the acupuncture condition reported significantly less vulvar pain and dyspareunia, as well as significantly greater improvements in sexual function. Considering that acupuncture is devoid of adverse effects, additional controlled studies are warranted.

## Interdisciplinary Treatments

An interdisciplinary model of care is espoused by many experts in the field, as per the recommendations of the Fourth International Consultation on Sexual Medicine for the treatment of vulvodynia [9]. One of the first steps involved in achieving optimal application and success of this model is to educate patients about the interdependency of biomedical, cognitive, affective, behavioral, and relationship factors in the onset and maintenance of their pain. Advantages of this model may include more engaged and hopeful patients and health-care professionals, increased coherence among the various professionals on the treatment team, multiple dimensions of provoked vestibulodynia being targeted simultaneously rather than sequentially, and higher patient treatment satisfaction.

There are only two published, uncontrolled quantitative studies evaluating a multimodal approach to the treatment of provoked vestibulodynia, with both reporting significant improvements in women's sexual function and pain [37, 38]. These multimodal treatments integrated sex therapy and physical therapy in a nonstandardized manner, such that not all participants received the same combination and duration of interventions. Spoelstra *et al.* also provided educational materials, included the partner when possible and appropriate, and in some cases, performed vestibulectomy, all in a stepwise fashion from what was considered to be the "least" to the "most" invasive treatments [37]. A retrospective qualitative study of 29 women with vulvodynia having taken part in a multidisciplinary treatment program suggests that 27 reported a significant benefit, with nine being pain free at post-treatment [50]. This program consisted of psychotherapy, physical therapy, and dietary recommendations. Another study using the same design was conducted among 19 women with vulvodynia who took part in a multimodal treatment comprised of group cognitive behavioral therapy, physical therapy, and regular medical appointments. Results indicated that participants reported increased knowledge and tools to manage their pain, improved psychological well-being, a sense of validation and support, and an enhanced sense of empowerment [51]. These positive and clinically relevant findings emphasize the need for randomized trials aimed at evaluating the efficacy of an integrated approach to care, over and above the efficacy of single modalities, and including a broad range of outcomes. To this effect, more randomized controlled trials assessing the outcome of single modalities, such as pelvic floor physical therapy, are necessary preliminary steps on the path to validate multimodal treatment

## Conclusions

Provoked vestibulodynia is a complex, multifactorial pain condition that results in significant sexual impairment and psychological distress for afflicted women; preliminary evidence suggests partners suffer negative consequences as well. Studies involving both clinical and population-based samples have shown that many psychosocial factors are associated with the onset and maintenance of provoked vestibulodynia, including anxiety, depression, posttraumatic stress disorder, child maltreatment, and other pain-related coping styles, such as catastrophizing, hypervigilance, and lower levels of self-efficacy. Psychological interventions targeting these factors, with a view to reducing pain and improving sexual function, have been shown to be efficacious. These interventions may need to be modulated based on the clinical presentation of the woman or couple. Although less well validated, alternative treatments seem promising and warrant further study given their lack of negative side effects and popular appeal.

## References

1 Aerts L, Bergeron S, Pukall CF, Khalifé. Provoked vestibulodynia: Does pain intensity correlate with sexual dysfunction and dissatisfaction? *J Sex Med*. 2016;13:955.

2 Bergeron S, Khalifé S, Dupuis M, McDuff. A randomized clinical trial comparing group cognitive-behavioral therapy and a topical steroid for women with dyspareunia. *J Consult Clin Psychol*. 2016;84:259.

3 Corsini-Munt S, Bergeron S, Rosen NO, *et al*. Feasibility and preliminary effectiveness of a novel cognitive-behavioral couple therapy for provoked vestibulodynia: A pilot study. *J Sex Med*. 2014; 11:2515.

4 Goldfinger C, Pukall CF, Thibault-Gagnon S, *et al*. Effectiveness of cognitive-behavioral therapy and physical therapy for provoked vestibulodynia: A randomized pilot study. *J Sex Med*. 2016;13:88.

5 Masheb RM, Kerns RD, Lozano C, *et al*. A randomized clinical trial for women with vulvodynia: Cognitive-behavioral therapy vs. supportive psychotherapy. *Pain*. 2009;141:31.

6 Pukall CF, Goldstein AT, Bergeron S, *et al*. Vulvodynia: definition, prevalence, impact, and pathophysiological factors. *J Sex Med*. 2016;13:291–304.

7 Bergeron S, Binik YM, Khalifé S, *et al.* Vulvar vestibulitis syndrome: Reliability of diagnosis and evaluation of current diagnostic criteria. *Obstet Gynecol.* 2001;98:45.

8 Bornstein J, Goldstein AT, Stockdale CK, *et al.* 2015 ISSVD, ISSWSH and IPPS consensus terminology and classification of persistent vulvar pain and vulvodynia. *Obstet Gynecol.* 2016;127:745.

9 Goldstein AT, Pukall CF, Brown C, *et al.* Vulvodynia: Assessment and treatment. *J Sex Med.* 2016;13:572.

10 Pukall CF, Bergeron S, Brown C, *et al.* Recommendations for self-report outcome measures in vulvodynia clinical trials. *Clin J Pain.* 2017;33(8):756.

11 Reed BD, Harlow SD, Sen A, *et al.* Prevalence and demographic characteristics of vulvodynia in a population-based sample. *Am J Obstet Gynecol.* 2012;206:170.e1.

12 Leclerc B, Bergeron S, Brassard A, *et al.* Attachment, sexual assertiveness, and sexual outcomes in women with provoked vestibulodynia and their partners: A mediation model. *Arch Sex Behav.* 2015;44:1561.

13 Crombez G, Dewitte MVE, van Lankveld JJDM. Understanding sexual pain: A cognitive-motivational account. *Pain.* 2010;152:251.

14 Elmerstig E, Wijma B, Berterö C. Why do young women continue to have sexual intercourse despite pain? *J Adolesc Health.* 2008;43:357.

15 Smith KB, Pukall CF. Sexual function, relationship adjustment, and the relational impact of pain in male partners of women with provoked vulvar pain. *J Sex Med.* 2014;11:1283.

16 Smith KB, Pukall CF. A systematic review of relationship adjustment and sexual satisfaction among women with provoked vestibulodynia. *J Sex Res.* 2011;48:166.

17 Smith KB, Pukall CF, Chamberlain SM. Sexual and relationship satisfaction and vestibular pain sensitivity among women with provoked vestibulodynia. *J Sex Med.* 2013;10:2009.

18 Rosen NO, Bergeron S, Sadikaj G, *et al.* Relationship satisfaction moderates the associations between male partner responses and depression in women with vulvodynia: A dyadic daily experience study. *Pain.* 2014;155:1374.

19 Rosen NO, Bergeron S, Sadikaj G, *et al.* Impact of male partner responses on sexual function in women with vulvodynia and their partners: a dyadic daily experience study. *Health Psychol.* 2014;33:823.

20 Rosen NO, Bergeron S, Leclerc B, *et al.* Woman and partner-perceived partner responses predict pain and sexual satisfaction in provoked vestibulodynia (PVD) couples. *J Sex Med.* 2010;7:3715.

21 Bois K, Bergeron S, Rosen NO, *et al.* Sexual and relationship intimacy among women with provoked vestibulodynia and their partners: Associations with sexual satisfaction, sexual function, and pain self-efficacy. *J Sex Med.* 2013;10:2024.

22 Rosen NO, Bois K, Mayrand M, *et al.* Observed and perceived disclosure and empathy are associated with better relationship adjustment and quality of life in couples coping with vulvodynia. *Arch Sex Behav.* 2016;45:1945.

23 Bois K, Bergeron S, Rosen N, *et al.* Intimacy, sexual satisfaction, and sexual distress in vulvodynia couples: An observational study. *Health Psychol.* 2016;35:531.

24 Awada N, Bergeron S, Steben M, *et al.* To say or not to say: Dyadic ambivalence over emotional expression and its associations with pain, sexuality, and distress in couples coping with provoked vestibulodynia. *J Sex Med.* 2014;11:1271.

25 Nguyen R, MacLehose R, Veasley C, *et al.* Comfort in discussing vulvar pain in social relationships among women with vulvodynia. *J Reprod Med.* 2012;57:109.

26 Nguyen RHN, Turner RM, Rydell SA, *et al.* Perceived stereotyping and seeking care for chronic vulvar pain. *Pain Med.* 2013;14:1461.

27 Nguyen RHN, Ecklund AM, MacLehose RF, *et al.* Co-morbid pain conditions and

feelings of invalidation and isolation among women with vulvodynia. *Psychol Health Med.* 2012;17:589.

28 Davis SNP, Bergeron S, Bois K, *et al.* A prospective 2-year examination of cognitive and behavioral correlates of provoked vestibulodynia outcomes. *Clin J Pain.* 2015;31:333.

29 Khandker M, Brady SS, Vitonis AF, *et al.* The influence of depression and anxiety on risk of adult onset vulvodynia. *J Womens Health.* 2011;20:1445.

30 Iglesias-Rios L, Harlow SD, Reed BD. Depression and posttraumatic stress disorder among women with vulvodynia: Evidence from the population-based woman to woman health study. *J Womens Health.* 2015;24:557.

31 Khandker M, Brady SS, Stewart EG, *et al.* Is chronic stress during childhood associated with adult-onset vulvodynia? *J Womens Health.* 2014;23:649.

32 Harlow B, Stewart EG. Adult-onset vulvodynia in relation to childhood violence victimization. *Am J Epidemiol.* 2005;161:871.

33 Leclerc B, Bergeron S, Binik Y, *et al.* History of sexual and physical abuse in women with dyspareunia: Association with pain, psychosocial adjustment, and sexual functioning. *J Sex Med.* 2010;7:971.

34 Corsini-Munt S, Bergeron S, Rosen NO, *et al.* A dyadic perspective on childhood maltreatment for women with provoked vestibulodynia and their partners: associations with pain and sexual and psychosocial functioning. *J Sex Res.* 2017;54(3):308.

35 King M, Rubin R, Goldstein AT. Current uses of surgery in the treatment of genital pain. *Curr Sex Health Rep.* 2014;6:252.

36 Goldstein A, Klingman D, Christopher K, *et al.* Surgical treatment of vulvar vestibulitis syndrome: Outcome assessment derived from a postoperative questionnaire. *J Sex Med.* 2006;3:923.

37 Spoelstra SK, Dijkstra JR, van el MF, *et al.* Long-term results of an individualized, multifaceted, and multidisciplinary therapeutic approach to provoked vestibulodynia. *J Sex Med.* 2011;8:489.

38 Backman G, Widenbrant M, Bohm-Starke N, *et al.* Combined physical and psychosexual therapy for provoked vestibulodynia – An evaluation of a multidisciplinary treatment model. *J Sex Med.* 2008; 45:378.

39 Pukall CF, Mitchell LS, Goldstein AT. Non-medical, medical, and surgical approaches for the treatment of provoked vestibulodynia. *Curr Sex Health Rep.* 2016;8:240.

40 Bergeron S, Corsini-Munt S, Aerts L, *et al.* Female sexual pain disorders: A review of the literature on etiology and treatment. *Curr Sex Health Rep.* 2015;7:159.

41 Pukall CF. Primary and secondary provoked vestibulodynia: A review of overlapping and distinct factors. *Sex Med Rev.* 2016;4:36.

42 Heddini U, Bohm-Starke N, Nilsson K, *et al.* Provoked vestibulodynia – Medical factors and comorbidity associated with treatment outcome. *J Sex Med.* 2012;9:1400.

43 Bergeron S, Binik YM, Khalifé S, *et al.* A randomized comparison of group cognitive-behavioral therapy, surface electromyographic biofeedback, and vestibulectomy in the treatment of dyspareunia resulting from vulvar vestibulitis. *Pain.* 2001;91:297.

44 Bergeron S, Khalife S, Glazer H, *et al.* Surgical and behavioral treatments for vestibulodynia – Two-and-one-half-year follow-up and predictors of outcome. *Obstet Gynecol.* 2008;111:159.

45 Brotto LA, Basson R, Smith KB, *et al.* Mindfulness-based group therapy for women with provoked vestibulodynia. *Mindfulness.* 2015;6:417.

46 Desrochers G, Bergeron S, Khalifé S, *et al.* Provoked vestibulodynia: Psychological predictors of topical and cognitive-behavioral treatment outcome. *Behav Res Ther.* 2010;48:106.

47 Curran S, Brotto L, Fisher H, *et al.* The ACTIV study: Acupuncture treatment in provoked vestibulodynia. *J Sex Med.* 2010;7:981.

48 Pukall C, Kandyba K, Amsel R, *et al.* Effectiveness of hypnosis for the treatment of vulvar vestibulitis syndrome: A preliminary investigation. *J Sex Med.* 2007;4:417.

49 Schlaeger JM, Xu N, Mejta CL, *et al.* Acupuncture for the treatment of vulvodynia: A randomized wait-list controlled pilot study. *J Sex Med.* 2015;12:1019.

50 Munday P, Buchan A, Ravenhill G, *et al.* A qualitative study of women with vulvodynia II. Response to a multidisciplinary approach to management. *J Reprod Med.* 2007;52:19.

51 Brotto LA, Yong P, Smith KB, *et al.* Impact of a multidisciplinary vulvodynia program on sexual functioning and dyspareunia. *J Sex Med.* 2015;12:238.

21

# Musculoskeletal Management of Pelvic and Sexual Pain Disorders

*Sara K. Sauder, Fiona McMahon, and Amy Stein*

### Abstract

The ideal candidate for pelvic floor physical therapy intervention is the patient who has musculoskeletal dysfunction or has been treated by her clinician for pathology but has not experienced pain resolution. The pathophysiology of pelvic floor dysfunction involves disruption to the functional anatomy of the pelvic floor and can be the primary or secondary cause of a range of painful conditions. Pelvic floor physical therapists are important and often essential members of the medical team caring for women with sexual pain.

**Keywords:** *pelvic floor physical therapy; pelvic floor muscle dysfunction; manual therapy; biofeedback; vulvar pain; sexual pain; vulvodynia; sexual dysfunction; women's health physical therapy; vestibulodynia; dyspareunia; pelvic floor muscles*

Ideal candidates for pelvic floor physical therapy referral are pelvic pain patients with musculoskeletal dysfunction or those who have been treated by clinicians for pelvic pathology but have not experienced symptom resolution.

The pathophysiology of pelvic floor dysfunction involves impairment in the functional anatomy of the pelvic floor, which can be the primary or secondary cause of a wide range of painful conditions.

Dysfunction in the myofascial system can result in painful myofascial trigger points and shortened tissues throughout the body, including the pelvic floor. Neural tension, entrapment between structures, or mechanical pressure on nerves can create acute and chronic pain preventing optimal pelvic floor function.

## Introduction

Approximately 50% of all American adults are currently affected by painful musculoskeletal diseases, disorders, or injuries [1]. Furthermore, the musculoskeletal system may contribute to a majority of chronic pelvic and sexual pain symptoms [2, 3]. Over half of the estimated 10 million women with sexual pain go without proper diagnosis or adequate treatment. It is likely that the lack of recognition by medical professionals of pelvic musculoskeletal disorders contributes to this gap in care [4]. Undiagnosed musculoskeletal pain can lead to comorbidities that may make diagnosis and treatment difficult.

Physical therapists (physiotherapists) specialize in the assessment and treatment of functional deficits of the musculoskeletal system. The purpose of physical therapy intervention is to return patients to optimal function. Treatment goals are determined by both the patient and the physical therapist in order to meet the patient's specific needs and goals.

*Textbook of Female Sexual Function and Dysfunction: Diagnosis and Treatment*, First Edition. Edited by Irwin Goldstein, Anita H. Clayton, Andrew T. Goldstein, Noel N. Kim, and Sheryl A. Kingsberg.
© 2018 John Wiley & Sons Ltd. Published 2018 by John Wiley & Sons Ltd.

For example, penetrative sexual intercourse may be an endpoint for one patient but not another.

Specifically, pelvic floor physical therapists focus on structural impairments of the spine, sacrum, hips, pelvis, pelvic floor muscles, connective tissue and nerves. Functional deficits may include difficulty with sitting, standing, or walking; pain or difficulty with sexual activity; and difficulty with bowel and bladder function. The personal and sensitive nature of these complaints, as well as a patient's uncertainty as to the cause of her symptoms, can make it uncomfortable for her to engage in frank discussions with her providers. This hesitancy may lead to a delay in seeking appropriate care, which may, in turn, cause an acute dysfunction to progress to a chronic problem.

Ideal candidates for pelvic floor physical therapy referral are patients with pelvic floor musculoskeletal dysfunction or those who have been treated by clinicians for pelvic pathology but have not experienced symptom resolution. Clinicians can identify appropriate patients by palpating the vulva, performing a digital examination of the vaginal and rectal muscles, and performing a moist cotton swab test on the vestibule. If the patient reports reproduction of any of her sexual pain symptoms with this examination, she is likely affected by pelvic floor dysfunction [5]. Box 21.1 details the recommended components of a pelvic floor muscle screening examination.

Physical therapy begins with a detailed history of a woman's bowel, bladder, and sexual function along with the details of any episodes of pain. The physical therapist determines the possible underlying neural and musculoskeletal factors contributing to a patient's pain, as this informs the objective assessment. For example, if the physical therapist hypothesizes that the spine is involved, then this might be one of the first areas to be examined. Similarly, if the pelvic floor muscles are likely driving the patient's symptoms, then the therapist will prioritize a pelvic floor examination. The evaluation is mainly performed at the first appointment; however, components of the evaluation are likely to extend throughout several follow-up appointments. Classically, the physical therapist assesses and treats at the same time.

Depending on the diagnosis, pelvic floor treatments may last only a few sessions or, for complex symptoms or impairments, they may continue a year or more. Some diagnoses, such as stress incontinence and some types of dyspareunia, do not require more than a few treatments. Treatment of sexual dysfunction, urogenital or pelvic pain, however, may be quite involved and resolution of symptoms may take months or even years. Despite this, in some cases physical therapy can be the most effective means of managing pain over the long term, with the least risk for adverse side effects.

## Pelvic Floor Anatomy

Pelvic floor physical therapists evaluate from the head to the toes, but pay special attention to the area between the diaphragm and knees. Within this area are the spine, pelvic bones, hips, pelvic floor muscles, connective tissue, pelvic nerves, and pelvic organs. The pelvic floor muscles form a sling laterally from one hip joint to the other and anteriorly to posteriorly from pubic symphysis to the sacrum and coccyx (Figure 21.1) Pelvic floor integrity is maintained by proper skeletal alignment and the

---

**Box 21.1 Nantes criteria for the diagnosis of pudendal neuralgia.**

- Pain in the area innervated by the pudendal nerve extending from anus to clitoris.
- Pain is more severe when sitting.
- Pain does not awaken patients from sleep.
- Pain with no objective sensory impairment
- Pain relieved by diagnostic pudendal block.

From Labat JJ [12].

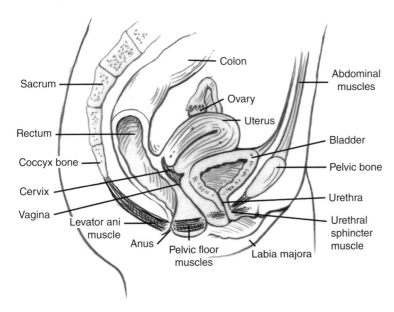

**Figure 21.1** Female urogenital system – mid-sagittal section. Used with permission from Amy Stein, DPT, BCB-PMD, *Heal Pelvic Pain*. New York: McGraw-Hill; 2009 [83].

coordinated actions of pelvic floor muscles, urethral and anal sphincters, lumbosacral plexus, ligaments, and connective tissues (also called the endopelvic fascia) [6].

Striated muscles, connective tissue, and ligaments provide mechanical support for pelvic organs. Pelvic floor muscles are made of Type 1 slow twitch and Type 2 fast twitch skeletal fibers [7]. This multimodal pelvic floor musculature assists with core stability and closure of the urogenital hiatus and is responsible for voluntary control of bowel, bladder, and sexual functions.

The individual pelvic floor muscles have unique clinical characteristics that the pelvic floor physical therapist considers. For example, the ischiocavernosus and bulbospongiosus can cause urinary urgency and frequency that may create distress and reduce interest in intimacy (Figure 21.2) [8]. The transverse perinei muscles are the site of most episiotomies and/or tearing during vaginal delivery. Even after the trauma has healed these muscles may develop significant scarring that can impede muscle expansion and cause pain with penetration. With overactivity or myofascial trigger points, the obturator

internus can contribute to pain with sitting, dyspareunia, and constipation. Spasm of the coccygeus and piriformis may mimic coccyx pain with sitting and sexual activity (Figure 21.3). Additionally, overactivity in muscles surrounding the urethra can create urethral discomfort, dysuria, and incomplete bladder voiding [9].

The pelvic floor muscles are primarily innervated by the pudendal nerve. This is the only nerve in the pelvic area that has motor, sensory and autonomic functions. The pudendal nerve has three branches: the dorsal clitoral, posterior labial (perineal), and inferior rectal. These branches provide sensory, motor, and sympathetic innervation to the vulva and vagina. Injury to the entire nerve or any of its branches may result in urogenital pain, dyspareunia, and female genital arousal disorder. In addition, because of the autonomic functions of the nerve, the patient may experience autonomic symptoms of increased heart rate and blood pressure, digestive difficulties leading to bloating, diarrhea and constipation, urinary symptoms of incomplete emptying and difficulty initiating, and sexual function problems with orgasm

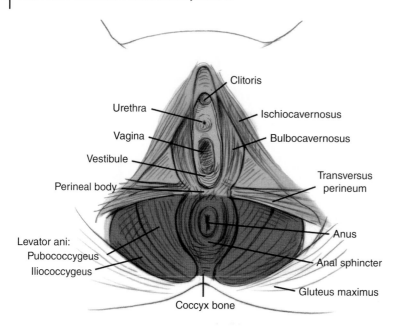

**Figure 21.2** Female pelvic floor anatomy. Used with permission from Amy Stein, DPT, BCB-PMD, *Heal Pelvic Pain*. New York: McGraw-Hill; 2009 [83].

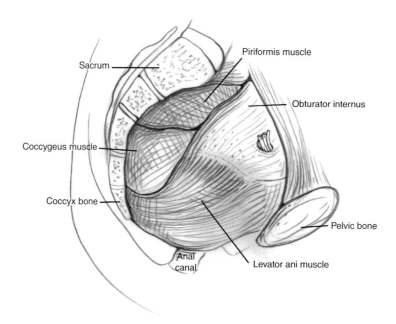

**Figure 21.3** Coccygeus, piriformis, and obturator internus muscles. Used with permission from Amy Stein, DPT, BCB-PMD, *Heal Pelvic Pain*. New York: McGraw-Hill; 2009 [83].

and lubrication [10, 11]. Pudendal nerve pain is often referred to as pudendal neuralgia, which is currently defined by the Nantes criteria (Box 21.1) [12]. Injuries to other nerves also contribute to pelvic and sexual pain [13]. These nerves include the ilioinguinal, iliohypogastric, genitofemoral, and posterior and lateral femoral cutaneous nerves. Careful

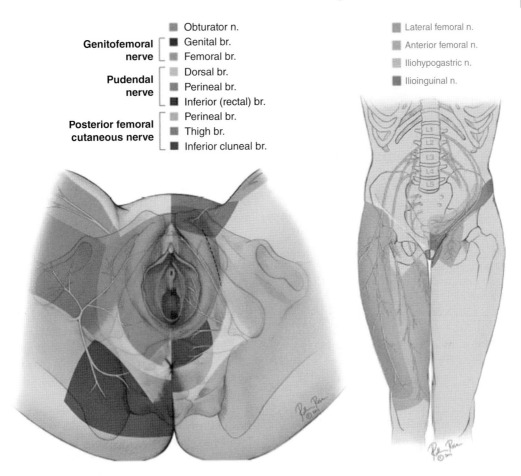

**Figure 21.4** Cutaneous nerves of the vulva, thigh, and groin. Used with permission from A. Lee Dellon, MD, PhD, from www.Dellon.com. (*See plate section for color representation of the figure*)

assessment of the sensory distributions of these nerves is important for effective treatment of pelvic pain syndromes (Figure 21.4).

Connective tissue is a key component of the pelvic floor and covers its structures. It is composed primarily of collagen and elastin. The collagen provides tensile strength, while the elastin provides flexibility [14]. More than 12 types of collagen have been identified in the human body [15]. The main structural components of pelvic connective tissue are Type I and Type III collagen. Type 1 is strong and organized into large fibers; Type III collagen is randomly organized branched fibers and is found in flexible fascia. Fascia is a type of connective tissue that is found throughout the abdominopelvic region.

Damage or an insult to the pelvic floor may injure the connective tissue or fascia, which then may become a primary or a secondary contributor to pelvic and sexual pain disorders, ranging from mild to significant in severity [16].

## Pathophysiology of Sexual Pain

The pathophysiology of pelvic floor dysfunction involves impairment in the functional anatomy of the pelvic floor. This can be the primary or secondary cause of a range of painful conditions. Any process that interrupts the integrity of pelvic neuromusculoskeletal or connective tissue can result in dysfunction of the bowel, bladder, and sexual activity, or problems with core stability or abdominopelvic organ support and function. Pelvic floor impairments leading to sexual pain include overactive pelvic floor muscles, skeletal abnormalities, myofascial restrictions, and inflammation. Neuromusculoskeletal impairments cause somatosensory stimulation that may result in inhibition or excitation of visceral functions; this effect is called the *somatovisceral reflex*. This reflex can cause diffuse pain throughout the pelvis and can contribute to dyspareunia.

The cause of overactive pelvic floor muscles is not always clear. Due to the physiology and biomechanics of the lumbosacropelvic region, muscle overactivity may result from chronic straining, poor postures in the sitting, standing, or toileting positions, dysfunctional gait patterns, previous sexual or physical abuse, or harmful repetitive movements from a sport or work activity. Overactive pelvic floor muscles may also result from childbirth injuries, infection, a traumatic event, cancer-related treatments, and abdominal or pelvic surgery. Autoimmune disorders and inflammatory conditions, including fibromyalgia, ulcerative colitis, interstitial cystitis, inflammatory bowel disorders, and endometriosis, can also contribute to pelvic floor muscle overactivity [7, 17, 18]. Regardless of the initial insult, disruption of appropriate movement patterns results in dysfunctional modifications of the pelvic floor musculature and connective, visceral, and neural tissues [19–21].

Biomechanical abnormalities due to musculoskeletal causes, such as scarring and adhesions, skeletal misalignment, tissue lengthening or shortening, and muscular asymmetry, may be the primary cause of myofascial trigger points, shortened myo-sarcomeres and connective, visceral, and neural restrictions from reduced range of motion [20]. Myofascial trigger points are hyperirritable points or nodules in skeletal muscle that possess high levels of inflammatory mediators and sensitized nociceptors [22].

Myofascial system dysfunction has been shown to be an important contributor to pelvic pain; up to 78% of women with chronic pelvic pain may suffer from some form of myofascial dysfunction [3].

Prolonged pelvic floor muscle contraction due to habit or lack of awareness can also cause myofascial trigger points and restrictions. Detrimental holding patterns may also be secondary to painful or noxious stimuli from various pelvic disorders, such as vulvodynia, vestibulodynia, persistent genital arousal disorder, bladder pain syndrome, irritable bowel syndrome, and incontinence [23]. These conditions contribute to muscle overactivity because of muscle guarding, shortening of skeletal sarcomeres and connective tissue, reduction in the mobility and range of motion of nerves, decreased blood flow, decreased tissue perfusion, and the development of myofascial trigger points [24, 25]. In turn, pelvic floor muscle overactivity can cause or contribute to pain in these disorders.

Muscle and connective tissue abnormalities and myofascial trigger points result in localized, referred, or radiating pain and tenderness [26]. As a result, the affected areas exhibit increased restrictions and decreased mobility, which further perpetuate the pain cycle. Common areas of myofascial pain and trigger points are in the back, thigh, gluteal, abdominal, and pelvic floor muscles. Altered connective tissue tension may result in tissue hypoxia leading to sensations of burning, itching, tingling, cold, shooting, and/or sharp pain [20, 27, 28]. Additionally, overactive pelvic floor muscles cause decreased blood flow through both muscle and mucosa, leading to hypoxia and excessive lactic acid production.

Chronic muscle overactivity can also affect the pannicular layer of fascia by limiting its mobility, creating pain with small movements. Fascia is sensitive due to its innervation and vascular supply. Fascial restrictions secondary to surgical trauma, limited muscle expansion, or scarring may limit movement that can lead to pain. Restrictions of the deepest layer of fascia, the visceral layer, can create widespread abdominopelvic pain and/or ambiguous or difficult to reproduce pain. An assessment of the fascial layers is performed in a physical therapy examination to determine if there is a visceral component to a patient's sexual pain [29].

Decreased mobility of the pelvic viscera due to adhesions and fascial restrictions may result in pain or altered function of the organ itself, as well as spasms in adjacent muscular tissue that further perpetuate the pain. The body may also perform compensatory movements to accommodate a reduced range of motion in a restricted organ system, exacerbating or creating additional musculoskeletal dysfunction [30]. Inflammatory visceral conditions can cause viscerosomatic reflexes that trigger visceral and nociceptive afferent neurons that contribute to myospasticity and palpable pelvic tissue texture changes [28]. The result is somatic dysfunction and potential nervous system upregulation [31, 32].

An upregulated nervous system, including central and peripheral sensitization, is common in patients with chronic pelvic and sexual pain. Central sensitization results from changes in the brain and spinal cord related to an increase in nociceptive sensitivity. These changes can be captured through electrophysiological and imaging techniques. Increases in excitability of the synaptic neurons in central nociceptive pathways result in hypersensitivity, hyperalgesia, and allodynia [33]. Peripheral sensitization is a form of functional plasticity of the nociceptor and results in increased sensitivity of peripheral nerve endings. The nociceptor becomes hypersensitive because the action potential of impaired nerve endings is decreased; therefore, a smaller stimulus is able to initiate a pain signal. Both of these types of upregulation of the nervous system may contribute to provoked and unprovoked sexual pain.

Hormonal deficiencies are a common cause of sexual pain in women of all ages. Any pharmaceutical agent or endocrine disorder that affects local sex hormone levels has the potential to create vulvovaginal pain [34].

An extensive discussion of this topic is given in Chapter 22. Specifically, decreased levels of estrogen and testosterone in the pelvic tissues may increase pain by causing epidermal thinning, leading to reduced pliability, tearing, inflammation, and infection. It is important for the pelvic floor physical therapist to recognize these findings and communicate them to the appropriate medical professional on the patient's team. Additionally, recognition of hormonal changes affecting the vulvovaginal tissues helps the therapist better qualify expectations and prognosis when counseling the patient.

## Musculoskeletal Evaluation

The authors believe that examining the external and internal pelvic neuromusculoskeletal structures and the pelvic floor is a necessary component of a routine pelvic examination. Box 21.2 summarizes a minimal screening examination for nonphysical therapists. A musculoskeletal evaluation is especially recommended prior to a diagnostic laparoscopy or hysterectomy in patients undergoing these procedures for chronic pelvic pain of unknown cause [4, 35]. In a recent study of almost 4000 women who had hysterectomies for chronic pelvic pain, fewer than 25% had endometriosis at the time of surgery. In those with a preoperative diagnosis of endometriosis, almost half did not actually have endometriosis at surgery [36]. In those patients without a clear surgical explanation for their pelvic pain, musculoskeletal causes may not have been adequately assessed pre-operatively, resulting in a treatment intervention that was likely to be inappropriate and ineffective.

A pelvic floor physical therapist's evaluation begins with an extensive subjective history taking, focusing on the patient's past and current pain symptoms, as well as bowel, bladder, and sexual function. It is imperative to uncover not just the current pain symptoms but also the symptoms present when sexual dysfunction began. The physical

---

**Box 21.2  Minimal screening pelvic floor neuromuscular examination for nonphysical therapists.**

Specific attention vaginally and/or rectally to evaluate muscles for:

- visible surface scarring
- tenderness
- tension: high, low, normal
- ability of patient to consciously release tight muscles
- tight muscle or connective tissue bands
- symmetry, hypertrophy, or atrophy.

Structures to include in evaluation:

- superficial vulvar muscles
- anal sphincter

- levator ani muscles
- obturator internus muscles
- ischial spine, for Tinel's sign at pudendal nerve
- ilio-inguinal, ilio-hypogastric and genitofemoral nerves at lower abdomen
- sacroiliac joints
- lumbosacral spine
- pubic symphysis
- groin
- observation of gait that may be abnormal with hip disorders.

---

therapist must ask questions that may initially appear unrelated to a patient's pain complaints. Determining bladder and bowel health status in a woman with sexual dysfunction is necessary because the pelvic floor muscles, connective tissue, vasculature, lymphatics and blood flow that are essential for normal sexual function also affect the bladder and bowels. Additionally, obtaining a history of any injuries is crucial to assist in determining if, for instance, a hernia or hip labral tear could be contributing to a woman's sexual pain complaints. Box 21.3 shows recommended questions to include in a physical therapy evaluation.

A thorough neuromusculoskeletal examination is then performed to determine if there are one or more underlying impairments causing the symptoms of sexual pain. This examination includes assessment of the bony alignment of the spine, pelvis, and hips in addition to assessment of muscles, connective tissues, and nerves. Muscle function is assessed through examination of length, tension, strength, endurance, and coordination. The primary muscles evaluated are the pelvic floor, hip, and core muscles, with other muscle groups examined as needed. An assessment of the fascial layers is also performed. Pelvic alignment is assessed for

symmetry to be sure that the muscles have appropriate and balanced tension to allow for optimal function. Improper pull of pelvic musculature secondary to pelvic obliquities will irritate nerves and affect blood and lymphatic vessels that, in turn, can create pain symptoms.

Inadequate hip range of motion, labral tears, or improper glide or impingement of the greater trochanter in the acetabulum may cause pelvic and sexual pain symptoms that seem unrelated to the actual hip joint; thus the hip needs to be specifically assessed [37]. Without a proper hip range of motion and joint stabilization, other muscle groups attempt to compensate [38]. This may lead to muscle overactivity in the pelvic floor, which may cause sexual dysfunction and sexual pain complaints.

Nerves are assessed via spinal joint mobilization, palpation, neural tensioning, and body mapping. The pelvic floor physical therapist determines if the source of nerve pain is at the spine by mobilizing spinal joints. The opening or closing of a spinal facet joint during flexion or extension can create pain along the distal distribution of a nerve [39]. Additionally, gentle percussion of a nerve is informative if it reproduces a patient's pain; this is a positive Tinel's sign [40]. Neural tension testing

---

**Box 21.3 Physical therapy evaluation questions.**

1) Do you have any urinary or fecal incontinence or difficulty controlling flatulence?
2) Do you have strong urinary or fecal urges?
3) Do triggers like running water or getting home from being out give you a sudden, intense urge to urinate?
4) When your urine/stool flow stops, does it feel as if your bladder/bowel is empty?
5) Does your urine flow straight into the toilet, curve to the side or does it hit your thigh or anus?
6) How frequently do you urinate during the day? Night?
7) Is urination or defecation uncomfortable or painful?
8) Do you have any vulvovaginal or anal itching or burning?
9) With sexual activity, do you have pain at penetration, deep pain or postorgasmic pain?
10) Do you have or have you had painful periods? When did it start and has it gotten better or worse?
11) Touch where your discomfort is. Does it change?
12) How do you cleanse your vulvovaginal area?
13) Have you had a hysterectomy or any other abdominopelvic surgery?
14) Are your ovaries intact?
15) When did your discomfort begin? Is it intermittent or constant?
16) If you were once able to orgasm, can you orgasm now? What stimulates an orgasm for you?
17) Is your discomfort constant?
18) What makes your discomfort better? Worse?
19) What is the lowest your discomfort gets on a scale of 1/10? What is the highest your discomfort gets on a scale of 1/10?
20) Do you think you will be able to resolve this discomfort?
21) What do you think is going on?
22) Does stress change your discomfort?
23) What medications are you taking? Any hormonal contraception or hormonal therapy?
24) Have you had an injury to your back, hip, or pelvis? What sports have you participated in?

---

involves placing a specific nerve into a state of tension to see if this reproduces a patient's pain complaint [41]. The nerve is then placed in a position of laxity via movement of a distal component, such as the head or foot, to assess whether the pain is reduced. This helps the therapist distinguish between either the muscle or the nerve as the source of the pain. Body mapping is a helpful means of assessing if a sexual pain runs along the course of a nerve [40]. The therapist compares the pain distribution to a dermatomal map to identify which nerves or spinal levels need to be addressed. Figure 21.4 shows cutaneous nerves of the vulva, thigh, and groin.

The pelvic floor physical therapist performs a brief vulvar screening examination in order to rule out intrinsic vulvar pathology. This includes retraction of the clitoral prepuce to assess for phimosis, separation and examination between the labia, and assessment of the vestibule for pain, allodynia, and inflammation. The physical therapist may consult with dermatology, gynecology, or urology colleagues if there are signs of pathology.

With patient consent, the therapist then performs an internal examination of the vagina and/or the rectum, depending on the patient's subjective history and complaints. The internal assessment allows the physical therapist to determine the health of the vaginal tissue and pelvic floor muscles [4, 20]. The therapist determines if the vaginal walls are supple and well lubricated or nonpliable, dry, and friable. Muscle tone and mobility is determined via gentle digital pressure into each muscle and gentle gliding across muscle fibers. The therapist assesses if the muscles are tense or lax and determines the presence or absence of discrete trigger points and tender points within specific muscles of the pelvic floor. As the patient bears down, the therapist evaluates the anterior, posterior, and lateral vaginal walls for laxity and the likelihood of pelvic organ prolapse, and assesses whether the patient is able to contract, relax, and lengthen the pelvic floor. The therapist also determines if a patient's pain complaint is reproducible. As mentioned previously, the pelvic floor muscles are capable of producing symptoms that mimic those from an organ or different area of the body. Without proper palpation, this important information would be missed.

## Physical Therapy Treatment of Pelvic and Sexual Pain Disorders

Evidence-based literature supporting the effectiveness of pelvic floor physical therapy for pelvic and sexual pain disorders is steadily increasing. Like research on other hands-on therapeutic modalities, studies have been hindered by the challenge of creating standardized treatment regimens and appropriate control and sham physical therapy groups. Despite this, emerging research has demonstrated the benefit of physical therapy in various pain syndromes, such as chronic low back pain and fibromyalgia, as well as pelvic floor dysfunction [42–44].

Research studies and expert opinion support the efficacy of physical therapy interventions for pelvic and sexual pain. In a study conducted by Anderson and colleagues, participants significantly reduced their use of pain medication over baseline following instruction in a self-trigger point release protocol using a therapeutic wand [45]. Additionally, Gentilcore-Saulnier demonstrated that pelvic floor physical therapy improved pelvic floor muscle control in women with pelvic pain symptoms [46]. In other studies, participants with provoked

vulvodynia had significant improvement in sexual pleasure and reduced pain with intercourse following physical therapy interventions or vulvar desensitization exercises in combination with cognitive behavioral therapy [47, 48]. Additional research supporting the use of pelvic floor physical therapy for the treatment of pelvic and sexual pain shows significant improvement in sexual function, anxiety, and pain intensity during intercourse [7, 44, 49–51]. Moreover, pelvic floor physical therapy is recommended by experts for the treatment of vulvodynia and interstitial cystitis/painful bladder syndrome [52–54].

Physical therapy intervention for the dysfunctional pelvic floor incorporates a comprehensive approach addressing specific tissue characteristics, strength, alignment, and neuromuscular control. Manual therapy is a hands-on approach to correct tissue restrictions, improve alignment, and enhance blood flow. Different manual techniques may be used to achieve different objectives. The manual physical therapy techniques covered in this chapter are myofascial release, joint mobilization, neural mobilization, scar tissue mobilization, visceral manipulation, and vestibule desensitization. Nonmanual techniques discussed include behavioral modifications, stress and anxiety management, exercise training, breathing practice, and bowel and bladder retraining. Adjunctive physical therapy modalities are also reviewed.

## Physical Therapy Treatment Techniques

### Myofascial Release and Trigger Point Release

As referenced in the pathophysiology section, myofascial and connective tissue restrictions and myofascial trigger points are common findings in pelvic and sexual pain disorders. Therefore, it is essential to address these findings as a first line of physical therapy treatment. The myofascia is a system of connective tissue that envelops all of the body's muscles and bones. Dysfunction in this system can result in painful myofascial trigger points and shortened tissues throughout the body, including the pelvic floor. The physical therapist identifies restrictions and trigger points by palpating for a local twitch response, for changes in myofascial tissue mobility, for tenderness and/or for referring pain. The myofascial release technique involves finding restrictions or lack of movement in tissues and then applying gentle pressure and stretch to these tissues. Myofascial trigger point release uses compression on the tender area or nodule and applying a sustained hold into the superficial or deep musculature. Both techniques assist in normalizing tissue mobility and the length-tension ratio of the sarcomeres [55, 56].

## Joint Mobilization

In cases of pelvic floor dysfunction, it is important to assess the range of motion in the joints of the spine, sacroiliac joints, and hips. Dysfunction in these joints can perpetuate dysfunction within the pelvic floor [57]. Joint mobilization is indicated when there is pain or lack of motion at a joint. The physical therapist distinguishes between physiologic motion of the joint and accessory motion of the joint. Physiologic motion is the grossly observable motion of the joint; an example is flexion of the hip joint. Accessory motion is the motion of the joint surfaces in relationship to one another. In the example of hip flexion, the accessory motion is the downward glide of the femoral head relative to the acetabulum. To improve range of movement, the therapist treats a restricted accessory motion to enhance the physiologic motion of the joint [58]. In a meta-analysis, Hing showed that joint mobilization with movement techniques is effective in decreasing pain in addition to increasing limb strength and range of motion of joints [59]. Joint mobilization has also been shown to act on the sympathetic nervous system, reducing sympathetic activity as measured by changes in heart rate, skin conductance, and blood pressure [60].

## Neural Mobilization

Several nerves provide sensory innervation to the pelvic floor, with the pudendal nerve providing autonomic, motor, and sensory innervation. In order to avoid irritation, nerves require adequate mobility through surrounding anatomical structures. Neural tension (the reduction in nerve mobility), entrapment between structures, or mechanical pressure on nerves can create acute and chronic pain that prevent optimal function of the pelvic floor. Treating the mechanical causes of neural tension is an objective of neural mobilization [61]. The physical therapist also treats the surrounding tissue to clear restrictions and ensure adequate blood flow to the nerve.

## Scar Tissue Mobilization

Scars within the pelvic and abdominal region may cause pain by preventing the proper movement of the pelvic and abdominal viscera, muscles, nerves, and fascia. Scar mobilization requires gentle movement of the scar to prevent and treat adhesions both at the surface and in deeper layers of the tissue [62]. Care is taken to avoid placing pressure directly on top of the scar during the proliferative phase of healing, so as to not stimulate the development of keloid scar tissue.

## Visceral Manipulation

Visceral manipulation restores an organ's ability to glide freely among adjacent structures in order to reduce pain and improve function. The research of Jean-Pierre Barral suggests that visceral manipulation may increase local serotonin, activity of smooth muscle, and local tissue metabolism [30]. Due to the complex interaction of the pelvic organs and pelvic muscles, visceral manipulation has the potential to offer profound relief to patients with pelvic floor dysfunction [63]. In a 2007 study, visceral manipulation significantly improved sexual function and quality of life in women experiencing vulvodynia [64].

## Vestibule Desensitization

Vestibule desensitization is a process in which the patient is presented with increasing mechanical pressure to the vestibule in order to increase the mechanical pain threshold. This allows her to experience vestibule palpation outside of the sexual experience. With this intervention, anxiety and fear that might come with intimacy are removed. This allows the patient to experience a potentially noxious stimulus without the expectation of penetration. A stimulus is first provided via gentle vestibule pressure with a moist cotton swab. As the patient accommodates to this mechanical input, it is no longer painful. She can then progress towards increased pressure at the vestibule and the vagina.

Cognitive behavioral therapy is an adjunct in the process of vulvar desensitization. It can help women manage fear of and response to pain. In a 2015 study, the use of vulvar desensitization techniques in combination with cognitive behavioral therapy produced significant improvement in the McCoy Female Sexuality Questionnaire, sexual pleasure, and vaginal lubrication [48].

## Bowel and Bladder Retraining

Pelvic floor muscle dysfunction can cause difficulty with bowel and bladder voiding, resulting in urgency, frequency, the sensation of incomplete emptying, postvoid dribbling, and incontinence [65, 66]. In the authors' experience, patients may engage in habits such as "just in case voiding", which can contribute to urgency and frequency and interfere with relaxed, pleasurable sexual activity. In addition, women with pelvic floor muscle overactivity may have difficulty with bowel function, leading to constipation, bloating, constipation, anal fissures, and the feeling of incomplete evacuation [41].

Working to remedy these dysfunctions is a key goal in the treatment of pelvic floor dysfunction.

Bowel and bladder retraining techniques encompass education and behavior modification to reduce urge and frequency. In addition to manual interventions, patients with bowel and bladder frequency are taught to gradually increase their intervoid interval. Therapists may teach interventions that help calm bowel and bladder urge, such as mental distraction, diaphragmatic breathing, and quick pelvic floor contractions.

## Exercise Training

Exercise improves mood and builds confidence and self-efficacy in women living with chronic pelvic pain [67]. Physical therapists evaluate their patients' current physical abilities and tolerances in order to create an effective and safe exercise plan. Exercise can retrain faulty movement patterns and strengthen weak muscles, which can improve the stability of the pelvic girdle.

## Breathing Practices

Breathing practice is a vital component of pelvic and sexual pain rehabilitation. Deep diaphragmatic breaths facilitate mobilization of the pelvic and abdominal contents and can reduce the anxiety experienced by many patients. Additionally, it is a tool to minimize pain [68, 69]. Physical therapists may work closely with mind–body practice instructors as patients may gain additional pain reduction benefits from therapies focusing on controlled breathing such as yoga, tai chi, qi gong, and meditation [70].

## Adjunctive Modalities

Many modalities can be used as adjuncts to the manual, strengthening, and neuromuscular interventions employed by pelvic floor physical therapists. They can aid in pain reduction, strengthening, and muscular coordination. In the authors' opinion, these modalities should not, however, be the sole interventions employed for patients with pelvic floor dysfunction.

## Biofeedback

Biofeedback allows the patient to assess the activity of her muscles in real time. Electromyography (EMG) biofeedback is commonly used to display the activity of muscles with digital feedback using a visual or auditory medium. Biofeedback can help patients learn when they are effectively performing pelvic floor muscle activation or relaxation, thereby allowing them to break the cycle of pain and reactive spasm [71]. In cases where pelvic floor muscle strength should be increased, biofeedback can give the patient feedback on the quality of their active pelvic floor muscle contractions. Whether a patient needs strengthening or relaxation, it is the authors' experience that she must have enough myofascial mobility to perform contraction and relaxation of the pelvic floor. Poor myofascial mobility may prevent her from successfully using biofeedback and increase her frustration.

## Vaginal Dilator and Wand use

Dilators and wands are tools that can stretch shortened pelvic floor tissues and muscles. They can also be used for vulvovaginal desensitization. Dilators are made from different materials, including silicone, plastic, and glass, that affect both their rigidity and slipperiness. Some patients may find softer silicone dilators more comfortable and others may opt for a more rigid variety. For patients suffering from introital dyspareunia, vestibulodynia, and vaginismus, dilators help to continue manual treatment and desensitization of pelvic tissues in between physical therapy visits. Dilators come in different diameters and are often sold as a set. If the patient's goal is to accommodate a partner's penis or a sex toy, she will gradually and progressively increase the size of dilators until a size similar to her goal is reached.

Women affected by cancer may have anatomic alterations in their vagina and surrounding myofascia due to surgery and/or pelvic radiation therapy; these changes often cause sexual pain and interfere with sexual function [37]. Vaginal dilators help to maintain or regain vaginal length and capacity. Success with these tools, especially in irradiated patients, may be higher with the help of a pelvic floor physical therapist.

Pelvic floor physical therapists may prescribe the use of dilators and wands in various ways for different functions. A patient with deep layer trigger points in muscles such as the coccygeus and obturator internus may benefit from sigmoid shaped pelvic wands, which allow her to more easily reach trigger points and myofascial restrictions deep within the pelvic bowl.

## Ultrasound

Ultrasound uses low frequency and intensity sound waves to generate thermal effects in treated tissue. The effects of ultrasound may improve blood flow and stimulate healing. Currently, the available research shows conflicting evidence on the effectiveness of ultrasound in the treatment of musculoskeletal pain disorders [72–74]. There are no trials that address the use of ultrasound for the treatment of overactive pelvic floor muscle dysfunction or pelvic pain. Therefore, the uncertain therapeutic benefit must be weighed against the cost of treatment when determining whether or not to use ultrasound.

## Electrical Stimulation

Electrical stimulation has two functions. At low intensities, electrical stimulation may be used for pain relief by blocking pain signals from reaching the brain; this is the mechanism of transcutaneous electrical stimulation. At higher intensities, electrical stimulation stimulates weak muscles to contract. Effective electrical stimulation for the treatment of pelvic pain can be done by placing leads over the S2-4 spinal levels [75]. Other options for lead placement include the T12-L2 spinal level and even as high as T6-T7. It is important that the physical therapist works closely with the patient to educate her and incorporate her feedback when deciding on lead placement for pelvic pain management.

### Dry Needling

In some states in the United States, physical therapists may legally perform dry needling. Dry needling is the insertion of thin monofilament needles, as used in the practice of acupuncture, into myofascial trigger points and other myofascial structures, to treat painful musculoskeletal disorders. The insertion of needles into trigger points can generate a local twitch response. It is hypothesized that the local twitch response provides a strong input back into the nervous system, which can break the cycle of holding, tension, and irritability within that trigger point [76]. Other hypotheses involve cholinergic, serotonergic, and endogenous opioid pathways [77]. In the pelvic floor muscles, dry needling is used on myofascial trigger points and tender points that have not responded to manual physical therapy.

### Mind–Body Practices

Physical therapists can help guide patients towards central and peripheral desensitization through progressive relaxation and guided imagery. The physical therapist can teach deep diaphragmatic breathing and can also emphasize the benefits of mind–body practices such as tai chi and yoga. All of these techniques downregulate the nervous system, so that patients can tolerate treatment more easily. Cardiovascular exercise, positive thinking, and proper sleep hygiene are other downregulating practices. This approach, in combination with physical therapy for tissue and biomechanical dysfunctions, is an effective biopsychosocial strategy for the pelvic pain patient. Hilton and Vandyken state, "Neurodynamic treatment, imagery, dynamic movement, theories, and cognitive behavioral approaches blend together with careful manual techniques to provide a treatment approach that is truly biopsychosocial and complies with the key tenants of the Neuromatrix Theory of pain." [78].

### Home Exercise Programs

Home exercise programs are essential to patients' success in physical therapy. A home program accelerates a patient's progress between physical therapy visits and empowers her to prevent symptom reoccurrence after discharge. Home exercise programs are individualized and consist of a combination of education and exercises to improve pain and sexual response.

## Treatments with Physician Collaboration

If a patient's pelvic pain or sexual dysfunction is recalcitrant and physical therapy techniques are not sufficient to eliminate symptoms, collaboration with a physician is necessary. The physician can prescribe oral medications that reduce muscle overactivity, anxiety, and neuropathic pain. The use of low-dose vaginal or rectal diazepam suppositories may also assist in relaxing an overactive pelvic floor [79]. Physicians may provide trigger point injections or dry needling of myofascial trigger points. In patients with severe pelvic floor muscle overactivity, botulinum toxin injections into specific resistant muscles may be useful [80]. The therapist may enhance the proposed treatment by attending the physician visit with the patient and demonstrating and confirming the areas in the pelvic floor that may benefit from these strategies.

## Treatment for Specific Sexual Pain Diagnoses

Sexual pain may stem from a combination of the following impairments: pelvic floor muscle overactivity, scarring, local or widespread inflammation, chronic infection, neural tension, abnormal breathing patterns, connective tissue restrictions, musculoskeletal abnormalities, or nervous system sensitization. Additionally, visceral diagnoses, such as interstitial cystitis or painful bladder syndrome, may be misdiagnosed or lumped into a cluster of diagnoses for sexual pain. As such, physical therapy interventions for sexual pain often need to systematically address more than one impairment at a time, and care is individualized for each patient.

## Vaginismus

Vaginismus is a commonly misunderstood sexual pain diagnosis. This disorder results from the combination of overactivity and spasm of the pelvic floor muscles and anxiety about impending touch/penetration of the vulva and vagina.

In women with vaginismus, the pelvic floor physical therapist typically does not do an internal examination or internal treatment for the first several appointments. The first few treatments may consist of developing trust with the patient, teaching her about her genital anatomy, external biofeedback, and manual work away from the vulva. In addition, the patient can be taught to do home exercises to relax her pelvic floor muscles using stretches, breathing techniques, and patient-initiated dilator use with a long-stemmed moist cotton swab.

Internal examination and internal manual therapy is only appropriate once the patient gives consent and when she can attain a relaxed state in treatments. This is

---

### Case 1

Sara is a 19-year-old female reporting inability to wear a tampon, undergo a gynecological examination, or have vaginal penetration with a finger or penis without severe pain. She reports she has never been able to insert anything into her vagina since her first attempt to do so at age 12.

**Examination** is remarkable for:

- patient displays adductor tension and uncontrolled pelvic floor muscles spasms with visual assessment of vulva;
- normal appearing genitalia;
- normal appearing hymen;
- diffuse pain throughout the posterior vestibule with a moist cotton swab but no significant pain lateral to the urethral meatus;
- inability to perform internal vaginal examination with therapist's finger;
- connective tissue restrictions at entire bony pelvis, bilateral adductors, and abdomen;
- right side pelvic innominate posteriorly rotated with right sacral side bend;
- hip and leg length normal.

**Assessment:** significant pelvic floor, adductor, and abdominal muscle overactivity

contributes to connective tissue restriction. These impairments are possibly leading to patient's pain in the posterior vestibule. Internal vaginal examination is not appropriate at this time secondary to the patient's inability to relax during evaluation.

**Treatment:**

- correct structural abnormalities of pelvis;
- scar massage to left side perineum and superficial vagina;
- treat pelvic floor muscle overactivity and tissue restrictions with manual therapy and via EMG biofeedback with relaxation exercises and diaphragmatic breathing and then progress to internal manual treatment techniques;
- treat connective tissue restrictions;
- educate patient in dilator home program and progress to larger dilator sizes

**Outcome:**

After twelve sessions, once a week, patient is able to use a medium plus dilator, use a tampon, and undergo gynecological examination with minimal to no discomfort.

demonstrated by a calm appearance on her face, a decrease in her attempts to adduct her thighs, and a reduction in the appearance of pelvic floor muscle spasms that are obvious by merely looking at the vulva. Additional treatments for the patient with vaginismus include a vaginal dilator program in which she uses progressively larger dilators, internal manual work with parameters that put the patient in charge of her discomfort, and biofeedback to retrain pelvic floor muscle and diaphragm holding patterns. If the patient has an intimate partner, it is key to bring the partner into treatment for education on the diagnosis, what they can do to help, and what they can expect during intimacy now and in the future. In cases in which psychosocial factors remain a significant barrier to patient progression, a referral for cognitive behavioral therapy is warranted.

## Vulvodynia

Vulvodynia is defined as vulvar pain of at least three months' duration, without clear identifiable cause, which may have potential associated factors [81]. Pelvic floor physical therapists treat vulvodynia based on what they discern is the neuromusculoskeletal root of the pain. If vulvar pain stems from a neuropathic origin, the therapist will assess the course of the involved nerve to determine if the pain is initiated proximally or distally. For example, in a patient who has a lumbar facet joint that restricts flexion, extension, or rotation, this restriction can create irritation along the entire route of the genitofemoral nerve. As the genitofemoral nerve innervates part of the vulva, it may be the source of the vulvodynia. An appropriate musculoskeletal assessment of the lumbar spine will reveal this to the therapist. Intervention options for correcting difficulty of spinal facet movement at a specific segment or segments will include either using a muscle contraction that will create movement in a joint, forced mobilization of the facet, or manipulation of the joint itself.

The pelvic floor muscles typically are contracted with minimal relaxation when the body is experiencing chronic pelvic pain, causing residual effects along an involved nerve. It is theorized that this is a protective mechanism, perhaps as a means of guarding reproductive organs. Therefore, it is often necessary to treat the muscle and fascia of the vulva in cases of neurogenic pain. In the above example, even after the dysfunction at the L1-L2 facet has resolved, the downstream sequelae of overactive pelvic floor muscles may not resolve spontaneously and may require intervention. The physical therapist must then use the techniques mentioned above to return the pelvic floor muscles to normal function.

Physical therapists teach their patients to perform active pelvic floor muscle relaxation exercises through breathing techniques and stretches in order to maintain the effects of physical therapy. In the above example, if the original upper lumbar dysfunction was created as a result of a repeated behavioral habit, such as a poor sleeping or sitting position, then these habits will be addressed and retrained.

This is an example of how to treat just one case of vulvodynia. Because sexual pain symptoms may superficially appear similar in different patients, it is imperative for the pelvic floor physical therapist to determine the root cause(s) of pain for each individual patient.

## Vestibulodynia

Under the umbrella of the vulvodynia classification is the more specific diagnosis of vestibulodynia, the term for pain confined to the vulvar vestibule. The vestibule, which is embryologically derived from the endoderm, is different from the rest of the vulva lateral to Hart's line (ectoderm) and from the vagina (mesoderm). It is this embryologic difference that underlies the vestibule's specific susceptibility to a sexual pain syndrome, emphasizing the need for proper examination of the vestibule.

## Case 2

Beth is a 42-year-old female reporting pain at left side of perineum during intercourse for one year. She reports a 5/10 "burning pain" with initial penetration, which worsens to 7/10 with repeated thrusting; it is not affected by bowel or bladder patterns. Sometimes she notices minimal amounts of bright red blood on her toilet paper when wiping after sex. Patient is still able to orgasm, but orgasms are shorter and less enjoyable and after orgasm she feels a strong urge to urinate. Patient also states she has pain with sitting which started after the birth of her second child.

**Exam** is remarkable for:

- negative moist cotton swab test of the vestibule;
- reproduction of symptoms with palpation of left side superficial and deep transverse perineal muscles;
- evidence of scarring of the perineum from a healed episiotomy extending towards the left;
- pelvic floor muscles globally overactive and tender to palpation; however, palpation does not reproduce patient's pain during intercourse;
- restriction in connective tissue mobility at entire bony pelvis;
- left side of pelvis (innominate bone) is elevated and coccyx is deviated to the left and side bent left;
- hip and leg length normal.

**Assessment:** scarring on the left side of perineum secondary to a episiotomy during her second vaginal delivery which extends into the vagina. This creates pain and tearing upon stretching during penetration and thrusting because of limited tissue mobility. Pelvic floor muscles are overactive due to this scarring and recurrent pain experienced from penetration. Because pelvic floor muscles are never completely relaxed they are weak. Therefore, the rhythmic contraction of these muscles during orgasms is not as strong and the orgasms are perceived as "muted". In addition, the inability of the pelvic floor muscles to relax after orgasm produces intense urinary urge sensations as the overactive pelvic floor muscles and fascia apply an external pull and pressure on the bladder.

**Treatment:**

- correct structural abnormalities in pelvis and coccyx;
- massage of the episiotomy scar tissue;
- treat pelvic floor muscle overactivity;
- treat connective tissue restrictions;
- educate patient in dilator home program.

**Outcome:**
After six weekly sessions, she no longer has pain with intercourse and has minimal and intermittent pain with sitting. Orgasms have returned to her pre-morbid intensity and satisfaction levels; no intense urinary urges occur after orgasm.

## Neuroproliferation-Associated Vestibulodynia

In a patient with vestibulodynia, it is necessary for the pelvic floor physical therapist to determine if she has had lifelong pain at the vestibule or if it is of new onset. The therapist must also determine if the patient has a history of inflammatory issues, such as a severe allergic reactions or chronic vulvovaginal candidiasis. A history of chronic inflammation or lifelong introital pain suggests vestibulodynia caused by a proliferation of nociceptors in the vestibular mucosa. In vestibulodynia resulting from neuroproliferative changes, allodynia will be present throughout the entire vestibule when examined with a moist cotton swab [82].

Patients with neuroproliferative vestibulodynia benefit from interventions that reduce the physical changes resulting from chronic pain. These interventions may include pelvic floor muscle relaxation, pelvic and skeletal alignment corrections, hip mobilizations, movement retraining, retraining of breathing patterns, connective tissue manipulation, and trigger point releases. In most cases of neuroproliferative vestibulodynia, the patient may benefit from consultation with a physician for further management, such as topical capsaicin or vulvar vestibulectomy. If a patient subsequently has a vestibulectomy, a postoperative pelvic floor physical therapy assessment is crucial to identify and reduce any remaining myofascial dysfunction.

### Vestibulodynia Caused By Overactive Muscles

Overactive pelvic floor muscles may also cause allodynia of the vulvar vestibule. However, in contrast to neuroproliferative vestibulodynia, women with vestibulodynia secondary to overactive pelvic floor muscles (specifically the puborectalis and pubococcygeus muscles) have pain only in the posterior vestibule [82]. In addition, it is important to educate the patient that the hypoxia and the resulting increase in lactic acid caused by the underlying overactive pelvic floor muscles induce a superficial burning in the vestibular mucosa. This is especially important as the allodynia at the vestibule "does not feel like a tight muscle" to most patients. The pelvic floor physical therapist may or may not notice a lifelong pattern of discomfort with attempted vaginal penetration be it sexual or nonsexual (i.e. with a tampon or speculum). It is possible for a girl to hold her pelvic floor muscles contracted as a response to constipation or anxiety, or as a behavioral habit. As she ages, it is unlikely that she will learn to relax her pelvic floor muscles on her own because she is usually unaware that she has been chronically contracting them. In other patients, the contracted pelvic floor muscle holding pattern may have begun much more recently. Perhaps the patient is a teacher who is unable to leave her classroom to urinate and chronically delays micturition. It is for these reasons that obtaining a thorough history is an essential part of a physical therapist's assessment.

The patient with vestibulodynia caused by overactive pelvic floor muscles may have allodynia and hyperalgesia in a single small area of the posterior vestibule or the entire posterior vestibule. Treatment interventions for patients with vestibulodynia caused by overactive pelvic floor muscles include pelvic floor muscle relaxation, pelvic and skeletal alignment corrections, hip mobilizations, movement retraining, correcting breathing patterns, connective tissue manipulation, and trigger point releases.

## Hormonally-Induced Dyspareunia

It is important for the pelvic floor physical therapist to recognize through history-taking and examination when hormonal changes cause or contribute to sexual pain. Although pelvic floor interventions cannot replace systemic or local hormone deficiencies, they may reduce the effects of low sex hormone levels, such as tearing and pain. Proper assessment of the clitoral glans, prepuce, labia minora, vestibule, urethra, and vagina will give the therapist information about the role of hormones in the patient's pain.

Pelvic floor physical therapy manual work to the vulvovaginal and rectal tissues promotes increased blood flow, which, in turn, brings increased oxygen and nutrition to fragile tissue, potentially improving its quality. Education about sexual position, assistive devices, lubricants, and vaginal moisturizers can be provided during treatments to assist in reducing the patient's sexual pain symptoms. Often women are unaware that their sexual pain is a result of a reduction of vulvovaginal sex hormones. In these situations, the therapist must discuss their objective findings and assessment with the patient's referring medical professional so that appropriate medical management can be provided.

## Conclusion

Neuromusculoskeletal problems cause or contribute to chronic pelvic and sexual pain disorders in many women. Patients suffering from these disorders benefit when health professionals screen for musculoskeletal

## Case 3

Maureen is a 54-year-old female with complaints of pain with sexual intercourse, urinary urgency and frequency, and mild urinary incontinence. She began to have painful intercourse five years ago; the pain was initially minimal but has progressively worsened to a 7/10. She began having urinary urgency and frequency one year ago and has had mild urinary incontinence for six months. She says she needs to urinate twice an hour, but if she drinks coffee or wine she urinates three times an hour; sometimes she does not make it to the bathroom in time and has some incontinence. She also reports mild incontinence with laughing or coughing. The combination of dyspareunia, urinary urgency, frequency, and incontinence has severely decreased her interest in sexual intercourse. She has been menopausal for three years. She has not been treated with systemic or local hormones.

**Examination** is remarkable for:

- labia minora with partial resorption, partial clitoral phimosis, small glans clitoris, inability to retract prepuce to visualize clitoral corona;
- reproduction of urinary urge with palpation of bulbospongiosus and ischiocavernosus internally and externally;
- reproduction of painful intercourse with palpation of deep vaginal pelvic floor muscles;
- globally bilateral vaginal pelvic floor muscles severely overactive;
- diffuse pain throughout vestibule with q-tip test;
- connective tissue restrictions at entire bony pelvis, bilateral adductors, and abdomen;
- no pelvic obliquities;
- hip and leg length normal.

**Assessment:** visible signs of vulvovaginal atrophy and scarring that warrant a consultation with a gynecologist for possible treatment and to rule out vulvar dermatoses. She likely has painful intercourse, urinary urgency, frequency, and incontinence due to genitourinary syndrome of menopause, pelvic floor muscle overactivity, and connective tissue restrictions.

**Treatment:**

- patient referred to a physician for possible hormonal therapy;
- treat pelvic floor muscle overactivity and vulvar trigger points with manual therapy techniques;
- treat clitoral phimosis with gentle stretching techniques and educate patient how to do this at home;
- treat connective tissue restrictions;
- educate patient in dilator home program with a small plus dilator and progress to larger dilator sizes;
- teach patient how to re-educate bladder to allow for longer periods between urination.

**Outcome:**
She was prescribed a compounded topical estradiol 0.01%/testosterone 0.1% gel to apply on the vulva and vestibule. She had elimination of her urinary incontinence after six weeks of topical hormone use and weekly physical therapy intervention. By the third week of physical therapy she was able to wait one hour between urination breaks; by the fourth weeks she was able to wait 1.5 hours and after eight weeks of treatment, she was able to wait two hours between urination breaks and reported no more than 2/10 discomfort with sexual intercourse. After twelve weeks of physical therapy intervention, her dyspareunia had resolved.

disorders in their medical history and physical examination and refer to skilled pelvic floor physical therapists for a thorough evaluation. Physical therapy intervention consists of a variety of effective modalities that improve impairments and reduce pain from pelvic floor dysfunction. Pelvic floor physical therapists are valuable and often essential members of the medical team caring for women with sexual pain.

# References

1   United States Bone and Joint Initiative. *The Burden of Musculoskeletal Diseases in the United States (BMUS)*, 3rd edn. Rosemont, IL: United States Bone and Joint Initiative. 2014. http://www.boneandjointburden.org; last accessed 2 January 2018.

2   Mieritz RM, Thorhauge K, Forman A, *et al*. Musculoskeletal dysfunctions in patients with chronic pelvic pain: A preliminary descriptive survey. *J Manip Physiological Therap.* 2016;39:616–622.

3   Pastore E, Katzman W. Recognizing myofascial pelvic pain in the female patient with chronic pelvic pain. *J Obstet Gynecol Neonatal Nurs.* 2012; 41:680–691.

4   Gyang A, Hartman M, Lamvu G. Musculoskeletal causes of chronic pelvic pain: what a gynecologist should know. *Obstet Gynecol.* 2013;121:645–650.

5   Peters KM, Carrico DJ. Frequency, urgency, and pelvic pain: Treating the pelvic floor versus the epithelium. *Cur Uro Rep.* 2006;7:450–455.

6   Rosenbaum TY. Pelvic floor involvement in male and female sexual dysfunction and the role of pelvic floor rehabilitation in treatment: a literature review. *J Sex Med.* 2011;4:4–13.

7   FitzGerald MP, Payne CK, Lukacz ES, *et al*. Randomized multicenter clinical trial of myofascial physical therapy in women with interstitial cystitis/painful bladder syndrome and pelvic floor tenderness. *J Urol.* 2012;187:2113–2118.

8   Corona-Quintanilla DL, Zempoalteca R, Arteaga L, *et al*. The role of pelvic and perineal striated muscles in urethral function during micturition in female rabbits. *Neurourol Urodyn.* 2014;33:455–460.

9   Jung J, Ahn HK, Huh Y. Clinical and functional anatomy of the urethral sphincter. *Int Neurourol J.* 2012;16:102–106.

10  Reitz A, Schmid DM, Curt A, *et al*. Autonomic dysreflexia in response to pudendal nerve stimulation. *Spinal Cord.* 2003;41:539–542.

11  Neill JD. *Knobil and Neill's Physiology of Reproduction*, 3rd edn. Amsterdam: Elsevier; 2006.

12  Labat JJ, Riant T, Robert R, *et al*. Diagnostic criteria for pudendal neuralgia by pudendal nerve entrapment (Nantes criteria). *Neurourol Urodyn.* 2008;27:306–310.

13  Elkins N, Hunt J, Scott KM. Neurogenic pelvic pain. *Phys Med Rehabil Clin N Am.* 2017;28(3):551–569.

14  Young B, Heath W. *Wheater's Functional Histology*. 4th edn. London: Harcourt Publishers Limited; 2000, pp. 296–297.

15  Burgeson R. Genetic heterogeneity of collagen. *Invest Derm.* 1982;79:25.

16  Norton PA. Pelvic floor disorders: the role of fascia and ligaments. *Clin Obstet Gynecol.* 1993;36:926–938.

17  Weiss JM. Chronic pelvic pain and myofascial trigger points. *The Pain Clinic.* 2000;2:13–18.

18  Weiss JM. Pelvic floor myofascial trigger points: manual therapy for interstitial cystitis and the urgency-frequency syndrome. *J Urol.* 2001; 166:2226–2231.

19  Baker PK. Musculoskeletal origins of chronic pelvic pain. *Obstet Gynecol Clin North Am.* 1993;20;719–742.

20  FitzGerald MP, Kotarinos R. Rehabilitation of the short pelvic floor. I: Background and patient evaluation. *Int Urogynecol J Pelvic Floor Dysfunct.* 2003;14:261–268.

21  FitzGerald MP, Kotarinos R. Rehabilitation of the short pelvic floor. II: Treatment of the patient with the short pelvic floor. *Int Urogynecol J Pelvic Floor Dysfunct.* 2003;14:269–275.

22  Moldwin R, Fariello J. Myofascial trigger points of the pelvic floor: associations with urological pain syndromes and treatment strategies including injection therapy. *Curr Urol Rep.* 2013;14:409–417.

23  Philpott H, Nandurkar S, Lubel J, Gibson PR. Food, fibre, bile acids and the pelvic floor: An integrated low risk low cost approach to managing irritable bowel

syndrome. *World J Gastroenterol.* 2015;21:11379–11386.

24  Pukall CF, Smith KB, Chamberlain SM. Provoked vestibulodynia. *Womens Health.* 2007;3:583–592.

25  Haefner HK, Collins MD, Davis GD, *et al.* The vulvodynia guideline. *J Lower Genital Tract Dis.* 2005;9:40–51.

26  Travell J, Simons D. *The Trigger Point Manual*, Vol 1. Baltimore, MD: Williams & Wilkin; 1983, pp. 31–36.

27  Travell J, Simons D. *The Trigger Point Manual*, Vol 2. Baltimore, MD: Williams & Wilkin; 1992, pp. 110–131.

28  Prendergast S, Weiss J. Screening for musculoskeletal causes of pelvic pain. *Clin Obstet Gynecol.* 2003;46:773–782.

29  Horton RC. The anatomy, biological plausibility and efficacy of visceral mobilization in the treatment of pelvic floor dysfunction. *J Pelvic Obstet Gynaecol Physiother.* 2015;117:5–18.

30  Barral JP, Mercier P. *Visceral Manipulation.* Seattle, WA: Eastland Press; 2005.

31  Van Buskirk RL. Nociceptive reflexes and the somatic dysfunction: a model. *J Am Osteopath Assoc.* 1990;90:792–794, 797–809.

32  Hilton S, Vandyken C. The puzzle of pelvic pain – a rehabilitation framework for balancing tissue dysfunction and central sensitization, part I: Pain physiology and evaluation for the physical therapist. *J Womens Health Phys Ther.* 2011;35:103–113.

33  Woolf C. Central sensitization: Implications for the diagnosis and treatment of pain. *Pain.* 2011; 152(3 suppl):S2–S15.

34  Goldstein AT, Belkin ZR, Krapf JM, *et al.* Polymorphisms of the androgen receptor gene and hormonal contraceptive induced provoked vestibulodynia. *J Sex Med.* 2014;11:2764–2771.

35  Prather H, Camacho-Soto A. Musculoskeletal etiologies of pelvic pain. *Obstet Gynecol Clin N Am.* 2014;41:433–442.

36  Mowers EL, Lim CS, Skinner B, *et al.* Prevalence of endometriosis during abdominal or laparoscopic hysterectomy for chronic pelvic pain. *Obstet Gynecol.* 2016 Jun;127:1045–1053.

37  Coady D, Kennedy V. Sexual health in women affected by cancer: focus on sexual pain. *Obstet Gynecol.* 2016;128:775–791.

38  Tu FF, Holt J, Gonzales J, Fitzgerald CM. Physical therapy evaluation of patients with chronic pelvic pain: A controlled study. *Am J Obstet Gynecol.* 2008;198: e1–e7.

39  Binder DS, Nampiaparampil DE. The provocative lumbar facet joint. *Curr Rev Musculoskelet Med.* 2009;2:15–24.

40  Tu FF, Hellman K, Backonja M. Gynecological management of neuropathic pain. *Am J Obstet Gynecol.* 2011;205:435–443.

41  Faubion SS, Shuster LT, Bharucha AE. Recognition and management of nonrelaxing pelvic floor dysfunction. *Mayo Clin Proc.* 2012;87:187–193.

42  Chou R, Huffman L. Non-pharmacologic therapies for acute and chronic low back pain: a review of the evidence for an American Pain Society/American College of Physicians clinical practice guideline. *Ann Intern Med.* 2007;147:492–504.

43  Hävermark A, Languis-Eklöf A. Long-term follow up of a physical therapy program for patients with fibromyalgia syndrome. *Scand J Caring Sci.* 2013;3:315–322.

44  Goldfinger C, Pukall CF, Gentilcore-Saulnier E, *et al.* A prospective study of pelvic floor physical therapy: pain and psychosexual outcomes in provoked vestibulodynia. *J Sex Med.* 2009;6:1955–1968.

45  Anderson R, Harvey R, Wise D. Chronic pelvic pain syndrome: reduction of medication use after pelvic floor physical therapy with an internal myofascial trigger point wand. *Appl Psychophysiol Biofeedback.* 2015; 40:45–52.

46  Gentilcore-Saulnier E, McLean L, Goldfinger C, *et al.* Pelvic floor muscle assessment outcomes in women with and

without provoked vestibulodynia and the impact of a physical therapy program. *J Sex Med*. 2010;7:1003–1022.

47 Goldfinger C, Pukall CF, Thibault-Gagnon S, *et al*. Effectiveness of cognitive-behavioral therapy and physical therapy for provoked vestibulodynia: A randomized pilot study. *J Sex Med*. 2016;13:88–94.

48 Lindström S, Kvist L. Treatment of provoked vulvodynia in a Swedish cohort using desensitization exercises and cognitive behavioral therapy. *BMC Womens Health*. 2015;15:108.

49 Hartmann D, Nelson C. The perceived effectiveness of physical therapy treatment on women complaining of chronic vulvar pain and diagnosed with either vulvar vestibulitis syndrome or dysesthetic vulvodynia. *J Womens Health Phys Ther*. 2001;25:13–18.

50 Gupta P, Gaines N, Sirls LT, Peters KM. A multidisciplinary approach to the evaluation and management of interstitial cystitis/bladder pain syndrome: an ideal model of care. *Transl Androl Urol*. 2015;4:611–619.

51 Morin M, Carroll M, Bergeron S. Systematic review of the effectiveness of physical therapy in women with provoked vestibulodynia. *Sex Med Rev*. 2017;5(3):295–322.

52 Goldstein AT, Pukall CF, Brown C, *et al*. Vulvodynia: assessment and treatment. *J Sex Med*. 2016;13:572–590.

53 Colaco M, Evans R. Current guidelines in the management of interstitial cystitis. *Transl Androl Urol*. 2015;4:677–683.

54 American College of Obstetricians and Gynecologists' Committee on Gynecologic Practice; American Society for Colposcopy and Cervical Pathology (ASCCP). Committee Opinion No. 673. Persistent vulvar pain. *Obstet Gynecol*. 2016;128:e78–e84.

55 McKenney K, Elder A, Elder C. Myofascial release as a treatment for orthpaedic conditions: a systematic review. *J Athl Train*. 2013;48:522–527.

56 Gordon AM, Huxley AF, Julian FJ. The variation in isometric tension with sarcomere length in vertebrate muscle fibres. *J Physiol*. 1966;184(1):170–192.

57 Kim M, Baek I, Goo B. The relationship between pelvic alignment and dysmenorrhea. *J Phys Ther Sci*. 2016;28:757–760.

58 Dutton M. *Dutton's Orthopaedic Examination, Evaluation, and Intervention*, 3rd edn. New York: McGraw-Hill Medical; 2012.

59 Hing W, Bigelow R, Bremner T. Mulligan's mobilization with movement: a systematic review. *J Man Manip Ther*. 2009;17:e40–e66.

60 Paungmali A, O'Leary S, Souvlis T, *et al*. Hypoalgesic and sympathoexcitatory effects of mobilization with movement for lateral epicondylalgia. *Phys Ther*. 2003; 83:374–383.

61 Ellis R, Hing W. Neural mobilization: a systematic review of randomized controlled trials with an analysis of therapeutic efficacy. *J Man Manip Ther*. 2008;16(1):8–22.

62 Arung W, Meurisse M, Detry O. Pathology and prevention of postoperative peritoneal adhesions. *World J Gastroenterol*. 2011;17:4545–4553.

63 Bergeron S, Binik YM, Khalife S, Pagidas K. Vulvar vestibulitis syndrome: a critical review. *Clin J Pain*. 1997;13:27–42.

64 Hartmann D, Strauhal MJ, Nelson CA. Treatment of women in the United States with localized, provoked vulvodynia: practice survey of women's health physical therapists. *J Reprod Med*. 2007;52:48–52.

65 Sinha S. Dysfunctional voiding: a review of the terminology, presentation, evaluation and management in children and adults. *Indian J Urol*. 2011;27:437–447.

66 Pedraza R, Nieto J, Ibarra S, Haas EM. Pelvic muscle rehabilitation: a standardized protocol for pelvic floor dysfunction. *Adv Urol*. 2014; 2014: 487436.

67 Curtis R, Windsor T, Mogle J, Bielek A. There's more than meets the eye: complex associations of daily pain, physical symptoms, and self-efficacy with activity in middle and older adulthood. *Gerontology*. 2017; 63:157–168.

**68** Stravrou S, Nicolaides N, Papageorgiou I, *et al.* The effectiveness of a stress-management intervention program in the management of overweight and obesity in childhood adolescence. *J Mol Biochem.* 2016;5:63–70.

**69** Shim L. Jones M, Prott G, *et al.* Predictors of outcome of anorectal biofeedback therapy in patients with constipation. *Aliment Pharmocol Ther.* 2011;33:1245–1251.

**70** Wren A, Wright M, Carson J, Keefe F. Yoga for persistent pain: new findings and directions for an ancient practice. *Pain.* 2011;152:477–480.

**71** Chiarioni G, Nardo A, Vantini I, *et al.* Biofeedback is superior to electrogalvanic stimulation and massage in treatment of levator ani syndrome. *Gastroenterology.* 2010;138:1321–1329.

**72** Robertson V, Baker K. A review of therapeutic ultrasound: effectiveness studies. *Phys Ther.* 2001;81:1339–1350.

**73** Morishita K, Karuasuno H, Yokoi. Effects of therapeutic ultrasound on range of motion and stretch pain. *J Phys Ther Sci.* 2014;24:711–715.

**74** Zhang C, Xie Y, Luo X. Effects of therapeutic ultrasound on pain, physical function and safety outcomes in patients with knee osteoarthritis: A systematic review and meta-analysis. *Clin Rehab.* 2016;30:960–971.

**75** Udoji M, Ness T. New directions in treatment of pelvic pain. *Pain Manag.* 2013; 3:387–394.

**76** Dunning J, Butts R, Mourad F, *et al.* Dry needling: a literature review with implications for clinical practice guidelines. *Phys Ther Rev.* 2014;19:252–265.

**77** Chou L, Kao M, Lin J. Probable mechanisms of needling therapies for myofascial pain control. *Evid Based Complement Alternat Med.* 2012;705327. http://dx.doi.org/10.1155/2012/705327; last accessed 2 January 2017.

**78** Hilton S, Vandyken C. The puzzle of pelvic pain – a rehabilitation framework for balancing tissue dysfunction and central sensitization, part II: A review of treatment considerations. *J Womens Health Phys Ther.* 2012;36:44–54.

**79** Carrico DJ, Peters KM. Vaginal diazepam use with urogenital pain/pelvic floor dysfunction: serum diazepam levels and efficacy data. *Urol Nurs.* 2011;31:279–284,299.

**80** Adelowo A, Hacker MT, Shapiro A, *et al.* Botulinum toxin type a (BOTOX) for refractory myofascial pelvic pain. *Female Pelvic Med Reconstr Surg.* 2013;19:288–292.

**81** Bornstein J, Goldstein AT, Stockdale CK, *et al.* 2015 ISSVD, ISSWSH and IPPS Consensus terminology and classification of persistent vulvar pain and vulvodynia. *Obstet Gynecol.* 2016;127:745–751.

**82** King M, Rubin R, Goldstein A. Current uses of surgery for the treatment of genital pain. *Curr Sex Health Rep.* 2014;6:252–258.

**83** Stein A. *Heal Pelvic Pain.* New York: McGraw-Hill; 2009.

22

# Medical Management of Dyspareunia and Vulvovaginal Pain

*Andrew T. Goldstein and Susan Kellogg Spadt*

### Abstract

Approximately 17–19% of women in the United States suffer from dyspareunia. Due to the multifactorial etiology of dyspareunia, it is critically important for the sexual medicine clinician to perform a comprehensive and methodical evaluation of the woman who presents with this issue. This chapter provides an overview of the components of the medical history, psychosocial history, physical examination, and laboratory tests that can guide the clinician's diagnosis and treatment of sexual pain. Once this thorough evaluation has been performed a more accurate differential diagnosis can be developed. The differential diagnosis will then guide a more targeted treatment strategy that will be discussed in this chapter.

**Keywords:** *vulvodynia; vestibulodynia; vulvar vestibule; dyspareunia; neuroproliferative; overactive pelvic floor muscle dysfunction; vestibulectomy; combined hormonal contraceptives*

In general, a woman with sexual pain will see several clinicians in an effort to evaluate and treat her condition. As a result, she may feel marginalized and patronized, which can add to the burden of her illness. Treatment should be chosen according to the characteristics of the individual case and the possible associated factors, rather than as a one-size-fits-all approach.

The use of combined hormonal contraceptive agents is highly associated with vestibulodynia, the most common cause of dyspareunia in premenopausal women. The authors endorse changing to a long acting reversible contraceptive (LARC) and treatment with topical cream comprised of estradiol 0.01% and testosterone 0.05–0.1% for women whose pain history supports the diagnosis of a hormonally associated vestibulodynia (e.g. use of combined hormonal contraceptives or GrNH Agonists; women after menopause or during lactation).

Pain throughout the entire vulvar vestibule may be associated with pathology within the mucosa of the vestibular endoderm, whereas pain confined solely to the posterior vestibule commonly suggests overactive pelvic floor muscle dysfunction. The authors recommend botulinum toxin Type A be used to augment pelvic floor physiotherapy in the treatment of women with with overactive pelvic floor muscle dysfunction.

## Introduction

As discussed in Chapter 18, a large number of women suffer from vulvovaginal pain and dyspareunia. A 2003 study showed that approximately 17–19% of women in the United States suffer from dyspareunia (i.e. pain experienced during penetrative sexual activities) [1]. As previously examined in Chapter 18, the International Society for the Study of Vulvovaginal Disease (ISSVD), The International Society for the Study of

*Textbook of Female Sexual Function and Dysfunction: Diagnosis and Treatment*, First Edition. Edited by Irwin Goldstein, Anita H. Clayton, Andrew T. Goldstein, Noel N. Kim, and Sheryl A. Kingsberg.
© 2018 John Wiley & Sons Ltd. Published 2018 by John Wiley & Sons Ltd.

Women's Sexual Health (ISSWSH), and the International Pelvic Pain Society (IPPS) recently developed a nomenclature to help differentiate among various causes of vulvar pain and vulvodynia (Figure 18.3) [2]. This nomenclature emphasizes that "treatment should be chosen according to the characteristics of the individual case and the possible associated factors, rather than as a one-size-fits-all approach". For instance, physical therapy could be recommended if musculoskeletal factors were suspected, whereas surgery could be recommended if neuroproliferation was identified as a primary contributing factor [2].

Due to the multifactoral etiology of dyspareunia, it is critically important for the sexual medicine clinician to perform a comprehensive and methodical evaluation of the woman who presents with this issue [3]. Therefore, the first half of this chapter provides an overview of the components of the medical history, psychosocial history, physical examination, and laboratory tests that can guide the clinician's diagnosis and treatment of sexual pain. Once this thorough evaluation has been performed, a more accurate differential diagnosis can be developed. The differential diagnosis will then guide a more targeted treatment strategy that will be discussed in the second half of this chapter. Two cases can be used to illustrate this evaluation and treatment approach.

- *Case 1*: A 28-year-old women initially develops introital dyspareunia, which over several months becomes a constant nonprovoked burning pain. A physical examination reveals significant atrophy, pain throughout the entire vestibule, and severe erythema at the glandular ostia. A thorough medical history reveals that the pain began three months after the patient began an anti-androgenic treatment for acne (spironolactone), and laboratory testing reveals that the patient's free testosterone level was less than 25% of the expected value of a woman her age. The combination of these data suggests that the patient has "hormonally associated vestibulodynia". An appropriate treatment regimen might be to stop the anti-androgenic medication and use topical hormones on the vulvar vestibule.

- *Case 2*: A 35-year-old woman reports the sudden onset of introital dyspareunia, vulvar burning, urinary frequency, and pain with defecation. Her examination reveals a retracted perineum, tenderness of the perineum to palpation, severe tenderness of the posterior vestibule (without tenderness in the anterior vestibule), and tight and tender levator ani muscles. All laboratory tests were normal. A thorough medical history elucidates that the pain began three months after the patient began an aggressive exercise regimen in preparation for her upcoming wedding. Further questioning reveals that she is having severe anxiety in anticipation of her marriage because her fiancé has been emotionally abusive and focused on her weight. The combination of these data suggests that her pain is "provoked vestibulodynia associated with overactive pelvic floor muscle dysfunction". In this situation, however, the patient would likely be better served by a treatment regimen consisting of cognitive behavior therapy, relationship counseling, and pelvic floor physical therapy, rather than a medical or surgical treatment.

## Evaluation

### Medical History

A patient's narrative of her illness provides information that is essential in the determination of the correct diagnosis of the presenting complaint. However, a woman's experience of dyspareunia is often more complicated and may be less "straight forward" than other medical conditions. In addition to pain, an affected woman may experience embarrassment, shame, guilt, loss of self-esteem, frustration, depression, and anxiety. Therefore, it is important for a clinician to use communication skills that enhance openness, comfort, trust, and confidence.

In general, a woman with sexual pain will see several clinicians in an effort to evaluate and treat her condition [2]. As a result, she may feel patronized, marginalized, or ostracized from these previous encounters, which can add to the burden of her illness. It is essential for the clinician to address these feelings in order to establish a constructive and trusting relationship. Furthermore, a clinician should refrain from being either too formal or too casual when obtaining the medical history. Eye to eye contact should be maintained. Providers should avoid being careless with words, as patients with high levels of distress may search for meaning in everything that is said. A clinician should not display extreme reactions such as surprise, grimaces, or laughter while the patient provides her narrative [4]. Privacy and assurances of confidentiality are essential when conducting the interview. Some patients may want a spouse, sexual partner, relative, or friend present during the interview or examination. While this may allow the patient to feel more comfortable, it might also inhibit the patient from disclosing pertinent aspects of her medical, social, relationship, or sexual history. When possible, there should be some time allotted for the patient and the clinician to discuss a sexual history privately [4].

While it is important to ask direct questions to obtain specific information, such as medication usage, it is equally essential to ask open-ended questions that allow a patient to describe her experience of the condition. This process can be facilitated by encouraging the patient to give as much detailed information as possible. Avoid the temptation to frequently interrupt the patient's narrative. Throughout the whole process, displaying empathy, understanding, and acceptance is essential. Repeating the information back to the patient to confirm the accuracy of her history is also an important component [4].

While each clinician must establish his/her own routine, the authors have found it especially helpful to provide a new patient the first 10 minutes of the interview to give her narrative of the experience of her condition. A useful prompt for this narrative might be, "Complete this sentence....I was feeling fine until..." Before she starts, she is asked to try to be as specific as possible and to try to follow a sequential timeline of her disease process. She is allowed to speak virtually uninterrupted for this time. Frequently, a patient will cry, and there may be moments of silence, but this can be cathartic and conveys the message that she will not be rushed, ignored, or devalued in the clinician–patient relationship. If there is not enough time to focus on a specific complaint during a single visit, the patient should be reassured of the importance of her problem and scheduled for a follow-up appointment to address that issue alone.

After completing the patient's history, it may be necessary to clarify her expectations. She may have several different complaints, so it will be important to determine which of these she feels is her chief complaint. For example, she may complain of generalized vulvar pain and burning, pain during intercourse, decreased libido, and difficulty achieving orgasm. While it is possible that a single intervention might address all of these issues, it is likely that a sequence of treatments will be needed.

After both an accurate history of present illness and chief complaint have been established, additional information should be gathered that may help the clinician narrow the differential diagnosis. Past medical, social, sexual, surgical, and medication history often provides essential information.

A list of questions that the authors have found valuable in the differential diagnosis of sexual pain can be found in Table 22.1 [4]. Validated questionnaires for specific disorders can also be used to aid in the diagnosis of some pain disorders, including irritable bowel syndrome [5], endometriosis [6], and interstitial cystitis/bladder pain

**Table 22.1** Useful questions when obtaining a sexual pain history.

| Do you have a history of: | Suggestive of what condition |
|---|---|
| Physical, sexual, and emotional abuse or anxiety? | overactive pelvic floor muscle dysfunction, VAG |
| Low back or hip pain? | overactive pelvic floor muscle dysfunction |
| Urinary urgency, frequency, hesitancy, or sensation of incomplete emptying? | overactive pelvic floor muscle dysfunction, IC |
| Chronic constipation, rectal fissures, pain with bowel movements | overactive pelvic floor muscle dysfunction, IBS |
| Oral contraceptive pill use (especially OCPs with 20 mµ or less of ethinyl estradiol, or the progestins norgestimate or drospirenone) preceding or during the onset of symptoms? | HPVD |
| Ovarian suppression by Lupron, Depo-Provera? | HPVD |
| Treatment of breast cancer with Aromitase inhibitors or Tamoxifen | HPVD |
| Decreased libido or decreased vaginal lubrication prior to the onset of dyspareunia? | HPVD |
| Perimenopausal or menopausal symptoms such as hot flashes and night sweats? | HPVD, AV |
| Contact allergies or skin sensitive to chemicals? | IPVD, NPPVD |
| Recurrent (culture positive) yeast infections? | IPVD, NPPVD |
| Persistent yellowish vaginal discharge? | DIV, LP, TRICH, STI, SA |
| Severe burning or an allergic reaction to a topical medication on the vulva or in the vagina? | IPVD, NPPVD |
| Burning after intercourse? | IPVD, NPPVD, HPVD, PVD, LP, LS, SA |
| Pain since first attempt at intercourse without any pain-free sex? | NPPVD, overactive pelvic floor muscle dysfunction |
| Pain with first tampon use? | NPPVD, overactive pelvic floor muscle dysfunction |
| Increased sensitivity of the umbilicus? | NPPVD |
| Postcoital spotting or bleeding? | VGF, LS, LP, DIV |
| Vulvar itching? | LS, LP, DIV, LSC, VIN, plasma cell vulvitis |
| Night-time scratching? | LS, LSC |
| Diarrhea? | IBS |
| Mid-cycle spotting or pain? | Endo |
| Pain is worse in sexual positions with deep thrusting? | Endo, IBS, adenomyosis |
| Vulvar ulcerations, tears, fissures? | RC, LS, LP, AV, LSC |
| Painful periods? | Endo |
| Chronic pelvic pain? | Endo, overactive pelvic floor muscle dysfunction, PID |
| Feeling of an obstruction in the vagina? | overactive pelvic floor muscle dysfunction, VAG, rectocele |
| Pain beginning after childbirth? | AV, VGF, overactive pelvic floor muscle dysfunction, HAPVD |
| Dribbling after urination? | Urethral diverticulum, overactive pelvic floor muscle dysfunction |

**Table 22.1** (Continued)

| Do you have a history of: | Suggestive of what condition |
| --- | --- |
| Changes in coloration or architecture of the labia or vulva? | LS, LP, female genital cutting |
| Decreased clitoral sensation? | LS |
| Frequent bicycle riding? | PN |
| Aggressive abdominal muscle strengthening or Pilates? | overactive pelvic floor muscle dysfunction |
| Pain mainly at the clitoris? | Postherpetic neuralgia, PN |
| Pain with sex is intermittent (i.e. sometimes it is pain free)? | overactive pelvic floor muscle dysfunction |
| Do you have oral lesions or bleeding gums? | LP, mucous membrane pemphigoid |
| History of high-risk human papilloma virus or cervical dysplasia? | VIN |

KEY: overactive pelvic floor muscle dysfunction = pelvic floor dysfunction; IC = interstitial cystitis; HAPVD = hormonally associated provoked vestibulodynia; NPPVD = neuroproliferative associated vestibulodynia; IPVD = Inflammation associated vestibulodynia; PN = pudendal neuralgia; LS = lichen sclerosus; LP = lichen planus; AV = atrophic vaginitis (Genitourinary Syndrome of Menopause); DIV = desquamative inflammatory vaginitis; PID = pelvic inflammatory disease; IBS = irritable bowel syndrome; VGF = vulvar granuloma fissuratum; endo = endometriosis; VIN = vulvar intraepithelial neoplasia; LSC = lichen simplex chronicus; VAG = vaginismus

syndrome [7, 8]. A recently developed validated instrument – Vulvar Pain Assessment Questionnaire – can also be extremely useful in the evaluation of dyspareunia as well as following progress of treatment [9].

## Psychosocial History

When a patient reports symptoms of dyspareunia or genital pain the questions should address [9]:

- pain characteristics, such as time since onset, temporal pattern, duration, location, quality, elicitors, intensity, and whether the pain is primary or secondary;
- sexuality: desire, arousal, orgasm, frequency of and satisfaction with sex, sexual repertoire, sexual distress;
- thoughts, emotions, behaviors, and couple interactions that accompany the pain experience, in particular, avoidance behaviors, conflict and negative, solicitous or facilitative partner responses, pain attributions, catastrophizing, hypervigilance, fear of pain, self-efficacy (i.e. the belief of one's

own ability to achieve a goal), anxiety and depression, all of which could positively or negatively affect the pain.

- comorbid mental health conditions and treatments; previous treatment attempts and outcomes; current relationship: strengths, areas of conflict including potential verbal and physical abuse, how they cope with the pain as a couple, emotional and nonsexual physical intimacy; childhood trauma including abuse and neglect, and any adult nonconsensual or negative sexual experience.

## Medication History

Many medications can cause dyspareunia. Therefore, it is essential to develop a timeline of medication use and compare it to the timeline of the patient's sexual pain history. In general, more than 90% of women take prescription medications; therefore, a discussion of the most commonly prescribed medications and their association with dyspareunia is warranted. In addition, it is important to note that patients frequently do not disclose use of herbal supplements to clinicians; thus, it is important to ask about herbs, vitamins, and alternative therapies when inquiring about medication history [10].

Antibiotics are one of the most common prescription medications used by women. While antibiotics do not directly cause sexual pain, long-term exposure does predispose women to alteration in the gut and vaginal flora, and chronic yeast infections, which may be a causative agent of the pain. Combined hormonal contraceptives (e.g. oral contraceptive pills, transdermal patch, vaginal ring) are the second most common prescription medication used by reproductive-aged women. The use of these agents is highly associated with vestibulodynia, the most common cause of dyspareunia in premenopausal women. Although not all women who use combined hormonal contraceptives develop sexual pain, in at least one case-control study, women who used oral contraceptives were 9.3 times more likely to develop vestibulodynia than controls [11]. Several authors suggest that women who use or have used low-dose ethinyl estradiol oral contraceptives are more likely to develop vestibulodynia [12]. The proposed mechanism linking combined hormonal contraceptives to sexual pain is that combined hormonal contraceptives use results in elevated sex hormone binding globulin and decreased free circulating testosterone, which may result in dysfunction of the androgen dependent mucin glands and atrophy of the endodermal mucosa of the vulvar vestibule, placing a woman at risk for chronic inflammation and dyspareunia [13].

Lastly, approximately 20% of reproductive-aged women use prescription medications for anxiety and depression. Psychotropic medications are frequently implicated as a cause of alterations in female sexual desire and lubrication. Both of these can contribute to dyspareunia due to their adverse effects on vaginal lubrication and sexual arousal [14].

It is important to recognize that some aspects of a patient's self-reported medical history may be inaccurate. For instance, it is common for a woman with chronic inflammation to self-diagnosis the cause as "chronic yeast infections". In reality, this may or may not be the cause of her signs and symptoms if the diagnosis has not been aided by clinical microscopy and/or culture [15]. Studies also suggest that clinician-aided diagnosis of candidiasis is frequently incorrect and lacks confirmatory fungal culture [16]. Clinically, the authors note that some women have a difficult time localizing their sexual pain. They may incorrectly identify the location of their dyspareunia; localizing it to the vagina while an examination reveals that the pain is originating from the vulva or bladder.

### Physical Examination

All women with dyspareunia should undergo a thorough physical examination. While this examination focuses primarily on the urogenital system, additional organ systems may need to be assessed depending on information gathered during the medical history. The goal of the physical examination is to gather data to determine the etiology of the sexual pain. This requires a meticulous and methodical examination. In addition, if the examiner can identify the correct location and reproduce a woman's pain, she feels validated as this shows her that her sexual pain is real and has a physical origin. In addition, it inspires confidence that the practitioner will be able to treat her pain.

It is useful if the patient watches the physical examination to establish a common nomenclature for the parts of the urogenital system. The authors use mirror examinations and/or a video colposcope linked to a monitor to show the patient our findings that are related to her experience of pain and to include her in the monitoring of treatment progress. It should be noted that consent should be obtained before taking any digital images [17].

During colposcopic examination of the vulva, commonly referred to vulvoscopy, important findings that can be observed include: infection, trauma, and dermatitis (Figure 22.1). Specifically, the observer should note any inflammation, induration, excoriation, fissures, ulceration, lichenification, hypopigmentation, hyperpigmentation, scarring, or architectural changes, which may be evidence of a dermatologic disease of the vulva (Figure 22.2). While erythema is a nonspecific finding, erythema near the ostia of the Bartholin and Skene glands is suggestive of vestibulodynia (Figure 22.3).

**Figure 22.1** Examination of the vulva with a colposcope.

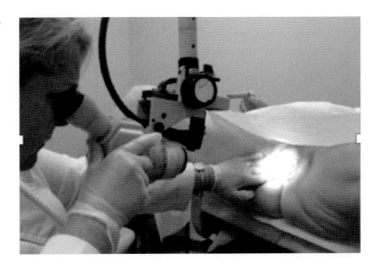

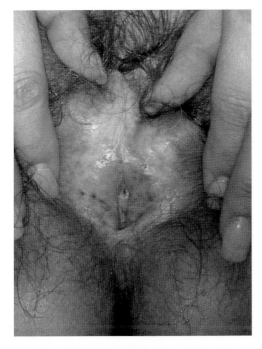

**Figure 22.2** Vulvar lichen sclerosus. Changes seen include complete resorption of the labia minora, complete phimosis of the glans clitoris, and narrowing of the introitus.

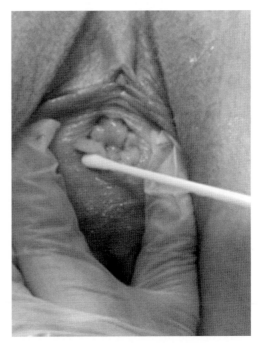

**Figure 22.3** Cotton swab test of the vulvar vestibule.

A sensory examination of the vulva is performed using a moistened cotton swab (called the "Q tip test") to determine if there are areas that exhibit an abnormal pain response. Women with sexual pain often exhibit localized or generalized "allodynia", the perception of pain upon provocation by a normally nonpainful stimulus and "hyperpathia", pain provoked by very light touch during the Q tip test. This examination should be performed systematically to ensure that all areas of the anogenital region are tested. Initially, the medial thigh, buttocks, and mons pubis are palpated. These areas are typically painless and this allows the patient to become comfortable with the examination. Then, labia majora, clitoral prepuce, perineum, and interlabial sulci should be evaluated. Pain in these areas would suggest a process that is affecting the whole anogenital region, including vulvar dermatoses, vulvovaginal infections, or neuropathic processes such as pudendal neuralgia. The labia minora are then gently palpated. Firstly, the medial labia minora are gently touched with the cotton swab lateral to Hart's line, which is the lateral boundary of the vulvar vestibule. The cotton swab is then used to gently palpate the vestibule at five locations: at the ostia of the Skene glands (lateral to the urethra), at the ostia of the Bartholin glands (4 and 8 o'clock on the vestibule), and at 6 o'clock at the fossa navicularis (Figure 22.4). Patients with vestibulodynia will frequently experience allodynia with the cotton swab palpation confined to the tissue of the vulvar vestibule but have normal sensation lateral to this anatomic landmark. If the pain is localized to the vestibule, it is important to determine if the pain affects the entire vestibule or just the posterior portion of vestibule. Pain throughout the entire vestibule may be associated with the possibility of an intrinsic pathology within the mucosa of the vestibular endoderm, whereas pain confined to the posterior vestibule suggests that the pain might be associated with a pathology extrinsic to the vestibule, most

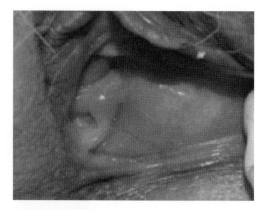

**Figure 22.4** Erythema of the ostia of the Bartholin gland in a patient with hormonally associated vestibulodynia.

commonly overactive pelvic floor muscle dysfunction [18].

A speculum examination of the vagina is the next step in the physical examination of a woman with dyspareunia. In general, a pediatric-sized Graves or Pederson speculum should be used and all efforts should be used to insert the speculum through the hymeneal ring without touching the vulvar vestibule. Initially, the vagina should be examined for evidence of abnormal vaginal discharge. A cotton swab should be used to collect some discharge for pH testing, wet mount, and potassium hydroxide (KOH) preparation. In addition, a culture should be obtained and sent for speciation and sensitivity. Important findings while visualizing the vagina include atrophy, erythema, erosions, ulcerations, abnormal discharge, or synechiae.

A manual examination is then performed with one finger instead of the usual two fingers. The examiner's index finger is inserted through the hymen without touching the vestibule. The urethra and bladder trigone are gently palpated. Intrinsic tenderness of the urethra may be suggestive of a urethral diverticulum or bladder pain syndrome/ interstitial cystitis, while tenderness of the bladder may be suggestive of either bladder pain syndrome/interstitial cystitis or endometriosis. The levator ani muscles are then palpated for hypertonicity, tenderness, weakness, and trigger points, which can be evidence of overactive pelvic floor muscle dysfunction (also known as levator ani syndrome or vaginismus). Because overactive pelvic floor muscle dysfunction is such an important and common cause of dyspareunia, an additional chapter in this textbook is devoted to the evaluation and treatment of overactive pelvic floor muscle dysfunction (Chapter 21).

The ischial spine is then located and the pudendal nerve is palpated as it enters Alcock's canal. Tenderness of the pudendal nerve is suggestive of pudendal neuralgia or pudendal nerve entrapment. Next, a bimanual examination is performed to assess the uterus and adnexa (ovaries and fallopian tubes). Abnormalities in the size, shape, or contour may be indicative of a leiomyoma. A diffusely enlarged, "boggy" and tender uterus may be evidence of adenomyosis. Tenderness of the adnexa can often be a sign of ovarian cysts, sexually transmitted infection, pelvic inflammatory disease, or endometriosis. A rectovaginal examination is then performed to assess the rectovaginal septum and the posterior cul-de-sac. Thickening or nodularity of the septum, nodularity of the uterosacral ligaments, or obliteration of the posterior cul-de-sac are suggestive of endometriosis. Traumatic neuromas can also be a source of significant pain in women who have had prior vaginal surgery, including repair of lacerations or episiotomies incurred during childbirth.

## Testing

### Wet Mount and Cultures

As previously discussed, vaginal discharge should be examined by wet preparation, pH, and potassium hydroxide testing. Specifically, vaginal discharge should be obtained on two cotton swabs from the upper third of the vagina, and the pH of the discharge should be tested. One swab is used to make a slide with saline and the other swab is combined with potassium hydroxide. The wet mount should be examined with a microscope on both low and high power magnification. The saline slide is examined for normal squamous epithelial cells, increased white blood cells (more than one white blood cell per epithelial cell), pathogens such as hyphae (yeast cells), trichomonas, parabasal cells, clue cells, and normal flora such as lactobacilli. As microscopic examination frequently misses candidiasis and trichomoniasis, a culture obtained at the time of vaginal inspection should be sent for speciation and sensitivity. In addition, if there is significant leukorrhea, a swab should be obtained for an immunochromatographic assay for trichomonas.

## Histology

A vulvar or vaginal biopsy should be obtained if there are specific findings on colposcopic examination of the vulva suggestive of a dermatoses, intraepithelial neoplasia, or neoplasia. It is unlikely, however, that the biopsy will prove useful if the physical findings are solely nonspecific erythema. After prepping the area with iodopovidone solution, the biopsy should be obtained at the edge of any ulcerations or erosions if present using a 4 mm punch biopsy or small Tischler biopsy forcep. Biopsies can be closed with one or two stitches of absorbable suture such as 4-0 Vicryl-rapide (Ethicon, Inc., Somerville, NJ) to aid in wound healing.

The authors recommend that all vulvovaginal biopsies should be sent with a description of the physical findings and a differential diagnosis to the attention of a pathologist who specializes in dermatologic disorders (a dermatopathologist). When persistent or extensive vulvovaginal ulcerations are present, a second biopsy may be obtained and sent in Michel's transport media for direct immunofluorescence to rule out the immunobullous diseases such as mucous membrane pemphigoid [19]. This additional biopsy should only be carried out when the more common sources of ulceration, such as genital herpes, have been ruled out.

## Serum Testing

Serum hormone testing can be useful in women with dyspareunia. Because hormonal abnormalities can be involved in vestibulodynia and vaginal pain, blood should be obtained for serum estradiol, total testosterone, free testosterone, albumin, prolactin, sex hormone binding globulin, and follicle stimulating hormone. An elevated prolactin level can cause anovulation and atrophic changes. Herpes type-specific serology should be obtained in women with symptoms of generalized vulvar burning or tingling, or in those with pain concentrated in the clitoris (clitorodynia).

## Additional Testing

Referrals for additional tests should be based on findings during the history and physical examination. Radiographic or ultrasonographic imaging may be appropriate to evaluate the uterus, ovaries, pelvis, or lumbosacral spine (particularly if sacroiliac joint dysfunction is suspected in relation to pelvic floor hypertonus). Specifically, a 3 Telsa MRI of the pelvis may reveal entrapment of the pudendal nerve in women with unilateral vulvar pain or clitorodynia. A MRI of the sacrum and lumbar spine is appropriate in women with an abnormal genital sensory examination. Diagnostic laparoscopy may be necessary if there is significant evidence of endometriosis or utero-ovarian pathology that does not respond to initial conservative management. Colonoscopy, barium enema, and/or a CT scan with contrast may be used to rule out pathology of the lower gastrointestinal tract if deep thrusting dyspareunia is present along with dyschezia, hematochezia, or symptoms consistent with inflammatory bowel disease. Cystoscopy (with or without hydrodistention) may be used to evaluate any unexplained microscopic or gross hematuria or aid in the diagnosis of interstitial cystitis/bladder pain syndrome. An electromyelogram may be used to assess the tone and strength of the levator ani muscles when there is evidence of overactive pelvic floor muscle dysfunction.

## Treatment

Unfortunately, there are few randomized, placebo controlled trials that have examined treatments for vestibulodynia. In addition, even though some of the existing studies were well designed when they were conducted, none differentiated among the different subtypes of vestibulodynia as outlined in the 2015 nomenclature. As such, it is possible that some treatment options would have shown better efficacy if they targeted only a specific subgroup of vulvar pain/vulvodynia. For example, one could hypothesize that capsaicin – which blocks the release of substance-P to desensitize the sensory nerves located in the vestibular mucosa – would work better in a subgroup of women with "neuroproliferative associated vestibulodynia" than in a mixed cohort of women that have vestibulodynia secondary to other causes (e.g. hormonal, inflammatory, musculoskeletal, etc.). However, it is still worth reviewing the previously published studies to illustrate the many different approaches that have been taken to treat vestibulodynia. In addition, it may allow us to contemplate future trials that will target specific subgroups of vestibulodynia with treatments targeting particular associated pathologies.

In the past, the typical treatment plan for a woman with dyspareunia and/or vulovovaginal pain started with treatments that are considered noninvasive (e.g. psychological treatments, physical therapy), and then, depending on treatment response, progressed to medical treatments (lidocaine, gabapentin, topical hormones, etc.), and then to surgical intervention if the pain is confined to vestibule. Treatment progression was usually based on "trial and error" [20]. More recently, the authors have favored a more algorithmic approach, deciding on specific treatments based on history, physical examination finding and laboratory tests

(Figure 22.5) [18]. Lastly, some have argued that concurrent or integrative (i.e. multidisciplinary) treatments, if possible, might be more efficacious in terms of outcome [20].

## Nonmedical Treatments

Despite their widespread use in the multimodal treatment of other chronic pain conditions, nonmedical treatments are

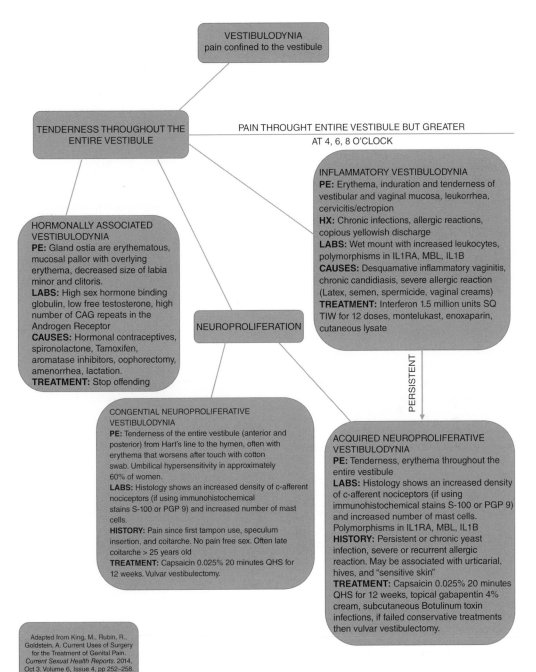

**Figure 22.5** Vulvar pain diagnostic and treatment algorithm.

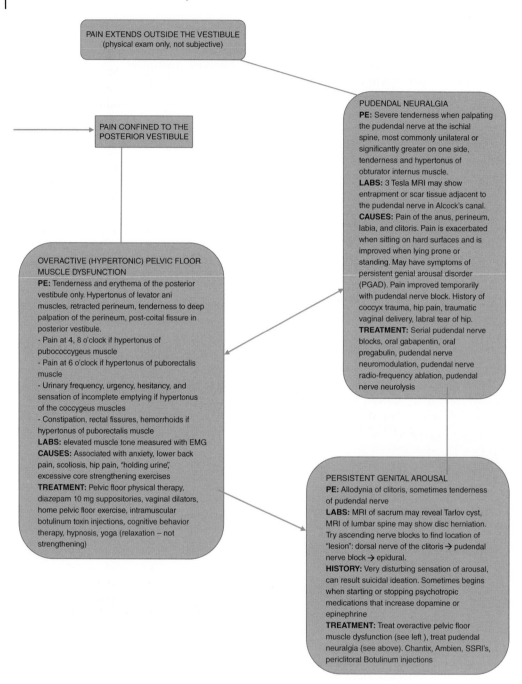

**Figure 22.5** (Continued)

sometimes absent from algorithms published in the medical literature. These treatments can be instrumental in the comprehensive multidisciplinary treatment of women with sexual pain and include: cognitive behavioral therapy, pelvic floor physiotherapy (physical therapy), and alternative treatments.

## Interdisciplinary Treatments

There are only two published, uncontrolled quantitative studies evaluating a multimodal approach to the treatment of genital pain, with both reporting major improvements in women's sexual function and pain [21, 22]. These multimodal treatments integrated sex therapy and physiotherapy in a nonstandardized manner, such that not all participants received the same combination and duration of interventions. Another retrospective qualitative study evaluated 29 women with vulvodynia who had taken part in a multidisciplinary treatment program consisting of psychotherapy, physiotherapy, and dietary advice. Of the 29 women, 27 reported a significant benefit, including nine women who were pain free at the end of the interventions [23]. Another study of 19 women with vulvodynia who had multimodal treatment included group cognitive behavioral therapy, physical therapy, and regular medical appointments. Participants reported increased knowledge and tools to manage the pain, improved psychological well-being, a sense of validation and support, and an enhanced sense of empowerment [24]. Though promising, the findings of these studies emphasize the need for randomized trials aimed at evaluating the efficacy of an integrated approach to care, over and above the efficacy of single treatments.

## Medical Treatments

### Lidocaine

Local anesthetics such as lidocaine exert their analgesic activity via the blockade of sodium channels on peripheral nociceptors and by blocking transmission of discharges from peripheral sensory nerves. Both neuroproliferation and sensitization of the vestibular nociceptors have been suggested as possible mechanisms of the pain in vestibulodynia. Therefore, the theory behind the use of local anesthetics is to achieve long-lasting desensitization of these nociceptors [7]. However, as the only double-blind, randomized, placebo controlled trial using lidocaine failed to show any benefit of this medication and the majority of the noncontrolled trials showed efficacy in the range of 50%, the authors do not recommend lidocaine as a long-term management option for vestibulodynia [7].

### Capsaicin

The rationale for the use of capsaicin in the treatment of vulvodynia is based on increased vanilloid receptor innervation found in women with this condition. Capsaicin binds to the vanilloid receptor receptors located in the peripheral terminals of nociceptors [25]. After hyperesthesia to the initial capsaicin exposure, capsaicin produces a long-lasting desensitization to burning and pain [26]. One prospective and one retrospective case series have evaluated the efficacy of capsaicin cream in vestibulodynia [27, 28]. Neither were controlled studies. However, despite the significant discomfort experienced by the patients with the use of capsaicin, the majority reported a significant reduction in dyspareunia. Therefore, despite the flaws in the available literature, the authors feel that capsaicin should be offered to patients suspected of having neuroproliferative associated vestibulodynia prior to undergoing vulvar vestibulectomy.

### Botulinum Toxin Type A

Botulinum toxin Type A (Botox®) inhibits the release of glutamate and substance-P from nociceptive neurons [29]. Current hypotheses suggest that the inhibition of these nociceptors may improve peripheral and central sensitization associated with vulvodynia. In addition, botulinum toxin Type A blocks the release of acetylcholine at the neuromuscular junction causing localized muscle paralysis [30]. This effect may be useful in the treatment of overactive pelvic floor muscle dysfunction. The efficacy of botulinum toxin Type A has been evaluated in one double-blind placebo controlled randomized controlled trial, two case series, and two case reports [7]. While the one randomized controlled trial of botulinum toxin Type A showed no improvement as compared to placebo, the noncontrolled studies have shown very significant efficacy. In one open label study in women of women who had failed conservative therapy for overactive pelvic floor muscle dysfunction, 83% reported dyspareunia after 24 weeks after injection of up to 300 units of botulinum toxin Type A [31]. Therefore, given the results of the majority of studies and the clinical experience of the authors, we recommend botulinum toxin Type A be used to augment pelvic floor physiotherapy in the treatment of women with dyspareunia and vestibulodynia associated with overactive pelvic floor muscle dysfunction.

### Corticosteroids

Despite the fact that most studies show elevated inflammatory cytokines in the vestibular mucosa of women with vestibulodynia, the majority of data suggests that topical corticosteroids are minimally effective in treating vestibulodynia [7]. Therefore, due to the lack of efficacy of low dose corticosteroids and potential side effects of high potency corticosteroids, the authors do not recommend topical corticosteroids for the management of dyspareunia or vestibulodynia.

### Interferon

Interferon is a signaling protein that downregulates the expression of proinflammatory cytokines [32]. Additionally, interferon is potent mast cell inhibitor and it has been suggested that mast cells have a role in the initiation of neuroproliferative associated vestibulodynia [33]. One randomized control trial, three case series, and one case study have examined the efficacy of interferon in vestibulodynia [7]. The majority of these studies found modest improvement with submucosal vestibular interferon injections. Though more studies are needed, the authors believe that interferon may play a role if treatment of inflammation associated vestibulodynia if this treatment is initiated shortly after the onset of symptoms.

### Hormonal Treatments

In a nonplacebo controlled study, Burrows and Goldstein showed that a topical cream that combined estradiol 0.01% and testosterone 0.1% reduced visual analogue pain scores from 7.5 to 2.0 in 50 consecutive women with vestibulodynia in whom the initiation of combined oral contraceptive pills was associated with vestibulodynia onset [34]. In a randomized controlled trial, Foster *et al.* showed that topical estradiol reduced vulvar pain sensitivity in menopausal women with mixed vulvovaginal complaints [35]. Lastly, Yount and colleagues reported that 88% of 201 women treated with estradiol alone or in combination with biofeedback had at least a 70% reduction in their pain [36]. Therefore, the authors endorse topical cream comprised of estradiol 0.01% (or topical estriol 0.03%) and testosterone 0.05–0.1% for all women who have vestibulodynia that affects the entire vestibule. This is especially true if the history supports the diagnosis of a hormonally associated vestibulodynia, such as history of combined hormonal contraceptives use, hormonal control of endometriosis, oophorectomy, lactation, when treated with GRNH agonists, perimenopause, or menopause.

### Systemic Medications

Leo and Dewani conducted a literature review regarding the effectiveness of oral antidepressant medication in treating vulvodynia [37]. Their review included two randomized controlled trials, one quasi-experimental trial, seven nonexperimental studies, and three case reports. The majority of the cases discussed in the reports reviewed received tricyclic antidepressant treatment. The results of randomized controlled trials of systemic tricyclic antidepressants provide evidence that they should not be used for vestibulodynia. Therefore, despite the widespread use of tricyclic antidepressants, a first-line treatment for vulvodynia, we recommend that antidepressant medication not be used for the management of vestibulodynia.

Anticonvulsant therapy has been recommended in the treatment of vulvodynia. However, convincing evidence to support this therapeutic option is lacking. Spoelstra and colleagues performed a review of the available peer-reviewed literature, including two case reports, three retrospective studies, two nonrandomized prospective studies, and one open-label pilot trial study [38]. Given the mixed results of these studies and potential side effects, the authors of this chapter concur with their recommendation to wait for the results of an National Institutes of Health-funded multicentered randomized controlled trial to be completed before recommending the use of anticonvulsants for vulvodynia [39].

## Surgical Treatment

As discussed earlier, one subcategory of vestibulodynia is a neuroproliferative associated vestibulodynia in which there is up to a 10-fold increase in the density of C-afferent nociceptors in the vulvar vestibular endoderm [40]. Due to the increased density of C-afferent nociceptors, women with neuroproliferative-associated vestibulodynia experience allodynia and hyperpathia at the vulvar vestibule. In women with neuroproliferative-associated vestibulodynia who have failed conservative treatment with topical capsaicin, vulvar vestibulectomy with vaginal advancement can be performed to remove the abnormal vestibular endoderm. Since this first published report in 1983, there have been over 40 published peer-reviewed papers examining variations of vulvar vestibulectomy [41]. A 2010 meta-analysis of 33 previous studies revealed that vulvar vestibulectomy provided significant relief of dyspareunia in 78.5% of patients, some relief in 88.8% of patients, and no relief in 12.2% [42]. In the nine studies that reported improvement in sexual function as a measure of surgical success, all nine reported significant improvement in sexual function following vestibulectomy.

Woodruff and Parmley were the first authors to describe vulvar vestibulectomy in 1983 [43]. Their procedure consisted of the excision of a semicircular segment of perineal skin, the mucosa of the posterior vulvar vestibule, and the posterior hymeneal ring. Three centimeters of the vaginal mucosa was then undermined and approximated to the perineum. Since this original procedure, several variations of the procedure have been described to help decreased complications, such as dehiscence of the vaginal advancement flap as well as to improve operative success [41]. Of all the variations, the authors of this chapter strongly believe that the best version of this procedure is a complete vulvar vestibulectomy with vaginal advancement. This procedure includes the excision of the mucosa of the entire vulvar vestibule, including the mucosa adjacent to the urethra [44]. By removing *all* of the vestibular mucosa, all of the hyperpathic areas are removed.

Complications of vestibulectomy occur, though they are infrequent. Specifically, complications include bleeding, infection, increased pain, hematoma, wound dehiscence, scar tissue formation, and Bartholin cyst formation. The risk of these complications can be reduced if appropriate surgical techniques are used. Since the risks of complication are low, they should be realistically presented when counseling patients about surgical treatment for vestibulodynia [42].

The authors want to emphasize that despite the very high success rates of surgery, the old adage that the success of surgery is made *before* walking into the operating room by choosing the appropriate surgical candidate is especially true in the case of vulvodynia. The surgery should only be performed in women with neuroproliferative-associated vestibulodynia. Women who have pain confined to the posterior vestibule, therefore, are typically *not* surgical candidates, as they most likely have vestibulodynia secondary to overactive pelvic floor muscle dysfunction. In addition, women who have allodynia of the entire vestibule should undergo a clinical trial of topical estradiol and testosterone cream (while off combined hormonal contraceptivess) to rule in or to exclude hormonally associated vestibulodynia.

### Emerging Therapies

Laser therapy for the treatment of dyspareunia and vulvovaginal pain is an area of developing research. In Murina's pilot study of 70 women treated with micro-ablative fractional $CO_2$ laser to the vulvar vestibule, improvement was reported in dyspareunia and pain scores, with gradual improvement occurring over four months of follow-up [45]. Two-thirds of women reported they were either "very improved" or "improved". No major adverse events were reported. Multicenter studies are underway. The authors await the results of further studies before making definitive recommendations

regarding the use of the fractional $CO_2$ laser for vulvovaginal pain.

## Conclusions

A comprehensive history and physical examination is essential in the evaluation and treatment of women with sexual pain disorders and/or vulvodynia. In addition, a thorough psychosocial evaluation must be included to fully understand the pain experience of women with dyspareunia. While past treatments were somewhat empirical in nature, the new vulvodynia nomenclature and subcategories of vulvodynia will enable clinician to implement a more targeted and logical treatment approach. In addition, the new nomenclature will facilitate the design of superior quality studies by researchers.

## References

1 West SL, Vinikoor LC, Zolnoun D. A systematic review of the literature on female sexual dysfunction prevalence and predictors. *Annu Rev Sex Res.* 2004;15:40–172.

2 Bornstein J, Goldstein AT, Stockdale CK, *et al.* 2015 ISSVD, ISSWSH, and IPPS Consensus Terminology and Classification of Persistent Vulvar Pain and Vulvodynia. *J Sex Med.* 2016;13:607–612.

3 Moynihan R. The making of a disease: female sexual dysfunction. *BMJ.* 2003;326:45–47.

4 Goldstein AT. Medical history, physical examination, and laboratory tests for the evaluation of dyspareunia. In: Goldstein A, Goldstein I (eds) *Female Sexual Pain Disorders: Evaluation and Management.* Wiley-Blackwell; 2009.

5 Wiklund IK, Fullerton S, Hawkey CJ, *et al.* An irritable bowel syndrome-specific symptom questionnaire: development and validation. *Scand J Gastroenterol.* 2003;38:947–954.

6 Fedele L, Bianchi S, Carmignani L, *et al.* Evaluation of a new questionnaire for the presurgical diagnosis of bladder endometriosis. *Hum Reprod.* 2007;22:2698–2701.

7 Goldstein AT, Pukall CF, Brown C, *et al.* Vulvodynia: Assessment and Treatment. *J Sex Med.* 2016;13:572–590.

8 Brewer ME, White WM, Klein FA, *et al.* Validity of Pelvic Pain, Urgency, and Frequency questionnaire in patients with interstitial cystitis/painful bladder syndrome. *Urology.* 2007;70:646–649.

9 Dargie E, Holden RR, Pukall CF. The Vulvar Pain Assessment Questionnaire inventory. *Pain.* 2016;157:2672–2686.

10 Glover DD, Rybeck BF, Tracy TS. Medication use in a rural gynecologic population: prescription, over-the-counter, and herbal medicines. *Am J Obstet Gynecol.* 2004;190:351–357.

11 Bouchard C, Brisson J, Fortier M, *et al.* Use of oral contraceptive pills and vulvar vestibulitis: a case-control study. *Am J Epidemiol.* 2002;156:254–261.

12 Greenstein A, Ben-Aroya Z, Fass O, *et al.* Vulvar vestibulitis syndrome and estrogen dose of oral contraceptive pills. *J Sex Med.* 2007;4:1679–1683.

13 Goldstein AT, Belkin ZR, Krapf JM, *et al.* Polymorphisms of the androgen receptor gene and hormonal contraceptive induced provoked vestibulodynia. *J Sex Med.* 2014;11: 764–771.

14 Clayton AH, Campbell BJ, Favit A, *et al.* Symptoms of sexual dysfunction in patients treated for major depressive disorder: a meta-analysis comparing selegiline transdermal system and placebo using a patient-rated scale. *J Clin Psychiatry.* 2007;68:1860–1806.

15 Ferris DG, Nyirjesy P, Sobel JD, *et al.* Over-the-counter antifungal drug misuse associated with patient-diagnosed vulvovaginal candidiasis. *Obstet Gynecol.* 2002;99:419–425.

16 Ledger WJ, Monif GR. A growing concern: inability to diagnose vulvovaginal infections correctly. *Obstet Gynecol.* 2004;103:782–784.

17 Berle I. Clinical photography and patient rights: the need for orthopraxy. *J Med Ethics.* 2008;34: 9–92.

18 King M, Rubin R, Goldstein A. Current uses of surgery for the treatment of genital pain. *Curr Sex Health Rep.* 2014;6:6.

19 Raghu AR, Nirmala NR, Sreekumaran N. Direct immunofluorescence in oral lichen planus and oral lichenoid reactions. *Quintessence Int.* 2002;33:234–239.

20 Landry T, Bergeron S, Dupuis MJ, Desrochers G. The treatment of provoked vestibulodynia: a critical review. *Clin J Pain.* 2008;24:155–171.

21 Backman H, Widenbrant M, Bohm-Starke N, Dahlof LG. Combined physical and psychosexual therapy for provoked vestibulodynia-an evaluation of a multidisciplinary treatment model. *J Sex Res.* 2008;45:378–385.

22 Spoelstra SK, Dijkstra JR, van Driel MF, Weijmar Schultz WC. Long-term results of an individualized, multifaceted, and multidisciplinary therapeutic approach to provoked vestibulodynia. *J Sex Med.* 2011;8:489–496.

23 Munday P, Buchan A, Ravenhill G, *et al.* A qualitative study of women with vulvodynia: II. Response to a multidisciplinary approach to management. *J Reprod Med.* 2007;52:19–22.

24 Sadownik LA, Seal BN, Brotto LA. Provoked vestibulodynia-women's experience of participating in a multidisciplinary vulvodynia program. *J Sex Med.* 2012;9:1086–1093.

25 Tympanidis P, Casula MA, Yiangou Y, *et al.* Increased vanilloid receptor VR1 innervation in vulvodynia. *Eur J Pain.* 2004;8:129–133.

26 Baron R. Capsaicin and nociception: from basic mechanisms to novel drugs. *Lancet.* 2000;356:785–787.

27 Steinberg AC, Oyama IA, Rejba AE, *et al.* Capsaicin for the treatment of vulvar vestibulitis. *Am J Obstet Gynecol.* 2005;192:1549–1553.

28 Murina F, Radici G, Bianco V. Capsaicin and the treatment of vulvar vestibulitis syndrome: a valuable alternative? *MedGenMed.* 2004;6:48.

29 Cui M, Khanijou S, Rubino J, Aoki KR. Subcutaneous administration of botulinum toxin A reduces formalin-induced pain. *Pain.* 2004;107:125–133.

30 Bentsianov B, Zalvan C, Blitzer A. Noncosmetic uses of botulinum toxin. *Clin Dermatol.* 2004;22:82–88.

31 Morrissey D, El-Khawand D, Ginzburg N, *et al.* Botulinum toxin A injections into pelvic floor muscles under electromyographic guidance for women with refractory high-tone pelvic floor dysfunction: a 6-month prospective pilot study. *Female Pelvic Med Reconstr Surg.* 2015;21:277–282.

32 Keisseier BC. The mechanism of action of interferon-β in relapsing multiple sclerosis. *CNS Drugs.* 2011;25(6):491–502.

33 Bornstein J, Cohen Y, Zarfati D, *et al.* Involvement of heparanase in the pathogenesis of localized vulvodynia. *Int J Gynecol Pathol.* 2008;27:136–141.

**34** Burrows LJ, Goldstein AT. The treatment of vestibulodynia with topical estradiol and testosterone. *Sex Med.* 2013;1:30–33.

**35** Foster DC, Palmer M, Marks J. Effect of vulvovaginal estrogen on sensorimotor response of the lower genital tract: a randomized controlled trial. *Obstet Gynecol.* 1999;94:232–237.

**36** Yount JJ, Solomons CC, Willems JJ, *et al.* Effective nonsurgical treatments for vulvar pain. *Women's Health Dig.* 1997;3:88–93.

**37** Leo RJ, Dewani S. A systematic review of the utility of antidepressant pharmacotherapy in the treatment of vulvodynia pain. *J Sex Med.* 2013;10:2497–2505.

**38** Spoelstra SK, Borg C, Weijmar Schultz WC. Anticonvulsant pharmacotherapy for generalized and localized vulvodynia: a critical review of the literature. *J Psychosom Obstet Gynaecol.* 2013;34:133–138.

**39** Brown CS, Foster DC, Wan JY, *et al.* Rationale and design of a multicenter randomized clinical trial of extended release gabapentin in provoked vestibulodynia and biological correlates of response. *Contemp Clin Trials.* 2013;36:154–165.

**40** Bohm-Starke N, Hilliges M, Falconer C, Rylander E. Increased intraepithelial innervation in women with vulvar vestibulitis syndrome. *Gynecol Obstet Invest.* 1998;46:256–260.

**41** Goldstein AT, Klingman D, Christopher K, *et al.* Surgical treatment of vulvar vestibulitis syndrome: outcome assessment derived from a postoperative questionnaire. *J Sex Med.* 2006;3:923–931.

**42** Tommola P, Unkila-Kallio L, Paavonen J. Surgical treatment of vulvar vestibulitis: a review. *Acta Obstet Gynecol Scand.* 2010;89:1385–1395.

**43** Woodruff JD, Parmley TH. Infection of the minor vestibular gland. *Obstet Gynecol.* 1983;62:609–612.

**44** Goldstein A. Surgical techniques: surgery for vulvar vestibulitis syndrome. *J Sex Med.* 2006;3:559–562.

**45** Murina F, Karram M, Salvatore S, Felice R. Fractional CO2 Laser Treatment of the vestibule for patients with vestibulodynia and genitourinary syndrome of menopause: a pilot study. *J Sex Med.* 2016;13:1915–1917.

**Part V**

**Future**

# 23

# Future Developments and Research

*James A. Simon*

### Abstract

Medication and device development for women's sexual health has lagged significantly behind both scientific advances and comparable innovations in men's sexual health. Testosterone therapy for hypogonadism is just one example. As such, women are forced to use male products at scaled down doses, or compounded products with their variabilities of formulation and absorption, and without the benefit of a package insert outlining any risks. While proprietary and confidentiality restrictions limit some of the thrilling developments reviewed here, the innovative landscape remains exciting. Future developments will, ultimately, depend upon the market and financial success of currently approved therapies.

**Keywords:** *future therapies; drug development for sexual dysfunction; regulatory pathways; Food and Drug Administration (FDA); clinical trials*

## Introduction: Historical and Regulatory Perspective

The history of product development in the treatment of female sexual dysfunction has been riddled with failures [1]. The difficulties include different regulatory criteria for men's versus women's products even for the same chemical entity (described later), as well as inappropriate efficacy evaluations carried over from treatments for male erectile dysfunction (e.g. counting sexual events, which are only tangentially associated with female sexual desire [2]). This section reviews the development landscape for several products in various therapeutic areas of women's sexual health. While the focus here is on pharmaceutical medications, a few devices for sexual dysfunction are also reviewed. The vantage point for this section is strictly a US

perspective. While other regulatory bodies (i.e. The European Medicines Agency) have not always agreed with the Food and Drug Administration (FDA) on the approval of female sexual therapies (e.g. Intrinsa®, discussed later), such disparities in approval are the exception.

Estrogens, whether endogenous or exogenous, are largely adjunctive for sexual benefits [3]. That is, without adequate estrogenization, sexual function can be significantly limited. Estrogen therapies (both systemic and local) are widely available to treat vulvar and vaginal atrophy (genitourinary syndrome of menopause). Systemic estrogen treatments are also FDA approved for vasomotor symptoms and prevention of bone loss to delay or reduce osteoporosis risk. Significant concerns about the long-term risks of such estrogen or estrogen and

*Textbook of Female Sexual Function and Dysfunction: Diagnosis and Treatment*, First Edition. Edited by Irwin Goldstein, Anita H. Clayton, Andrew T. Goldstein, Noel N. Kim, and Sheryl A. Kingsberg.
© 2018 John Wiley & Sons Ltd. Published 2018 by John Wiley & Sons Ltd.

progestin therapies continue to abound, despite evidence documenting safety in early menopausal women [4–8]. Because of such controversy regarding the risk/benefit balance of systemic hormonal treatments, testosterone therapies for women have languished in development following a series of regulatory failures.

A brief overview of testosterone's regulatory history will be illustrative and facilitate an understanding of other women's sexual health developments. Testosterone therapy has been the mainstay of "off-label" treatment for peri- and postmenopausal women with low sexual desire and other sexual dysfunctions (i.e. reduced clitoral sensitivity) [9–14]. Prior to the clinical development of testosterone patches for women (Intrinsa®, Proctor and Gamble), most clinical trials were investigator initiated, of limited sample size, and employed subcutaneous implants [15], intramuscular injections [16], or oral therapies [17, 18]. Each of these approaches had significant and distinct disadvantages: subcutaneous implants required a surgical procedure, albeit a minor one, every 4–6 months; intramuscular injections could be accompanied by supraphysiological serum testosterone concentrations and associated side effects (acne, hirsutism); oral medication had adverse effects on lipids and lipoproteins due to their "first-pass" liver metabolism. These testosterone therapies, however, did have positive effects on various aspects of female sexual functioning, especially in surgically menopausal women [18–21], who often have a profound testosterone deficiency. But similar results were also documented in naturally menopausal women [22]. These benefits included increases in the number of satisfying sexual events, improved sexual desire, (often with improved arousal/orgasm/pleasure scores, decreased sexual concerns, improved sexual responsiveness and better self-image), along with decreased sexual distress. All of these endpoints were documented using validated instruments. Yet, despite efforts to obtain FDA approval for testosterone therapy in

women, regulatory barriers and their associated costs have prevented approval.

Testosterone patches (Intrinsa®) failed to achieve FDA approval for treatment of hypoactive sexual desire disorder because of perceived safety concerns requiring long-term (i.e., 5 years) safety studies focused on cardiovascular disease (i.e. triggering of stroke and myocardial ischemia events) and breast cancer risks. These potential risks were assumed to be valid based on estrogen's risks, and the temporally simultaneous FDA-Intrinsa™ advisory committee and publication of the Women's Health Initiative estrogen-only arm [23]. With the absence of such risks in the clinical development program, Intrinsa® was deemed clinically effective by the FDA's advisory committee in 2004, based upon multiple randomized, placebo-controlled clinical trials in postmenopausal women. The concerns about cardiovascular and breast cancer safety, however, resulted in the withdrawal of the Intrinsa® application. Even in the absence of long-term safety data, the testosterone patch was approved for marketing in Europe by the European Medicines Agency based upon the exact same efficacy and safety data.

Transdermal testosterone gel for women (Libigel™; BioSante) also failed to achieve FDA regulatory approval for the treatment of hypoactive sexual desire disorder in postmenopausal women due to inadequate efficacy, presumably due to the very high placebo effect [24]. In a five-year FDA Special Protocol Assessment safety trial, there was no indication of increased risk for cardiovascular disease or breast cancer through approximately four years (unpublished data) before the company discontinued the study due to insufficient resources [25].

AndroFeme® (Lawley Pharmaceuticals Ltd.) is a 1% daily testosterone cream specifically formulated for use in women that is available in Australia. It has been shown to increase sexual motivation [26].

The therapeutic need for testosterone in women is currently being satisfied by the growing use of compounded testosterone products with little regulatory oversight and no package insert articulating the risks or the use of men's testosterone products of which there are now about 30 varieties, including generic formulations that are FDA approved for men. Male testosterone products require dose adjustment for female use (in general one-tenth of the male dose).

The disparity between the approval of testosterone products for men versus women stems largely from a completely different set of criteria for approval, and the cost differences thereof. Briefly speaking, men's testosterone products are approved for hypogonadism, indicated by a serum testosterone level that is below normal, and any associated symptoms. Approval requires safely returning the serum concentration of testosterone to the normal male range. Safety is adequately satisfied by a six-month safety study, although review and updating of this safety hurdle is underway at the FDA. In women, however, approval is for the complex biopsychosocial phenomena, hypoactive sexual desire disorder (Chapters 5 and 6). For development of testosterone products for use in women, the therapy must: (i) restore testosterone concentrations into the normal female range; (ii) effectively treat the specific symptom of low desire; and (iii) reduce the distress of having low desire. That is, efficacy in women must satisfy three different endpoints at once, while documenting safety during a five-year study.

## The Marketplace

Large amounts of capital are necessary for the development of medications or devices and the initial marketing of a newly FDA-approved product is extremely costly. This is particularly critical in a new therapeutic category like women's sexual health, where public and practitioner education must also be advanced. The Intrinsa® testosterone patch was approved for marketing in the then European Union, but was withdrawn in 2010 for financial (i.e. business) reasons. Sales of the product in several European countries were hampered by: (i) approval only for surgically menopausal women, (ii) prior authorization by the government was strictly enforced, and (iii) costs of the product were set too high by the manufacturer, a deterrent both to the patient attempting to buy it "out of pocket", and to private insurers considering adding it to their formulary.

A sample of future products in development is listed here [27]. Products are listed in alphabetical order.

### AMAG Pharmaceuticals

AMAG Pharmaceuticals acquired the exclusive US rights to bremelanotide from Palatin Technologies, Inc. in early 2017. Palatin was developing targeted, receptor specific peptide therapeutics for the treatment of various diseases with significant unmet medical need and commercial potential. In this context, AMAG-Palatin is developing bremelanotide, a melanocortin peptide agonist, specifically, a MC4r agonist, for sexual dysfunction. This on-demand, self-administered auto-injector therapy is used in anticipation of sexual activity. Bremelanotide targets endogenous pathways involved in sexual desire and arousal. Following a successful phase 2B randomized, placebo-controlled, dose ranging clinical trial in more than 1200 premenopausal women with acquired, generalized hypoactive sexual desire disorder, Clayton *et al.* [28] reported highly significant benefits on desire, arousal, and orgasm. Also noted were statistically significant decreases in desire-related distress and increases in sexual events and patient satisfaction. Bremelanotide was generally well tolerated. The most common adverse events were nausea, headache, and flushing (generally described by study participants as mild/moderate). More recently, the results of two phase 3 efficacy trials and the open label roll-over safety extension study were reported [29]. These so called RECONNECT studies also showed statistically significant and clinically meaningful improvement when compared to placebo in sexual desire and distress. About 60% of enrolled study subjects on bremelanotide completed the trial, and about 80% of patients that completed the Phase 3 efficacy studies elected to participate in the open label roll-over safety extension study. Side effects were similar to those reported in Phase 2B.

At a similar time to its acquisition of Palatin, AMAG also acquired from Endoceutics, Inc. the marketing rights to a vaginal dehydroepiandrosterone product, prasterone (aka Vaginorm$^{TM}$ or Intrarosa$^{TM}$). Prasterone is a steroid indicated for the treatment of moderate to severe dyspareunia, a symptom of vulvar and vaginal atrophy, due to menopause. As preliminary studies for the treatment of vulvovaginal atrophy [30, 31] suggested a benefit for other sexual dysfunctions, Endoceutics is embarking on a separate study in women without vulvovaginal atrophy to assess Intrarosa's$^{TM}$ benefit for hypoactive sexual desire disorder.

### Emotional Brain

Based on the early writings of Drs John Bancroft [32] and Michael A. Perelman [33] suggesting that loss of sexual desire could result from two entirely different phenomena, either too much inhibition or not enough stimulation, Emotional Brain, Inc. embarked on the development of a personalized medicine approach to the treatment of hypoactive sexual desire disorder, using two separate clinical treatments. These two treatments are based upon the documented time from a rise in serum testosterone to a clinically recognized increase in sexual desire [34], and then either increasing stimulation or decreasing inhibition to sexual cues. Described in detail in three separate consecutive published manuscripts [35–37], the two resulting products, Lybrido and Lybridos, consisted of formulations to increase excitation and decrease inhibition, respectively. Testosterone/sildenafil (Lybrido), as its constituents would suggest, increases the brain's response to sexual cues and enhances genital sexual response. Testosterone/buspirone (Lybridos) increases the brain's response to

sexual cues and reduces the inhibitory response to such cues. To document this dual control concept, and the efficacy of the two therapies, Emotional Brain conducted a double-blind, randomized, placebo-controlled trial with Lybrido and Lybridos in 56 patients suffering from hypoactive sexual desire disorder. Each study subject served as her own control, with all study subjects receiving Lybrido, Lybridos, or matching placebo for one month each during three consecutive months. The order of the three treatments was randomized with a one-week washout between them. Sexual satisfaction was assessed following each sexual event using the sexual arousal response self-assessment questionnaire. Women with low sensitivity to sexual cues and hypoactive sexual desire disorder reported significantly more sexual satisfaction during sexual events when using Lybrido compared to placebo, while women with high inhibition to sexual cues and hypoactive sexual desire disorder reported significantly more sexual satisfaction during sexual events when using Lybridos compared to placebo. At the time of writing, these results are still unpublished, as is the proprietary instrument to ascertain whether a woman with hypoactive sexual desire disorder has high inhibition or low excitation. Such discrimination would be required to assess which of the two products would best serve the women with hypoactive sexual desire disorder. Phase 3 trials are planned.

### S1 Biopharma

S1 Biopharma, Inc. is developing Lorexys®. An investigational new drug application (IND) for this therapy, a combination product consisting of bupropion and trazodone as a treatment for hypoactive sexual desire disorder in women, was filed with the FDA in 2012. Bupropion, (Wellbutrin®, and others) is a norepinephrine and dopamine reuptake inhibitor prescribed for more than 20 years in the treatment of major depression and smoking cessation, and used off-label to treat sexual side effects of selective serotonin reuptake inhibitors. Bupropion is mildly activating and is usually dosed in the morning to avoid sleep disturbances. It has been demonstrated to improve sexual function in women with hypoactive sexual desire disorder when used alone at relatively high doses [38]. Trazodone (Desyrel®, Oleptro®, and others) is an antidepressant of the serotonin antagonist reuptake inhibitor class acting as a 5-$HT_{2A}$ receptor antagonist and a moderate 5-HT reuptake inhibitor. Trazodone also has anxiolytic and sleep-inducing (hypnotic) effects. Psychosexual side effects of trazodone reported in women include increased libido, priapism of the clitoris and spontaneous orgasms [39–41]. A small clinical trial of trazodone has demonstrated prosexual effects as well [42]. Using both these agents together in a time release formulation is thought to "cancel out" the alerting (bupropion) and sedating (trazodone) side effects while the prosexual effects are additive.

In the so-called Phase 2a Trial 1000, two dose combinations of Lorexys® were compared to bupropion in an open label, three-way, cross-over design of 30 premenopausal women with hypoactive sexual desire disorder. The results of this trial were presented at the 4th International Consultation on Sexual Medicine 2015 in Madrid, Spain. Compared to bupropion alone, the Lorexys® treatment group had a significantly greater number of responders based on multiple assessments (desire domain of the Female Sexual Function Index, Female Sexual Distress Scale Revised, and the Patient Global Impression of Change). Moderate sedation was the most common side effect (unpublished). More extensive trials are planned.

## Strategic Science & Technologies, LLC

Strategic Science & Technologies, LLC has a proprietary topical drug delivery technology (KNOSIS™), which provides targeted local delivery of active pharmaceutical ingredients. Targeted local delivery has several advantages according to the company: (i) significantly lower systemic exposure resulting in an improved safety profile, (ii) faster onset of action, (iii) avoidance of first-pass metabolism and potential inactivation of the drug by the liver, and (iv) more sustained and controlled delivery of the drug over time, leading to less fluctuation or sudden spikes in circulating drug levels.

Strategic Science & Technologies is developing a prescription product for female sexual arousal disorder using topical sildenafil and Strategic Science & Technologies' proprietary technology containing 5% sildenafil citrate by weight. Due to the skin's highly protective barrier, the stratum corneum, topical delivery approaches have been mostly limited to small, uncharged molecules. KNOSIS™ overcomes these challenges using two novel features: (i) by producing a hostile biophysical environment for the active pharmaceutical ingredient, thereby increasing its free energy and creating a positive chemical potential, which drives the active pharmaceutical ingredient into the skin; and (ii) by preventing the formation of hydrogen bonds between the active pharmaceutical ingredient and the stratum corneum, which can inhibit the ability of the active pharmaceutical ingredient to permeate into the tissue.

Results from preclinical functional and molecular biology studies have shed light on an analogous nitric oxide–cyclic guanosine monophosphate biological pathway present in female genital tissue. Deduced by means of immunohistochemistry methods in female tissue sections, the phosphodiesterase type 5 isoenzyme is expressed in vascular smooth muscle cells of human clitoral corpus cavernosum, the vagina, and the labia minora [43–45]. Collectively, these structures play a central role in mediating the female genital arousal response, thus providing the basis of support for the development of Strategic Science & Technologies' topical sildenafil for this critical unmet medical need.

A Phase 1 pharmacokinetic and safety trial with topical sildenafil clearly demonstrated successful delivery of sildenafil across the vulvar skin and vaginal epithelium and into the systemic circulation. No significant systemic or dermal adverse effects were seen with applications of 1–2 g of topical sildenafil, considered sufficient to deliver a therapeutic dose of sildenafil (data unpublished).

Strategic Science & Technologies recently completed a Phase 2 proof-of-concept study in premenopausal and postmenopausal women with female sexual arousal disorder. The Phase 2, double-blind, placebo-controlled, two-way cross-over clinical trial evaluated the efficacy and safety of topical sildenafil in women with female sexual arousal disorder following a single 2 g dose (71 mg sildenafil) applied to the local vulvar-vaginal target site. The study enrolled a total of 31 women with female sexual arousal disorder, 15 premenopausal and 16 postmenopausal, and assessed genital response using a vaginal photoplethysmograph and perceived sexual arousal with a Likert-scale questionnaire and arousometer device (data pending/unpublished, Dr. Cindy Meston, University of Texas at Austin). Secondary objectives included time to onset of action and safety.

## Other Companies and Products

Tefina$^{TM}$, an intranasal "on demand" testosterone gel, is being developed by Acerus Pharmaceuticals Corp., a Canadian pharmaceutical company (formerly Trimel Pharma). Tefina$^{TM}$ is intended for the treatment of women with acquired orgasmic disorder. The gel is a 0.6 mg nasal application of testosterone (2–6 h before sexual activity). Tefina$^{TM}$ has been studied in a Phase 2, double-blind, placebo-controlled study of 253 pre- and postmenopausal women experiencing acquired female orgasmic disorder, characterized by a markedly reduced intensity of orgasmic sensations, or by a marked delay in, marked infrequency or absence of orgasm, that has persisted for a minimum duration of approximately six months and causes clinically significant distress in the individual. Conducted in the United States, Canada, and Australia, study participants were randomized to one of three dosage strengths (0.6 mg, 1.2 mg, 1.8 mg) or a matching placebo, and treated over the course of 84 days. The primary endpoint of the study was to compare the nasal testosterone gel to placebo on the occurrence of orgasm. Secondary endpoints included the change from baseline in sexually-related distress due to female orgasmic disorder, and the change in sexual functioning and sexual event satisfaction. According to a press release (28 May 2014 from Trimel Pharmaceuticals Corp.), Tefina$^{TM}$ 0.6 mg (the lowest of three doses tested) led to a statistically significant increase in the average number of orgasms during the 84-day treatment period of 2.3 versus 1.7 for the placebo arm (p = 0.0015). The secondary endpoints were noted to have improved, but no data were reported. Tefina$^{TM}$ was described as "well tolerated" with no reported serious adverse events. To date this study has not been published.

Femprox® is an alprostadil-based 0.4% topical cream applied directly to the clitoris and G-spot before coitus. It was developed for the treatment of female sexual interest/arousal disorder. It contains prostaglandin E1 as the active ingredient and a proprietary permeation enhancer (NexACT), which facilitates the delivery of the drug into the circulation. Apricus Biosciences has completed nine clinical studies to date, including a 98 patient Phase 2 study in the United States, and a near 400 patient Phase 3 study in China demonstrating a statistically significant dose-dependent increase in sexual function (assessed by the Female Sexual Function Index), while reducing sexually-related distress with mild topical irritation as the only adverse event [46]. Femprox® exerts a local, relaxant effect on vulvar and clitoral blood vessels in women, leading to increased blood flow. The resultant increase in vaginal lubrication and sensory feedback is believed to produce a clinically significant increase in sexual arousal in women with female sexual arousal disorder or female sexual interest/arousal disorder.

Mona Lisa Touch® Laser developed by Deka M.E.L.A. Srl in Italy and sold in the United States by Cynosure/Hologic has been FDA cleared for the treatment of vaginal atrophy due to menopause and the resulting symptoms. Recently, preliminary data for use of this laser have been published for the treatment of vulvovestibulitis syndrome and dyspareunia unrelated to menopausal changes. These preliminary results suggest significant benefits for vulvovestibulitis syndrome associated pain and improved sexual function [47].

Lasofoxifene (Pfizer Inc., Sermonix Pharmaceuticals Inc.), a selective estrogen receptor modulator (e.g. tamoxifene, toremifene, raloxifene, ospemifene), failed to achieve regulatory approval for osteoporosis prevention and vulvovaginal atrophy in 2006, and osteoporosis treatment in 2009, due to FDA concerns over benefit/risk for those indications, despite significant fracture reduction and a 70% decrease in breast cancer risk. Lasofoxifene has demonstrated efficacy for vulvovaginal atrophy and improved sexual function in several clinical studies [48].

Development continues for this agent for breast cancer resistant patients, a population that can often benefit from vulvovaginal atrophy/genitourinary syndrome of menopause treatment without estrogens, and which may also have hypoactive sexual desire disorder.

Almost 10 years ago, initial reports of radiofrequency treatments for vaginal laxity appeared in the literature [49]. Viveve, Inc. continues these investigations in hopes of obtaining FDA approval for this indication. Vaginal laxity can be a sexual problem for some women and their male partners. Lack of adequate friction and indirect stimulation of the clitoris can result from laxity. Because radiofrequency energy can be "tuned" to provide a depth of penetration associated with protein denaturation and resultant new collagen development, it is thought that this treatment can lead to vaginal tightening and improved sexual function including orgasmic function [50]. Several small preliminary studies appear to confirm the benefits of this approach, including one with 12 months of "long-term" safety data [51–53].

# References

1 Simon JA. Implementing a successful clinical development program for female sexual dysfunctions (aka how to navigate a regulatory minefield). *Maturitas.* 2011;69(2):97–98.

2 Kingsberg SA, Althof SE. Satisfying sexual events as outcome measures in clinical trial of female sexual dysfunction. *J Sex Med.* 2011;8(12):3262–3270.

3 Nastri CO, Lara LA, Ferriani RA, *et al.* Hormone therapy for sexual function in perimenopausal and postmenopausal women. *Cochrane Database Syst Rev.* 2013(6):CD009672.

4 Kaunitz AM, Manson JE. Failure to treat menopausal symptoms: a disconnect between clinical practice and scientific data. *Menopause.* 2015;22(7):687–688.

5 Marko K, Simon J. Clinical trials in menopause: a review. *Menopause.* 2018; 25(2):217–230.

6 Manson JE, Goldstein SR, Kagan R, *et al.* Why the product labeling for low-dose vaginal estrogen should be changed. *Menopause.* 2014;21(9):911–916.

7 Langer RD. The evidence base for HRT: what can we believe? *Climacteric.* 2017;20(2):91–96.

8 Worsley R, Bell RJ, Gartoulla P, Davis SR. Prevalence and predictors of low sexual desire, sexually-related personal distress and hypoactive sexual desire dysfunction in a community based sample of midlife women. *J Sex Med.* 2017;14(5):675–686.

9 Somboonporn W, Davis S, Seif MW, Bell R. Testosterone for peri- and postmenopausal

women. *Cochrane Database Syst Rev.* 2005(4):CD004509.

10  Abdallah RT, Simon JA. Testosterone therapy in women: its role in the management of hypoactive sexual desire disorder. *Int J Impot Res.* 2007;19(5):458–463.

11  Hubayter Z, Simon JA. Testosterone therapy for sexual dysfunction in postmenopausal women. *Climacteric.* 2008;11(3):181–191.

12  Krapf JM, Simon JA. The role of testosterone in the management of hypoactive sexual desire disorder in postmenopausal women. *Maturitas.* 2009;63(3):213–219.

13  Pollycove R, Simon J. Female sexual dysfunction and testosterone therapy: essentials for gynecologists. In: Plouffe L Jr., Rizk B (eds) *Androgens in Gynecological Practice: Managing the Basics.* Cambridge University Press; 2015, pp. 38–53.

14  Davis SR, Wahlin-Jacobsen S. Testosterone in women – the clinical significance. *Lancet Diabetes Endocrinol.* 2015;3(12):980–992.

15  Davis SR, McCloud P, Strauss BJ, Burger H. Testosterone enhances estradiol's effects on postmenopausal bone density and sexuality. *Maturitas.* 2008;61 (1–2):17–26.

16  Sherwin BB, Gelfand MM. The role of androgen in the maintenance of sexual functioning in oophorectomized women. *Psychosom Med.* 1987;49(4):397–409.

17  Lobo RA, Rosen RC, Yang HM, *et al.* Comparative effects of oral esterified estrogens with and without methyltestosterone on endocrine profiles and dimensions of sexual function in postmenopausal women with hypoactive sexual desire. *Fertil Steril.* 2003;79(6):1341–1352.

18  Simon J, Braunstein G, Nachtigall L, *et al.* Testosterone patch increases sexual activity and desire in surgically menopausal women with hypoactive sexual desire disorder. *J Clin Endocrinol Metab.* 2005;90(9):5226–5233.

19  Shifren JL, Braunstein GD, Simon JA, *et al.* Transdermal testosterone treatment in women with impaired sexual function after oophorectomy. *N Engl J Med.* 2000;343(10):682–688.

20  Braunstein GD, Sundwall DA, Katz M, *et al.* Safety and efficacy of a testosterone patch for the treatment of hypoactive sexual desire disorder in surgically menopausal women: a randomized, placebo-controlled trial. *Arch Intern Med.* 2005;165(14):1582–1589.

21  Nachtigall L, Casson P, Lucas J, *et al.* Safety and tolerability of testosterone patch therapy for up to 4 years in surgically menopausal women receiving oral or transdermal oestrogen. *Gynecol Endocrinol.* 2011;27(1):39–48.

22  Shifren JL, Davis SR, Moreau M, *et al.* Testosterone patch for the treatment of hypoactive sexual desire disorder in naturally menopausal women: results from the INTIMATE NM1 Study. *Menopause.* 2006;13(5):770–779.

23  Anderson GL, Limacher M, Assaf AR, *et al.* Effects of conjugated equine estrogen in postmenopausal women with hysterectomy: the Women's Health Initiative randomized controlled trial. *JAMA.* 2004;291(14):1701–1712.

24  Snabes M, Simes S, Zborowski J. A Clear Pathway to Approval for Libigel® Treatment of Postmenopausal Women with Hypoactive Sexual Desire Disorder (HSDD). ISSWSH Annual Meeting, Jerusalem, Israel; 2012.

25  White WB, Grady D, Giudice LC, *et al.* A cardiovascular safety study of LibiGel (testosterone gel) in postmenopausal women with elevated cardiovascular risk and hypoactive sexual desire disorder. *Am Heart J.* 2012;163(1):27–32.

26  El-Hage G, Eden JA, Manga RZ. A double-blind, randomized, placebo-controlled trial of the effect of testosterone cream on the sexual motivation of menopausal hysterectomized women with hypoactive sexual desire disorder. *Climacteric.* 2007;10(4):335–343.

27 Kingsberg SA, Clayton AH, Pfaus JG. The female sexual response: current models, neurobiological underpinnings and agents currently approved or under investigation for the treatment of hypoactive sexual desire disorder. *CNS Drugs.* 2015;29(11):915–933.

28 Clayton AH, Althof SE, Kingsberg S, *et al.* Bremelanotide for female sexual dysfunctions in premenopausal women: a randomized, placebo-controlled dose-finding trial. *Womens Health (Lond).* 2016;12(3):325–337.

29 Clayton A, Kingsberg S, Simon J, *et al.* Efficacy of the Investigational Drug Bremelanotide for Hypoactive Sexual Desire Disorder: Results From the RECONNECT Studies. American Society of Psychopharmacology Annual Meeting (ASCPP-NCDEU); Miami Beach, FL; 2017.

30 Bouchard C, Labrie F, Derogatis L, *et al.* Effect of intravaginal dehydroepiandrosterone (DHEA) on the female sexual function in postmenopausal women: ERC-230 open-label study. *Horm Mol Biol Clin Investig.* 2016;25(3):181–190.

31 Labrie F, Archer D, Bouchard C, *et al.* Lack of influence of dyspareunia on the beneficial effect of intravaginal prasterone (dehydroepiandrosterone, DHEA) on sexual dysfunction in postmenopausal women. *J Sex Med.* 2014;11(7):1766–1785.

32 Bancroft J, Graham CA, Janssen E, Sanders SA. The dual control model: current status and future directions. *J Sex Res.* 2009;46(2–3): 121–142.

33 Perelman MA. The sexual tipping point: a mind/body model for sexual medicine. *J Sex Med.* 2009;6(3):629–632.

34 Tuiten A, Van Honk J, Koppeschaar H, *et al.* Time course of effects of testosterone administration on sexual arousal in women. *Arch Gen Psychiatry.* 2000;57(2):149–153; discussion 155–156.

35 Bloemers J, van Rooij K, Poels S, *et al.* Toward personalized sexual medicine (part 1): integrating the "dual control model" into differential drug treatments for hypoactive

sexual desire disorder and female sexual arousal disorder. *J Sex Med.* 2013;10(3):791–809.

36 Poels S, Bloemers J, van Rooij K, *et al.* Toward personalized sexual medicine (part 2): testosterone combined with a PDE5 inhibitor increases sexual satisfaction in women with HSDD and FSAD, and a low sensitive system for sexual cues. *J Sex Med.* 2013;10(3):810–823.

37 van Rooij K, Poels S, Bloemers J, *et al.* Toward personalized sexual medicine (part 3): testosterone combined with a Serotonin1A receptor agonist increases sexual satisfaction in women with HSDD and FSAD, and dysfunctional activation of sexual inhibitory mechanisms. *J Sex Med.* 2013;10(3):824–837.

38 Segraves RT, Clayton A, Croft H, *et al.* Bupropion sustained release for the treatment of hypoactive sexual desire disorder in premenopausal women. *J Clin Psychopharmacol.* 2004;24(3): 339–342.

39 Gartrell N. Increased libido in women receiving trazodone. *Am J Psychiatry.* 1986;143(6):781–782.

40 Pescatori E, Engelman JC, Davis G, Goldstein I. Priapism of the clitoris: a case report following trazodone use. *J Urol.* 1993;149(6):1557–1559.

41 Battaglia C, Venturoli S. Persistent genital arousal disorder and trazodone. Morphometric and vascular modifications of the clitoris. A case report. *J Sex Med.* 2009;6(10):2896–2900.

42 Eraslan D, Ertekin E, Ertekin BA, Ozturk O. Treatment of insomnia with hypnotics resulting in improved sexual functioning in post-menopausal women. *Psychiatr Danub.* 2014;26(4):353–357.

43 Ückert S, Oelke M, Waldkirch E, *et al.* Cyclic adenosine monophosphate and cyclic guanosine monophosphate-phosphodiesterase isoenzymes in human vagina: relation to nitric oxide synthase isoforms and vasoactive intestinal polypeptide-containing nerves. *Urology.* 2005;65(3):604–610.

44 Ückert S, Oelke M, Albrecht K, *et al.* Immunohistochemical description of cyclic nucleotide phosphodiesterase (PDE) isoenzymes in the human labia minora. *J Sex Med.* 2007;4(3):602–608.

45 Ückert S, Oelke M, Albrecht K, *et al.* Expression and distribution of key enzymes of the cyclic GMP signaling in the human clitoris: relation to phosphodiesterase type 5 (PDE5). *Int J Impot Res.* 2011;23(5):206–212.

46 Zhang M, Liao QP, Yao C, *et al.* [Multicenter randomized, double-blind, placebo-controlled trial of prostaglandin E1 cream for female sexual arousal disorder]. *Beijing Da Xue Xue Bao.* 2010;42(6):727–733.

47 Murina F, Karram M, Salvatore S, Felice R. Fractional $CO_2$ laser treatment of the vestibule for patients with vestibulodynia and genitourinary syndrome of menopause: a pilot study. *J Sex Med.* 2016;13(12): 1915–1917.

48 Kingsberg S, Simon J, Symons J, Portman D. Lasofoxifene as a Treatment for Sexual Dysfunction in Postmenopausal Women. 21st Annual Fall Scientific Meeting Sexual Medicine Society of North America (SMSNA); Las Vegas, NV; 2015.

49 Millheiser LS, Pauls RN, Herbst SJ, Chen BH. Radiofrequency treatment of vaginal laxity after vaginal delivery: nonsurgical vaginal tightening. *J Sex Med.* 2010;7(9): 3088–3095.

50 Alinsod RM. Transcutaneous temperature controlled radiofrequency for orgasmic dysfunction. *Lasers Surg Med.* 2016;48(7):641–645.

51 Sekiguchi Y, Utsugisawa Y, Azekosi Y, *et al.* Laxity of the vaginal introitus after childbirth: nonsurgical outpatient procedure for vaginal tissue restoration and improved sexual satisfaction using low-energy radiofrequency thermal therapy. *J Womens Health (Larchmt).* 2013;22(9): 775–781.

52 Krychman M, Rowan CG, Allan BB, *et al.* Effect of single-treatment, surface-cooled radiofrequency therapy on vaginal laxity and female sexual function: the VIVEVE I randomized controlled trial. *J Sex Med.* 2017;14(2):215–225.

53 Vicariotto F, DE Seta F, Faoro V, Raichi M. Dynamic quadripolar radiofrequency treatment of vaginal laxity/menopausal vulvo-vaginal atrophy: 12-month efficacy and safety. *Minerva Ginecol.* 2017;69(4):342–349.

# Index

Page locators in **bold** indicate tables. Page locators in *italics* indicate figures.

*Textbook of Female Sexual Function and Dysfunction: Diagnosis and Treatment*, First Edition. Edited by
Irwin Goldstein, Anita H. Clayton, Andrew T. Goldstein, Noel N. Kim, and Sheryl A. Kingsberg.
© 2018 John Wiley & Sons Ltd. Published 2018 by John Wiley & Sons Ltd.

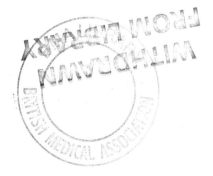